CLINICAL PHYSIOLOGY OF THE VENOUS SYSTEM

BASIC SCIENCE FOR THE CARDIOLOGIST

1. B. Swynghedauw (ed.): *Molecular Cardiology for the Cardiologist.* Second Edition. 1998 ISBN 0-7923-8323-0
2. B. Levy, A. Tedgui (eds.): *Biology of the Arterial Wall.* 1999 ISBN 0-7923-8458-X
3. M.R. Sanders, J.B. Kostis (eds.): *Molecular Cardiology in Clinical Practice.* 1999 ISBN 0-7923-8602-7
4. B.Ostadal, F. Kolar (eds.): *Cardiac Ischemia: From Injury to Protection.* 1999 ISBN 0-7923-8642-6
5. H. Schunkert, G.A.J. Riegger (eds.): *Apoptosis in Cardiac Biology.* 1999 ISBN 0-7923-8648-5
6. A. Malliani, (ed.): *Principles of Cardiovascular Neural Regulation in Health and Disease.* 2000 ISBN 0-7923-7775-3
7. P. Benlian: *Genetics of Dyslipidemia.* 2001 ISBN 0-7923-7362-6
8. D. Young: *Role of Potassium in Preventive Cardiovascular Medicine.* 2001 ISBN 0-7923-7376-6
9. E. Carmeliet, J. Vereecke: *Cardiac Cellular Electrophysiology.* 2002 ISBN 0-7923-7544-0
10. C. Holubarsch: *Mechanics and Energetics of the Myocardium.* 2002 ISBN 0-7923-7570-X
11. J.S. Ingwall: *ATP and the Heart.* 2002 ISBN 1-4020-7093-4
12. W.C. De Mello, M.J. Janse: *Heart Cell Coupling and Impuse Propagation in Health and Disease.* 2002 ISBN 1-4020-7182-5
13. P.P.-Dimitrow: *Coronary Flow Reserve – Measurement and Application: Focus on transthoracic Doppler echocardiography.* 2002 ISBN 1-4020-7213-9
14. G.A. Danieli: *Genetics and Genomics for the Cardiologist.* 2002 ISBN 1-4020-7309-7
15. F.A. Schneider, I.R. Siska, J.A. Avram: *Clinical Physiology of the Venous System.* 2003. ISBN 1-4020-7411-5

KLUWER ACADEMIC PUBLISHERS – DORDRECHT/BOSTON/LONDON

CLINICAL PHYSIOLOGY OF THE VENOUS SYSTEM

by

Francisc A. Schneider, M.D., Ph.D,
Professor of Physiology
Western University "Vasile Goldiş"Arad
University of Medicine and Pharmacy
Timisoara

Ioana Raluca Siska, M.D., Ph.D.,
Assistant Professor of Physiology
University of Medicine and Pharmacy
Timisoara

Jecu Aurel Avram, M.D., Ph.D.,
Professor of Surgery and Phlebology
University of Medicine and Pharmacy
Timisoara

KLUWER ACADEMIC PUBLISHERS
BOSTON / DORDRECHT / LONDON

Distributors for North, Central and South America:
Kluwer Academic Publishers
101 Philip Drive
Assinippi Park
Norwell, Massachusetts 02061 USA
Telephone (781) 871-6600
Fax (781) 681-9045
E-Mail: kluwer@wkap.com

Distributors for all other countries:
Kluwer Academic Publishers Group
Post Office Box 322
3300 AH Dordrecht, THE NETHERLANDS
Telephone 31 786 576 000
Fax 31 786 576 254
E-Mail: services@wkap.nl

Electronic Services <http://www.wkap.nl>

Library of Congress Cataloging-in-Publication Data

A C.I.P. Catalogue record for this book is available
from the Library of Congress.

1-4020-7411-5
Clinical Physiology of the Venous System by Schneider, Siska, Avram

Printed on acid-free paper.

Printed in the United States of America.

TABLE OF CONTENTS

CHAPTER 4.
REGULATION OF THE VENOUS TONE 77

CHAPTER 6

We dedicate this book to the memory of
Professor Pius Brânzeu, the founder of
the Romanian School of Phlebology

INTRODUCTION

The circulatory system is made up of the heart and a vast array of vessels: arteries, capillaries and veins. The veins are vessels through which the blood flows from various organs or parts of the body to the heart. Phlebology is the study of the venous system and its diseases. Although this definition of what we call today the venous system is no more than five centuries old, the sufferings of the veins go back to man's prehistory.

0.1. HISTORICAL ACCOUNT

Centuries of civilization have yielded numerous documents pertaining to mankind's interests in veins (1, 2, 9).

Neolithic engravings discovered in Tassili caves (Sahara) show people with swollen and bandaged lower legs. Phoenicians and Egyptians were the first to mention venous varices in the 2nd millennium BC (in Eber's papyrus). As records of Hippocrates' work show, venous stasis and venous ulcer were among the major concerns of physicians in the third and fourth century BC. Venous diseases also preoccupied physicians in Greek and Roman antiquity.

The medical treatises of Galen of Pergamon (129-201) and of Ibn Sina-Avicenna (980-1037) contain descriptions and treatments for the venous diseases of the lower limbs. Galen's concept concerning the circulation of the blood - according to which the veins transport the blood to all the organs - was taken over by Vesalius, and was the accepted view until the 16th century. But Vesalius was the first to accurately illustrate the anatomy of the veins, in "De Humani Corporis Fabrica", published in 1543.

Before him, it was Leonardo da Vinci who, in his drawings, clearly illustrated the superficial veins of the lower limbs and arms. Eustachio (1520-1574) described the azygos veins and inferior vena cava.

In 1603, Fabricios d'Aguapendente named the valves of the veins and elaborated a theory according to which the function of these valves was to slow down the circulation of the blood.

Harvey's work, "Exercitatio Anatomica De Motu Cordis et Sanguinis", published in 1628, combines physiology and anatomy. The accurate description of the venous system clearly demonstrates the blood flow and the valvular arrest of the venous circulation.

In the 17th century, venous stasis and varicose veins were attributed to blows, contusions, excessive effort, or prolonged standing position, whereas in the 15th century, when Galen's theory of humours dominated medical thoughts, varicose elongation, tortuosity and deletion were attributed to the weight of the stagnant blood on the venous walls. In those times, physicians were convinced that varicosities contained black bile and that healing of the ulcer would have been catastrophic.

The correct observations of Fabry (1589) and Bodie (1846), crystallized in the observations of Trendelenburg (1890) concerning the functions of the superficial and communicating veins, the venous valves and the interplay of the muscle pump, elucidating the roles of veins.

In the twentieth century clinical observations and operations (Nobili, Unger, Keller, Mayo, Babcock, etc), physiological studies and non-invasive determinations of venous filling recovery time, venous pressure recovery time, direct imaging by duplex scan, resonance imaging, continuous wave Doppler instrument for venous testing, color flow scanning and magnetic resonance imaging allowed a correct understanding of the anatomy and functions of the venous system.

In the field of applied physiology of the venous system, Romanian physicians played an important part. Foremost among them are Marin Popescu, who was the first to point out the myogenic automatism of the portal vein (11), and Pius Brânzeu, who carried out the first transplants of valved veins in the post-traumatic syndrome of lower limbs (3).

The physiological significance of the veins has been reevaluated only in the last two decades. Scientists have recognized that veins comprise a multifunctional system. Some of these show close similarities with arterial functions, whereas others are specific for veins. Specific venous functions include the adaptive role in the maintenance of orthostatic tolerance of the organism and cardiovascular reactions during exercise. Today, autologous venous grafts are frequently used as prostheses of affected arteries.

The growing interest in clinical physiology of the venous system is connected with the very high incidence of varicosity, thrombophlebitis, phlebosclerosis, orthostatic intolerance and other vein diseases.

0.2. EMBRYOLOGY AND DEVELOPMENT OF VENOUS SYSTEM

Blood vessels are among the first organs to develop during embryogenesis and are essential for organogenesis and nutrition of the embryo.

Veins and arteries are morphologically, functionally, and molecularly very different. This distinction is established during vasculogenesis, angioblast precursors for the trunk vein and artery are spatially mixed in the lateral posterior mesoderm. The venous - arterial decision is guided and preceded by an increase in expression of the venous - gene marker and diminution of expression of the arterial - gene marker, adjudicating a venous versus arterial decision (14).

There is an essential and early developmental distinction between vein and artery, in addition to those differences later imposed by blood pressure (15). Initially, mesodermal cells differentiate in situ into early hemangioblasts and form cellular aggregates - blood islands, in which the inner cell population develops into hematopoietic precursors and primitive endothelial cells (5, 6).

The second stage is a form of primordial vascular network (13). Lumen formation of the primitive capillaries may result from endothelial vascularization or from a continuation of the pre-existing lumen through the joining of the distal endothelial cells and intracellular lumen formation. These processes are controlled by growth factors and growth-inhibitory metabolites (4).

In the third stage, the primitive vascular plexus develops into an interconnecting network by splitting the preexisting vessel in daughter vessels by endothelial sprouting (10).

In this process, periendothelial cells play important roles, concerning sprouting, remodeling, and production of specialized extracellular matrices.

The blood vessels seem to be initially surrounded by a fibronectin-rich matrix, which is later incorporated into the basal lamina along with interalia laminin.

Several layers of fibronectin-expressing cells can be seen around larger vessels (12).

In the microvasculature, around endothelial tubes are perycites, which may be involved in capillary blood flow regulation and maintenance of a selective permeability barrier for plasma constituents. Another property of pericytes is their plasticity in differentiating into smooth muscle cells.

The next phase in development is the acquisition of a media for the larger vessels, when the vascular network expands. The adventitia of these vessels has a similar embryonic contribution on the media, suggesting a common origin of fibroblasts and smooth muscle cells (8).

Anastomoses appear and disappear, capillaries fuse and give rise to arteries or veins, and the direction of the blood flow may reverse several times. The tunica media of the vessels appear after a stable vascular pattern has been formed.

The fourth stage occurs during the organogenetic period, after the outset of circulation, when a tree of veins, capillaries and arteries are remodeled by metabolic demands of the growing embryo.

The early embryonic veins are segregated into two groups, visceral and somatic. The visceral group comprises the derivatives of the vitelline and umbilical veins; the somatic group includes all remaining veins. All of them develop initially with a symmetric bilateral array of channels - the cardinal venous complexes, divided into a precardinal vein for the rostral part, and the postcardinal vein for the caudal part. These form the superior and the inferior vena cava, where veins converge. Pulmonary veins drain into the precardinal complex.

The primitive tubular symmetric heart receives its venous return through the right and the left sinusal horns.

The symmetric bilateral array of channels is changed by growth and differentiation of the nervous system, of the skeleton and musculature, the cardiac asymmetry and venous return to the right part; by repositioning of the heart, lung and gut, and venous involvement, by the developing liver, pancreas, spleen etc (5).

0.3. ANATOMICAL FEATURES

Because the heart is a pair of muscular pumps, there is a minor loop - the pulmonary circulation, and a major loop - the systemic circulation. A single artery – aorta, from the systemic circulation, and the pulmonary trunk, from the minor loop, emerge from the heart, giving origin by successive branching to hundreds of arteries. By further branching, these produce about $4x10^6$ arterioles in systemic circulation and four times as many capillaries. About a similar number of venules converge into each other, forming veins, but more numerous, and finally forming the superior and the inferior vena cava, which open in the heart. An identical pattern is found in the pulmonary circulation, but the number of vessels is smaller.

The veins, as a whole, form three main systems: pulmonary, systemic and portal (7).

Pulmonary veins, usually four, two from each lung, return oxygenated blood from pulmonary capillary networks in the left atrium.

Systemic veins are divided into:

- Cardiac veins, which drain directly into the heart.
- Veins draining into the superior vena cava are divided into three groups:
  - veins of the head and neck
  - veins of the upper limbs
  - veins of the thorax.
- Veins draining into the inferior vena cava, are divided into two groups:
  - veins of the abdomen and pelvis
  - veins of the lower limbs.

The portal vein includes the veins draining the abdominal part of the digestive tube, spleen, pancreas and gallbladder. It conveys the blood to the liver, ending in the sinusoids, which converge in the hepatic veins and finally in the inferior vena cava.

Two or more capillaries converge in a postcapillary venule, with oval or polygonal endothelial cells supported by basal lamina and a delicate adventitia of collagen fibers, fibroblasts and pericytes. Venules do not acquire musculature until a new convergence. The veins have a relatively thin wall in comparison with the arteries of similar size. The amount of muscle is considerably less than in the arteries, while collagen and elastic fibers are their predominant components.

The orientation of the muscle cells is variable. In the arm and leg veins the musculature is circularly. In the iliac vein, the brahiocephalic vein, the vena cava, portal vein and renal vein, the musculature is longitudinal.

Muscular tissue is absent in maternal placental veins, the dural venous sinuses and pial veins, the retinal veins, the veins of trabecular the bone, and the venous spaces of erectile tissue.

REFERENCES

1. Avram J. "Short history of phlebology and perforant veins". In *Surgery of perforant veins*, J Avram, ed. Editura Hestia, Timisoara - Romania, 2000 [in Romanian]
2. Bergan JJ. "Historical highlights in treating venous insufficiency". In *Venous disease*, JJ Bergan, ed. Saunders, 1991
3. Brânzeu P, *Great performances in surgery*, Editura de Vest, Timisoara - Romania, 1997 [in Romanian]
4. Carmeliet P. Mechanism of angiogenesis and arteriogenesis. Nature Med 2000; 6: 389-395
5. Collins P. "Embriology and development". In *Gray's Anatomy*, PL Williams, ed. Churchill Livingstone, 1995
6. Flamme I, Risau W. Induction of vasculogenesis and hematopoiesis in vitro. Development 1992; 116: 435-439
7. Gabella G. "Cardiovascular system". In *Gray's Anatomy*, PL Williams, ed. Churchill Livingstone, 1995
8. Gittenberger-de Groot AC, DeRuiter MCBergwerff M, Poelman RI. Smooth muscle origin and its relationship to heterogeneity in development and disease. Arterioscl Thromb Vasc Biol 1999; 19: 1589-1594
9. Monos E, Berczi V, Nadasy G. Local control of veins. Physiol Rev 1995; 75: 611-666
10. Patan S, Alvarez MJ, Schittny JC, Burri PH. Interssusceptive microvascular growth: a common alternative to endothelial sprouting. Arch Histol Cytol 1992; 55: 65-75
11. Popescu M. Physiology and pharmacodynamics of portal vein. Bul de l'Acad de Med de Roumanie 1940; 1-3: 6-8 [in French]
12. Risau W. Mechanism of angiogenesis. Nature 1997; 386: 671-674
13. Wilting J, Christ B. Embrionic angiogenesis: a review. Naturwissenshaften 1996; 83: 153-164
14. Yancoupoulos GD, Klagsbrun M, Folkman J. Vasculogenesis, angiogenesis and growth factors: ephrins enter the fray at the border. Cell 1998; 93: 661-664
15. Zhong TP, Childs S, Leu JP, Fishman MC. Gredlock signalling pathway fashions the first embryonic artery. Nature 2001; 414: 216-220

PREFACE

I visited Arad, a small and pleasant city next to Timisoara, located west of Romania, some years ago. I am so glad that during my visit to this city Professor Schneider and I discussed the development of this wonderful book. It is a real privilege for me to introduce Professor Francisc Schneider, head of the Physiology Department of the University Vasile Goldis in Arad, Romania, and his coworkers Ioana Raluca Siska and Jecu Aurel Avram. They are active and creative people, who maintain and bring to life good science and research in Romania. This volume bespeaks the rebirth of physiology in Romania and its long scientific tradition. Every seasoned vascular physiologist certainly remembers Marin Popescu who was the first to demonstrate in 1940 the myogenic regulation of the portal vein tone and the contribution of Pius Branzeu to vein transplantation. The present book is an excellent overview on the physiology and pathophysiology of veins. There is currently no equivalent in the marketplace. The authors have succeeded to write a comparable summary on what is known to be a difficult topic.

This volume on the venous system complements "Biology of the Arterial Wall" which was published in the Basic Science for the Cardiologist book series a few years ago by B. Levy and A. Tedgui. Obviously the two types of vessels are quite different, not only in terms of anatomy and physiology, but also in terms of tone regulation and capacity to produce cytokines and coagulation elements. An interesting aspect of vein physiology is the

transformation of vein structure when veins are used as grafts. This volume also includes vein pathophysiology, an enormous problem in terms of cost and a major target for pharmaceutical companies. This area of medicine is frequently forgotten or neglected despite its relevance in current clinical practice. The reader will find at the end of the book an interesting and useful chapter that summarizes all the particular forms of phlebitis. This chapter is unique to this volume. The book includes an important bibliography and for the reader pressed for time, several take home messages at the beginning of each chapter.
The first three chapters cover hemodynamic and biological functions of the veins at both the organ and cell levels. Chapter 4 describes tone regulation. The last five chapters are devoted to pathophysiology; information on varicose veins and thromboembolic disease both from a diagnostic and therapeutic point of view; and venous insufficiency and congenital abnormalities.

Bernard Swynghedauw, PhD, MD
Series Editor: *Basic Science for the Cardiologist* book series
Directeur de Recherches émérite à l'INSERM
Past president of the Federation of European Physiological Societies (FEPS)

ABBREVIATIONS

ACE = angiotensin-converting enzyme
ACh = acetylcholine
ANG = angiotensin
APC = activated protein C
APG = air pletysmography
AT = antithrombin
ATIII = antithrombin III

AV = arterio-venous

AVC = arterio-venous communication
BK = bradykinin
CaCB = calcium channel blockers
CaD = caldesmon

CaM = calmodulin
CaMK II = Ca^{2+}-calmodulin protein-kinase II
CaP = calponin
CGRP = calcitonin gene-related peptide
COX = cyclooxygenase
CT = computer tomography
CVI = chronic venous insufficiency
DAG = diacylglycerol
DVT = deep venous thrombosis
EC = endothelial cell(s)
ECE = endothelin-converting enzyme
EDHF = endothelium-derived hyperpolarizing factor
ER = estrogen receptors
ET-1 = endothelin-1
FGF = fibroblast growth factors
GC = guanilate cyclase
GSV = great saphenous vein
HMWK = high molecular weight kininogen
HUVEC = human umbilical vein endothelial cells
ICAM = intercellular adhesion molecules
ICV = inferior cava vein
IGF = insulin-like growth factor
IL = interleukin
IMA = internal mammary artery
IPG = impedance pletismography

ROS = reactive oxygen species
rtPA = recombinant tissular plasminogen

IP_3 = inositol triphosphate
LC = light chain
LDL = low density lipoproteins
LMWH = low molecular weight heparin
LSV = low saphenous vein
LT = leukotriene
MAPK = mitogen activated protein kinase
MAPKK = mitogen activated protein kinase kinase
MLCK = myosin light chain kinase
MLCP = myosin light chain phosphatase
MMP = matrix metalloproteinase
MRA = magnetical resonance angiography
MRI = magnetical resonance imaging
NA = noradrenaline
NANC = non-adrenergic non-cholinergic
NE = norepinephrine
NO = nitric oxide
NOS = nitric oxide synthase
NPY = neuropeptide Y
PAF = platelet-activating factor
PAI = plasminogen activator inhibitors
PAR-1 = protease-activated receptor-1
PDGF = platelet-derived growth factor
PE = pulmonary embolism

PGI_2 = prostacyclin
PKA = protein kinase A
PKC = protein kinase C
PKG = protein kinase G
PLA_2 = phospholipase A_2
PLC = phospholipase C
PLD = phospholipase D

PPG = photopletismography
PR = progesterone receptors
PS = pentasacharides
PTS = postthrombotic syndrome
PVC = central venous pressure
RAS = renin-angiotensin system

activator
SCV = superior cava vein
SEPS = subfascial endoscopic perforant surgery
SMC = smooth muscle cells
SOD = superoxide dismutase
SPG = strain gauge pletismography
SR = sarcoplasmic reticulum
SV = saphenous vein
TAFI = thrombin-activatable fibrinolysis inhibitor
TF = tissue factor
TFPI = tissue factor pathway inhibitor
TGF-β1 = transforming growth factor-β1
TIE/TEK = tyrosine kinase with immunoglobulin and epidermal growth factor homology domains
TIMP = tissue inhibitors of MMP
TNFα = tumor necrosis factor-alpha
t-PA = tissue plasminogen activator(s)
Tr T = thrombin time
TT = traveler's thrombosis
TxA_2 = thromboxane A_2
UFH = unfractioned heparin
u-PA = urokinase-type plasminogen activator
VCAM = vascular cell adhesion molecules
VEGF = vascular endothelial growth factor
VSMC = vascular smooth muscle cells
VV = varicose veins
vWF = von Willebrand's factor

CHAPTER 1

HYDRODYNAMIC AND RHEOLOGIC LAWS APPLIED TO THE VENOUS CIRCULATION

TAKE HOME MESSAGES

- To understand the circulation it is necessary to apply the physical principles and equations for the blood flow.
- Blood is not a perfect fluid; it is the viscous one, with rheologic particularities.
- The relationship between blood flow, pressure and resistance is, in general way expressed in Ohm's law.
- Compliance of the veins relates closely to the passive and active biomechanical properties of their wall and to its physiological control.

To understand the circulation in the blood vessels it is necessary to apply the physical principles and equations to the flow of blood in the blood vessels.

Hydrodynamics describes the behavior of perfect fluids in horizontal rigid tubes. But blood vessels are not rigid they are not always horizontal and the blood is not a perfect fluid; it is viscous, with rheologic particularities.

It is important to know the mechanical relations between pressures and flow gradients, blood volume distribution, capacity, distensibility, compliance and resistance to flow in the vascular system, in its venous part.

The blood flows from areas of high pressure to areas of low pressure, determinate by the pumping of the ventricles – hydrodynamic pressure, because its pressure falls progressively due to vessels resistance.

1.1. HYDROSTATIC PRESSURE IN VEINS

Beside the hydrodynamic pressure, hydrostatic pressure occurs in the vascular system. The hydrostatic pressure is caused by the height of the blood column when posture is considered (2).

Hydrostatic pressure is expressed as force per unit area, considering the density (ρ), the gravitational acceleration (g) and the height (h) – Pascal law (ρgh).

The zero reference pressure level for the cardiovascular system is the position of the heart. With the person lying down, the head, heart and feet are all at the same level, and the hydrostatic pressure is the same. When the person is standing, the pressure rises by 1mmHg for each 13.6 mm distance below / or decreases above the heart. So, in an adult who is standing, the pressure in the vein of the feet is approximately +90 mmHg and in the sagital sinus is -30 mmHg (but the venous valves of the legs limit the rise of the pressure).

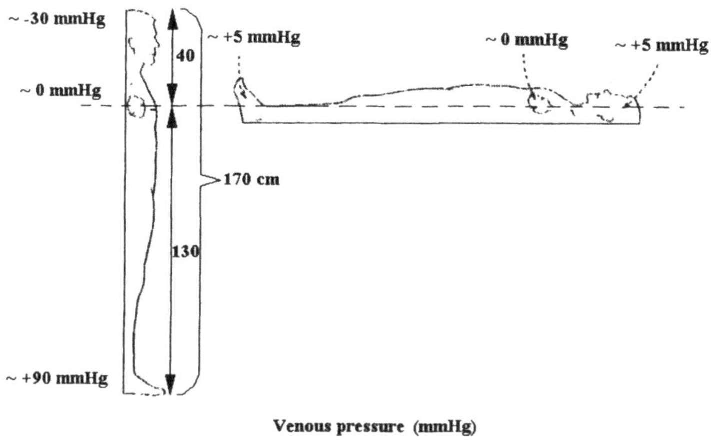

Fig.1.1. Effects of gravity on venous pressure.

1.2. FLOW, PRESSURE AND RESISTANCE

The flow through a vessel is determined by pressure difference between the two ends of the vessel and the vascular resistance. The relationship between flow, pressure and resistance is analogous, in a general way, to the relationship between the current (I), electromotive force (E) and resistance (R) in an electrical circuit expressed in Ohm's law (1):

$$E = IR$$

I = flow (Q)
E = pressure (ΔP)
R = resistance (R)

So:

$$Q = \frac{\Delta P}{R}; \qquad \Delta P = QR; \qquad R = \frac{\Delta P}{Q}$$

1.2.1. Pressure in Veins

Systemic blood reaches the venules at about 20 mmHg, so the arteriovenous gradient is about 90 mmHg. It falls steadily in the larger veins to about 5.5 mmHg in the veins outside the thorax. Blood from all systemic veins flows into the right atrium at approximately 0 mmHg.

In a rigid tube the difference in pressure between the two ends of the vessels determines the rate of flow, and not the absolute pressure in the vessel. But the vascular system is distensible, so when the pressure in the veins is increased, it dilates the veins and the result is increased blood flow. With the same pressure difference between the two ends of the veins, the blood flows increases in proportion to the fourth power of the diameter.

So, for example, an increase of relative diameter from 2, having a 16 ml/min.flow, to relative diameter 4, the flow becomes 256 ml/min (and with a decrease of the initial diameter 2 to 1, the flow decrease from 16 ml/min to 1 ml/min).

1.2.2. Distensibility and Compliance

Vascular distensibility (V.D.) is expressed as the increase in volume for 1 mmHg pressure.

$$\text{V.D.} = \frac{\textit{increase in volume}}{\textit{increase in pressure} \times \textit{initial volume}}$$

For example:

- initial volume = 10 ml;
- increase in pressure = 1 mmHg;
- final volume = 11 ml.

$$\text{V.D.} = \frac{1ml}{1mm \times 10ml} = 0.1 \text{ ml/mmHg } (10\%)$$

The veins are about 6-10 times as distensible as the arteries.

The total distensibility in any vascular areas is expressed by term compliance or capacitance:

$$\text{Vascular capacitance} = \frac{increase \quad in \quad volume}{increase \quad in \quad pressure} = \frac{\Delta V}{\Delta P};$$

or distensibility × volume.

The compliance of a vein is about 30 times that its corresponding artery, because it is about 10 times as distensible and it has a volume about 3 times as great.

The thin-walled venous vessels accommodate large volume changes with little change in pressure.

Venous compliance has a geometrical aspect (Fig. 2.): at low venous pressure, the veins are partially collapsed and are elliptical in cross section. Increases of the transmural pressure with an increasing venous volume, imposes a circular cross section (6).

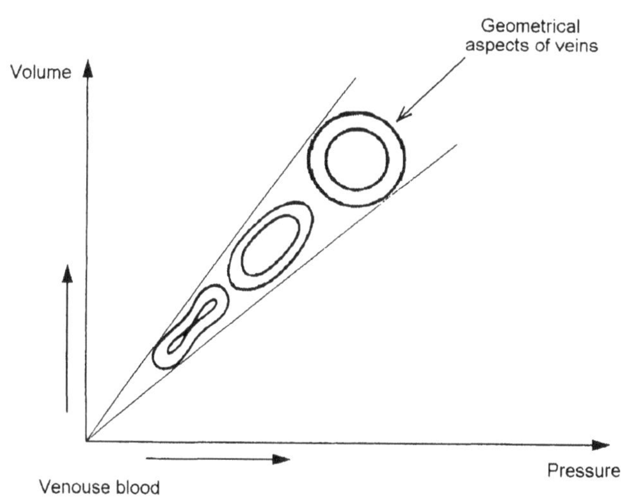

Fig.1.2. Geometrical aspects of veins.

Compliance of the veins relates closely to the passive and active biomechanical properties of their wall and to its physiological control (4).

1.2.3. Relation between Distending Pressure and Tension

The law of Laplace states that the distending pressure (P) in a distensible vessel is equal at equilibrium to the tension in the wall (T) divided by the radius (r).

$$P = \frac{T}{R}; T = P \times r.$$

P is actually the transmural pressure, expressed in dynes/cm^2.
T is expressed in dynes/cm, and r in cm.

Consequently, the smaller the radius of a blood vessel, the less the tension in the wall necessary to balance the distending pressure and it is less prone to rupture (the protective effect of small size in case of thin-walled and delicate vessels – Table 1.I.).

In the human aorta the tension at normal pressures is about 170,000 dynes/cm, in the vena cava it is about 21,000 and in the capillaries it is approximately 16 dynes/cm.

1.3. VELOCITY

Velocity (V) is proportional to flow (Q) divided by the area of the conduct (A):

$$V = \frac{Q}{A}; Q = \frac{\Delta P}{R}; A = \pi r^2$$

For the case in which blood flows in an unbranched tube of variable cross section, the flow will be equal to all cross sections, but the average velocity will vary according the Q/A.

The venous system is a branched network of tubes in which the characteristic branching pattern is that the total cross-sectional area of the branches is larger than the cross-sectional area of the terminal trunk (Table 1.I).

Table I.I.

	Lumen diameter	Wall thickness	Area
Capillaries	8 µm	0.50 µm	50.24 μm^2
Venules	20 µm	1.00 µm	314 μm^2
Veins	5	0.50 mm	19.625 mm^2
Vena cava	30	1.50 mm	706.5 mm^2

This means that the total cross-sectional area of the venous system decreases from the capillaries, venules, veins, to the cave veins. Correspondingly, the average blood flow velocity in small vessels is less than in large vein (7).

Table I.II.

	Number	Total cross-sectional area (cm^2)	Pressure (mmHg)	Blood velocity (cm/sec)
Capillaries	$8*10^9$	4500	20	0.018
Venules	10^9	4000	15	0.021
Veins	200	40	10	2.1
Vena cava	2	18	5	4.5

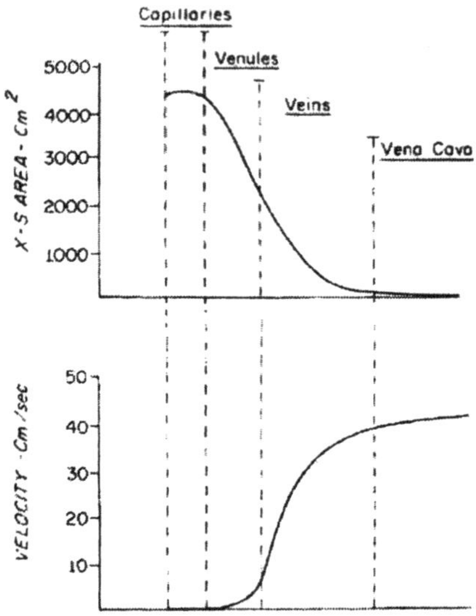

Fig.1.3. Relations between cross sectional area and velocity in veins.

1.4. RESISTANCE, CONDUCTANCE AND VISCOSITY IN THE VENOUS SYSTEM

Veins have a large cross-sectional area, so the resistance to flow is low, and the pressure drops about 15 mmHg from capillaries to the heart (in the supine individual). It is only a fraction of that from the aorta to the capillaries (about 80 mmHg).

Resistance is the impediment to blood flow in a vessel, but it cannot be measured and must be calculated from measurements of blood flow and pressure difference in the vessel (3).

If the pressure difference between two points in a vessel is 1 mmHg and the flow is 1 ml/sec, then:

$$R = \frac{\Delta P}{Q} = \frac{1}{1} = 1\text{PRU (peripheral resistance unit)},$$

or in CGS units:

$$R = \frac{dyne \times \sec}{cm^5} = \frac{1333 \times mmHg}{ml/\sec} = \text{PRU} \times 1333 = 1333\ \text{dyne} \times \sec \times \text{cm}^{-5}$$

At rest, if the rate of blood flow through the circulatory system is about 100 ml/sec, and the pressure difference from the systemic arteries to the systemic veins is about 100 mmHg, and then the resistance is 100/100=1 PRU. In pulmonary circulation, the difference from the pulmonary artery to the pulmonary veins is about 10 mmHg, so that the resistancc is 10/100 = 0.1 PRU.

The reciprocal of resistance is ***conductance*** (C).

$$C = \frac{1}{R}$$

Viscosity

The resistance to blood flow is determined not only by the radius of the blood vessels (vascular hindrance) but also by the viscosity of the blood (5). Viscosity is analogous to internal friction, the flow of one layer of fluid past another. Viscosity is the proportionality constant of shearing force per unit area – the shear stress. The rate of shear is expressed in poise. Water of 20°C has a viscosity of 0.01 poise or 1.0 centipoises (cp).

The viscosity of the blood is shear rate dependent, and is three to four times the viscosity of the water. The viscous properties of the blood are complex and are dependent on the concentration of red cells (the hematocrit). The hematocrit of a normal man averages about 42. When the hematocrit rises to 60 is polycythemie, and when hematocrit rises at 70, the blood viscosity become ten times that of water.

Another factor that affects blood viscosity is the concentration of proteins and their types in the plasma, but they are not significant, because the viscosity of blood plasma is about 1.5 times that of water.

Viscosity decreases with increasing shear rates. So, in the blood the viscosity is dependent on the rate of the flow and the vein diameter. In veins having a large diameter, at higher but no turbulent flow rates, the red cell stream is in the center of the vein, and near the margins of the vessel is a relatively cell free plasma. So the flow rate increase of the red cells in the axial stream is associated with a progressive decrease in apparent viscosity (sigma effect).

The apparent viscosity of the blood decreases with the decreasing diameter in veins smaller than 1.5 mm because there is a relatively unshared column behind the red cell particles (Fahreus -Lindquist effect).

So, the viscosity of the blood depends almost entirely on the concentration of red blood cells. In severe anemia, the blood viscosity may fall and decrease the resistance to blood flow in the peripheral vessels.

In polycytemia the viscosity increases, the flow of the blood through the vessels is often very sluggish and increases peripheral resistance.

As the Poiseuille equation shows:

$$Q = \Delta P \times \frac{\pi r^4}{8\eta l}$$

ΔP = pressure gradient
r = radius of the vessel
η = viscosity
l = the length of the vessel.

Rearranging the Poiseuille equation for resistance:

$$R = \frac{8\eta l}{\pi r^4}$$

The resistance of a vessel is directly proportional to the blood viscosity and length of the vessel but inversely proportional to the fourth power of the radius.

And the conductance (C) = $\frac{\pi r^4}{8\eta l}$

So, the resistance to blood flow is determined by the radius of the vessel and the viscosity of the blood, but the effect in vivo derivates from that predicted by the poiseuille formula, because the viscosity of the blood 7vessel.

REFERENCES

1. Berne RM, Levy MN. "Haemodynamics".In *Physiology*, RM Berne, MN Levy, ed. Mosby, 1998
2. Ganong WF. "Circulating-biophysical considerations". In *Review of Medical Physiology*, WF Ganong, ed. Lange Medical Publications, Los Altos, 1985
3. Guyton AC, Hall JE. "Overview of the circulation". In *Textbook of Medical Physiology*, AC Guyton, JE Hall, ed. Saunders, 1996
4. Monos E. Compliance of the veins - Local control mechanism. Med Razgl 1991; 30 (suppl 1): 129-132
5. Pop de Popa I, Socoteanu I, Badiu Gh. "Haemorrheologic aspects". In *Physiology and pathophysiology of haemodynamics*, I Teodorescu-Exarcu, ed. Editura Medicala, Bucuresti - Romania, 1985 [in Romanian]
6. Rowell LB. "The venous system". In *Human circulation: regulation during physical stress*, LB Rowell, ed. Oxford University Press, 1986
7. Scher AM, Feigl EO. "Pressure and hydrostatics". In *Textbook of Physiology*, HD Patton, AF Fuchs, B Hille, AM Scher, R. Schteiner, ed. Saunders, 1989

CHAPTER 2

VEINS AND THEIR FUNCTIONS

TAKE HOME MESSAGES

- Veins are not purely passive collectors and conducts; the rate of blood flow and pressure in veins assures the regulation of the cardiac function and the optimization of the circulatory system.
- Special regional functions concern the veins draining the brain, hart, liver, limbs and lungs.

2.1. VEINS AS CONDUCT

The primary function of the veins is to conduct the blood from the capillaries to the heart.

The blood enters the venules with an appreciable pressure residuum (vis à tergo) from the arterial side, after it has pressed through the capillaries. The resistance meets the pressure by flow from the veins themselves and from the heart itself (the vis à fronte).

But the veins are not purely passive collectors and conducts. In addition to the vis à tergo and the vis à fronte mechanisms, muscle, abdominal and thoracic pumps and venous valves favor the venous blood flow from areas of high pressure - from capillaries, to areas of low pressure

- to atriums. Pulsations of arteries nearby may also compress the veins. Muscular movements, together with the venous valves, aid venous return. When the muscles contracts, the increased muscular pressure compress and empties the veins. When the exercise is isometric, in a sustained contraction, the blood flow would is fully marked (4).

The systemic blood reaches the venules at a pressure of about 20 mmHg, so the arteriovenouse pressure gradient is about 90 mmHg. It falls steadily in the larger veins to about 5.5 mmHg, in the veins outside the thorax.

The blood from all the systemic veins flows into the right atrium. Therefore the pressure in the right atrium is called the central venous pressure. The normal central venous pressure is approximately 0 mmHg, with a lower limit of about –3 to –5 mmHg (equal to the pressure in the pericardial and interpleural spaces). It can rise to as high as 30 mmHg under heart failure or massive transfusion of blood (1).

The pressure in the great veins fluctuates with heart action. The right atrial pressure changes are transmitted to the great veins producing three characteristic waves in the jugular pulse: the "a" wave is due to atrial systole; the "c" wave is the transmitted manifestation of the rise in atrial pressure produced by the bulging of the tricuspid valve into the atria during isometric ventricular contraction; the "v" wave mirrors the rise in atrial pressure before the tricuspid valve opens during diastole (Fig.2.1.).

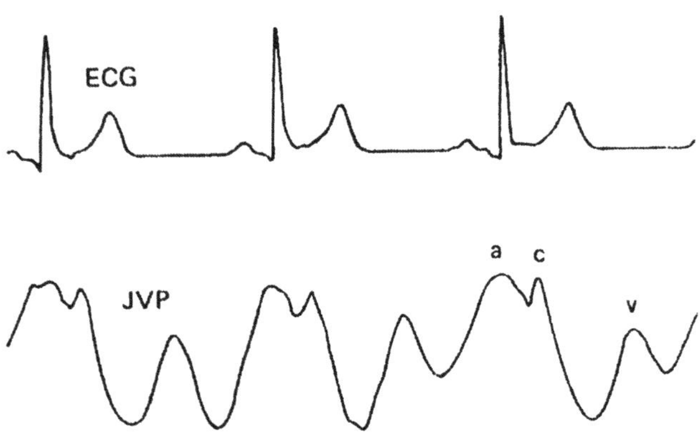

Fig.2.1. Variations of jugular pressure.

The veins within the thorax are exposed to a subatmospheric pressure that acts to aid return the blood to the thorax. Negative intrathoracic pressure during inspiration increases and the flow of blood in the thorax increases. Opposed effects are seen during expiration. When abdominal pressure is raised, this will cause an increase of blood return into the thorax (8).

In expire forcefully with the glottis closed, as in strain lifting a weight, the intrathoracic and abdominal pressure increase, and blood may initially be forced into the atrium, causing an increase in cardiac output, but in second time when the external pressure becomes high, the venous vessels are closed and the flow of the blood into the thorax and the cardiac output decrease.

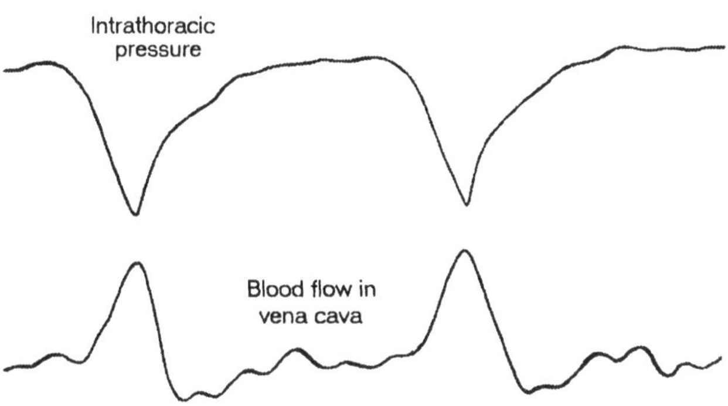

Fig.2.2. Relation between the intrathoracic pressures and the blood flow in the vena cava

In upright posture, the pressure equal to the height of the blood column from heart to foot, about 100 mmHg, is imposed on the veins of the foot. So, the veins of the legs are distended and the volume of blood in the veins below the heart increases by about 500 ml in an average 70-kg human, while the right atrial pressure and stroke volume decrease (11).

The "muscle pump" i.e. the compression of the vein by movement, is important in moving venous blood from the legs upright. It works together with the venous valves. Patients with varicose veins, whose valves are incompetent, they may have venous stasis and ankle edema (5). Pulsations of nearby arteries may also compress veins. Venous return is also aided in venoconstriction in the splanchnic region and in the skin. It is a major factor controlling cardiac output and possibly compensating mild hemorrhage.

There is a relationship between venous return, venous pressure and cardiac output. The passive properties of the venous system are of importance in cardiovascular control and in the return of blood from the capillaries to the heart.

2.2. VEINS AS A RESERVOIR

The veins act as a reservoir, a low-pressure storage system (capacity vessels), holding the greater amount of blood (64 %). When a person bleeds severely so that the arterial pressure begins to fall, pressure reflexes are elicited with sympathetic nerve signals to the veins, causing them to constrict and to deliver a part of the containing blood. Certain portions of the venous system are blood reservoirs. These include the spleen, the liver, the abdominal veins, the venous plexus of the skin, and the veins of the lungs.

Even slight increases in pressure cause the veins to store extra blood. In upright posture, the volume of blood in the veins below the heart increases by about 500 ml in an average 70 kg human. The extra volume of blood causes immediate elastic distension of the vein, but the smooth muscle tension correspondingly decreases. It is stress-relaxation or delayed compliance (6).

Two adaptations limit this translocation of blood: the venous valves and the muscular movements. This translocation of blood increases the orthostatic tolerance of the organism (orthostatic hypotension and the orthostatic edema are important problems).

2.3. VENOUS RETURN AND THE FILLING PRESSURE

The venous return to the right heart maintains the filling pressure, providing adaptation to the changing cardiac output requirements. The rate at which blood flows from the vascular tree, via venous system, into the right atrium (and determines the cardiac output) depends on the mean circulatory filling pressure. By definition, the mean systemic filling pressure is the pressure in all parts of the systemic circulation when there is no flow in the circulation. The normal mean systemic filling pressure is 7 mmHg (3.5 – 14 mmHg). The mean systemic filling pressure increases with an increase in blood volume. The grater the difference between the mean systemic filling pressure and the right atrial pressure (PRA) is, the greater becomes the venous return. When this is 0, there is no venous return (8).

So, the mean systemic filling pressure (PSF) represents a pressure pushing the blood into the veins from the periphery toward the heart in spite of the resistance to venous return (RVR):

$$\mathrm{VR} = \frac{PSF - PRA}{RVR}$$

In the normal human at rest the VR = 5 liters/min and the RVR = 1.4 mmHg/liter, because the PSF = 7 mmHg and PRA = 0 mmHg.

2.4. VENOUS RETURN AND REGULATION OF CARDIAC FUNCTION

The rate of the blood flow into the heart from the veins assures the regulation of the cardiac function, through the intrinsec ability of the heart to adapt, in two ways:

a) A stretch of the ventricle during filling increases the force of contraction by the mechanism of the Frank-Starling law. It is dependent on the volume of blood in the ventricle at the end of diastole – preload (the degree of stretch of the muscle when it begins to contract).

b) A stretch of the right atrial wall during filling increases the intrinsec heart rate by 10 to 20 percent. It is caused by the stretch of the sinus nod.

An additional 40 to 60 percent increase in rate is caused by the stretch receptors of the atria by the Bainbridge reflex.

2.5. THE ROLE IN THE OPTIMIZATION OF THE CIRCULATORY SYSTEM

Changes of the body position influence the hydrostatic level in blood vessels and induce adaptation of the capacitance of the venous system by myogenic response, segmental neural reflex, metabolic and humoral control (1).

The volume in the skeletal muscle veins is reduced during contraction, but in relaxation the pressure is reduced favoring a higher blood flow. This is known as "muscle pump" and is efficient because the venous pressure in the feet while walking remains about 25 mmHg, when the venous valve is competent. If a person is standing absolutely still, the venous pressure in the lower part of the leg will rise to 90 mmHg.

2.6. THE ROLE OF THE VENOUS SYSTEM IN EXCHANGE PROCESSES

Not only the capillaries, but also the venules, contribute to the exchange processes with extravascular space.
The exchange processes are (7):

- resorbtion of interstitial fluid;
- transportation of large molecules, especially in inflammation;
- leaving and return to the circulation of the polymorphonuclear leucocytes;
- distribution of circulating precursors of the effector lymphocytes.

2.7. THE ROLE OF THE VEIN IN SYNTHESIS OF BIOLOGICALLY ACTIVE SUBSTANCES, COAGULATION AND FIBRINOLYSIS

Due to their endothelium veins are also involved in:

1. Synthesis of vasodilatator substances (NO, prostacyclin);
2. Synthesis of vasoconstrictor substances (endothelin, angiotensin, tromboxane, PAF).

3. Maintain the nonthrombogenic blood-tissue interface (9).
4. Regulation of blood clotting by participation to coagulant pathways (von Willebrand factor).
5. Anticoagulant activity (PGI_2, thrombomoduline, glicoseaminoglican heparinlike, tissue factor pathway inhibitor), fibrinolytic activity (tissue type plasminogen activator - > tPA) and antifibrinolytic activity (plasminogen activator inhibitor type 1 –> PAI-1) (2, 3).

2.8. SPECIAL REGIONAL FUNCTIONS OF THE VEINS

2.8.1. Veins of the Head and Face

2.8.1.1. Veins of the Brain

The veins of the brain comprise cerebral, cereberal and brainstem veins. They have no valves and no muscular tissue, but have a layer of pia mater with a perivascular space. They pierce the arachnoid mater and the inner dural layer to open into the cranial venous sinuses.

The dural sinuses are venous channels between two layers of dura mater draining blood from the brain and cranial bones. The emissary veins make connections between the venous sinuses and the extracranial veins. These are significant in the spread of infection from extracranial foci to venous sinuses and in the possibility of infective thrombosis.

A unique feature of the cerebral circulation is that it lies within a rigid structure→the cranium. Because the intracranial contents are incompressible, any increase in arterial inflow must be associated with a comparable increase in venous outflow. So the internal jugular vein acts as a siphonage device (11).

Throughout the walls of the venous sinuses are the arachnoidal villi. Large conglomerates of these villi form arachnoidal granulations protruding into the sinus assuring absorption of cerebrospinal fluid. Normally, the villi allow cerebrospinal fluid to flow into the blood when its pressure is about 1.5 mmHg greater than the pressure of the blood in the venous sinuses. Under normal conditions, the pressure almost never rises more than a few mmHg higher than the pressure in the venous sinuses.

When the villi become blocked, the cerebrospinal fluid pressure rises, causing hydrocephalus.

2.8.1.2. Facial Veins

Facial veins develop temperature-dependent myogenic tone and contribute to the cranial thermoregulation. In contrast to the other veins, it possesses β_1-adrenergic receptors and contributes to the emotional blushing (7).

2.8.2. Cardiac Veins

The veins draining the heart, for the large majority, return in the right atrium through the coronary sinus, but some reach the right atrium by way of the anterior coronary veins. In addition, the Thebesius small veins open directly into all chambers of the heart. The coronary flow is greatest during ventricular diastole and least during systole, but phasic coronary venous flow is greatest during systole because ventricular contraction expels blood from the myocardium.

Under normal conditions, during diastole the pressure gradient for coronary perfusion is the difference between aortic pressure and the pressure in the coronary sinus. When the tissue pressure exceeds the venous outflow pressure, the arteriovenous gradient does not operate and the flow is proportional to the gradient between arterial pressure and tissue pressure.

2.8.3. Hepatic Veins

Hepatic veins convey blood from the liver to the inferior vena cava draining the blood from organs of digestion including the gastrointestinal tract (except the lower anal canal), liver, gall bladder, pancreas and spleen, into the hepatic portal vein.

The viscera and the liver receive about 30% of the cardiac output, about 1000 ml from the portal vein and 500 ml from the hepatic artery.

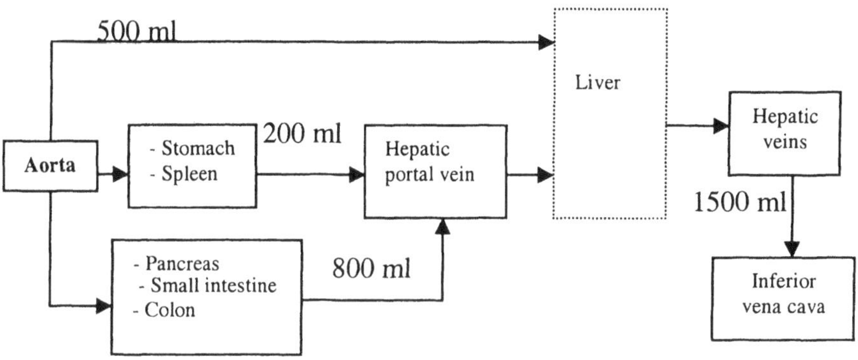

Fig.2.3.

In the liver, the portal vein ramifies like an artery, ending in the sinusoids; hepatic artery blood also enters the sinusoids.

The sinusoid blood flows into the central vein of each lobule and the central veins coalesce to form the hepatic veins, which drain into the inferior vena cava.

Portal venous pressure is normally about 10 mmHg, and hepatic venous pressure is approximately 5 mmHg. When portal venous pressure rises substantially – portal hypertension, the consequences are ascites, rupture of the splanchnic veins and collateral circulation, i.e. anastomoses between portal and systemic circulations of the left gastric vein, rectal veins, epigastric veins and retroperitoneal veins.

The portal vein contains nutrients that have been absorbed from the intestinal lumen, gastrointestinal and pancreatic hormones. They are carried directly into the liver, transformed, stored, and/or may pass into the general circulation.

The spleen and the large, distensible splanchnic veins can accommodate variable volumes of blood, and help to regulate central venous pressure and cardiac output (4).

2.8.4. Cutaneous Veins

There is a close association between the arteriolar and the venous plexus and an anastomotic connection between the arterioles and the venules. This permits an exchange of heat between the blood in the vessels at different temperatures flowing in opposite directions, for conservation or dissipation of heat (counter current heat exchange).

The blood flow in response to thermoregulatory stimuli can vary from 1 to as much as 150 ml / 100 g of skin per minute. These variations are possible because blood can be shunted through the anastomoses.
The cutaneous veins act as blood reservoirs.

2.8.5. Veins of the Limbs

They are grouped as superficial and deep, interconnected. The superficial veins are subcutaneous; arteries accompany the deep veins. Valves are more numerous in the lower limbs. The superficial veins of the upper limbs are usually visible when the muscle is contracted, driving the blood from the deep to the superficial veins, via *venae comitantes.*

The superficial veins of the lower limbs are the great saphenous and small saphenous. Perforating veins connect the great saphenous with the deep veins, but in these perforating veins the valves are arranged so as to prevent flow of blood from the deep to the superficial veins. At rest, pressure in the superficial veins is equal to the height of the column of blood. When the calf muscle contracts, blood is pumped proximally in the deep veins, while the valves in the perforating veins prevent the flow into the superficial veins. During relaxation blood can be aspirated from the superficial into the deep veins (5).

The connection between superficial and deep veins, especially in the lower limbs, permits heat exchange by counter-current, in order to participate in the thermal economy. Some actions have the opposite effect on the deep limb veins, draining chiefly skeletal muscles, and the cutaneous veins, because, for example, lowering temperatures causes a cutaneous venoconstriction but a muscle vasodilatation.

2.8.6. Veins of the Lungs

The lungs have both a pulmonary and a systemic circulation.

The systemic, bronchial venous circulation, conducts the blood from the bronchial airways and all the pulmonary structures, except the respiratory bronchioles and the alveolar walls, and it is less than 1% of the cardiac output. Bronchial veins do not receive all the blood conveyed by bronchial arteries; some enter the pulmonary veins.

The pulmonary circulation assures the gas transfer between the blood and the alveolar air. The pulmonary artery branches give an extensive capillary network in the alveolar wall. The capillaries unite to form larger alveolar microvessels that become venules; these join to form veins and finally four pulmonary veins drain into the left atrium.

The total volume of the pulmonary circulation is about 500 ml, the capillary volume is approximately equal to the stroke volume of the right ventricle, and the remainder is distributed almost equally between the arterial and venous vessels.

The pressure in the pulmonary circulation of a normal supine person is for the pulmonary artery 24-mmHg sistolic and 9 mmHg diastolic (a mean of 14 mmHg), in the capillaries – a mean of 10.5 mmHg, in venules a mean of 9 mmHg, and in left atrium, a mean of 8 mmHg.

The pulmonary hemodynamics is obtained by measuring the changes in the driving pressure. Driving pressure (DP) is the difference between mean pulmonary atrial pressure (P_{pa}) and mean left atrial pressure (P_{lat}).

$$DP = P_{pa} - P_{lat}$$

It is about 6 mmHg.

The pulmonary vascular resistance is less than 10% of that in the systemic vascular bed. At high lung volume the arteries and the veins are dilated and flow resistance is much less.

The effects of gravity are relatively greater in the pulmonary circulation than in the systemic circulation, because blood pressure is much lower. When a normal person lies down, the pulmonary blood volume increases and when the person stands up, his blood is discharged into the general circulation.

Because of their distensibility, the pulmonary veins are an important blood reservoir. There is nonuniform ventilation and nonuniform circulation in the lungs. Both the air and the blood supply to the alveoli vary greatly from one part of the lung to another. This variation is the effect of the lung volume and of the gravity.

Upright position causes a greater air and blood flow to the base than to the top of the lungs. The adult lung is about 30 cm high, so the effect of gravity in upright divides perfusion zones into three parts (10):

a) Zone 1, the lung apex that does not receive blood flow if the regional pulmonary artery pressure (a) is less than the alveolar pressure (A). In this case the venouse blood flow (v) is 0 (Pa<PA>Pv).
b) Zone 2, the middle part of the lung, where the pulmonary artery pressure exceeds the alveolar pressure, which exceeds the pulmonary venous pressure (Pa>PA>Pv). In this region, it is the arterial-alveolar pressure gradient that produces flow, not the arterio-venous gradient.
c) Zone 3 is the basal portion of the lung, where the pulmonary artery pressure exceeds the pulmonary venous pressure, which exceeds the alveolar pressure (Pa>Pv>PA).

REFERENCES

1. Berne RM, Levy MN. "The cardiovascular system". In *Physiology*, RM Berne, MN Levy, ed. Mosby, 1998
2. Crisnic D, Siska I, Crisnic M, Cocarla D, Schneider F. The role of venous endothelium in the fibrinolytic activity. Fiziologia-Physiology 2001; 11: 25-30
3. Fukao H, Matsuo O. Antithrombotic regulation in human endothelial cells by fibrinolytic factors. Semin Thromb Hemost 2000; 26: 33-38
4. Ganong WF. "Circulation". In *Review of Medical Physiology*, Ganong WF, ed. Lange Medical Publications, 1985
5. Guyton AC, Hall JE. "Overview of the circulation". In *Textbook of Medical Physiology*, AC Guyton, JE Hall, ed. Saunders, 1996
6. Haulica I. "Physiology of the vascular system" In *Human physiology*, I Haulica, ed. Editura Medicala, Bucuresti - Romania, 1996 [in Romanian]
7. Monos E, Berczi V, Nadasy G. Local control of veins. Physiol Rev 1995; 75: 611-666
8. Scher AM "The circulation". In *Textbook of Physiology*, HD Patton, AF Fuchs, B Hille, AM Scher, R. Schteiner, ed. Saunders, 1989
9. Serban M, Schramm W. Clinical haemostasiology. Editura Brumar, Timisoara - Romania, 2001[in Romanian]
10. Staub NC. "The respiratory system". In *Physiology*, RM Berne, MN Levy, ed. Mosby, 1998
11. Teodorescu-Exarcu I, Badiu Gh. "Physiology of venous circulation". In *Physiology and pathophysiology of haemodynamics*, I Teodorescu-Exarcu, ed. Editura Medicala, Bucuresti - Romania, 1985 [in Romanian]

CHAPTER 3

VENOUS WALL - MORPHOLOGICAL AND FUNCTIONAL ASPECTS

TAKE HOME MESSAGES

- Similar to arteries, venous wall presents three tunics: **intima, media and adventitia.**
- In some regions, **venous intima** extends into the lumen valves, which prevent gravitational backflow of blood.
- Venous endothelial cells are involved in:
  - regulation of venous tone
  - control of coagulation and fibrinolysis
  - vascular remodeling process
  - immune surveillance, response to tissue injury or infection.
- Differences between arterial and venous vessels with respect to many endothelial functions were noted.
- **Venous smooth muscle** morphology and function are similar to those of arterial smooth muscle.
- In most veins, **adventitia** contains loose connective tissue, elastic and collagen fibers, and smooth muscle fibers, and represents the greatest part of the venous wall.

The dimensions of arteries and veins, unlike those of the microvascular components, are largely species-related and depend primarily on the total blood volume. Unlike arteries, a correspondence between the size and structure in veins cannot be systematically established.

Veins are arbitrarily classified as small, medium, and large. Small veins have a diameter that may vary from 0.2 to 1 mm. Medium-size veins measure approximately 1 to 10 mm in diameter, their wall thickness representing one-tenth of the vascular diameter. In humans, the large veins are larger than 9 to 10 mm, and their wall is extremely thin (one twentieth of their vascular diameter).

The three basic tunics - intima, media and adventitia - can be recognized in the wall of veins, but their boundaries are less distinct than in arteries. Generally speaking, the veins of the upper regions of the body are essentially draining veins that return blood to the heart by gravity and their walls contain mostly elastic fibers and collagen fibers. The veins of the lower regions of the body are predominantly propulsive veins that propel the blood to the heart by contracting their muscle fibers (177).

3.1. VENOUS ENDOTHELIUM

The endothelium is a confluent monolayer of thin, flattened, rhomboid-shaped cells lining the intimal surface of all blood vessels, including veins. In the adult human, the endothelium is composed of approximately 1 to 6 x 10^{13} cells. The net mass of the endothelium is 1 kg and has a surface area of approximately 5,000 m^2 (Jaffe, 1984, quoted by 185).

Until the late 1960s, the conventional wisdom in cardiovascular circles was that endothelium was a relatively inert nonthrombogenic cellular barrier. The electron microscopic studies of Palade in 1953 and the physiologic studies of Gowan in 1959 concerning the interaction between lymphocytes and endothelial cells of postcapillar venules stimulated numerous studies that led to the current view of endothelium as a dynamic and heterogeneous "organ" (59). In 1966, Florey considered the endothelium "more than a sheet of nucleated cellophane" (60).

The detailed study of endothelial functions first became feasible with the development in the 1970s of *in vitro* endothelial cells cultures, appreciation of endothelial cell roles being largely based on the behavior of cultured human umbilical vein endothelial cells (HUVEC)(89).

3.1.1. Microscopic Aspects

Small veins present a thin intima (endothelium lying on a very thin subendothelial connective tissue layer, which increases with the vessel size).

The intima of *medium-size veins* is rather poor, being made up of short polygonal endothelial cells and a thin basal lamina. The subendothelial layer contains delicate collagen and scattered elastic fibers. The poorly defined elastica interna is found in veins that conduct blood against the force of gravity (veins draining the extremities). The intima extends into the lumen pairs of semilunar folds, called valves, which are formed by connective core covered on both surfaces by endothelium. Valves only occur in veins of more than 2 mm diameter, their role being to prevent gravitational backflow of blood. At this level the venous wall is thick (177).

The intima of *large veins* has the same configuration as in the medium-sized veins. Endothelial cells (EC) are linked together by tight junctions and gap junctions, the latter being less frequent than those found in arteries. The basal lamina is thin, and the elastica interna is largely fenestrated or fragmented. Some large veins have well defined valves (177).

Endothelium is highly differentiated to mediate and monitor the extensive bidirectional exchange of small molecules and to restrict some of the transport of macromolecules. Three major types of intercellular junctions have been identified in endothelial cells: tight junctions, gap junctions and adherens junctions. Endothelial junctions are formed by transmembrane proteins, linked to cytoplasmic and cytoskeletal proteins (43, 44, 45, 100).

Morphological studies indicate that the endothelial junctions are generally less elaborate in veins than in arteries; the loosest junctional organization occurs in venules, while the strongest is found in arterioles.

In vivo, endothelial cells are attached to the surface of blood vessels by their interactions with the underlying subendothelium, which consists of a highly organized matrix of molecules that includes collagen, elastin, fibronectin, laminin, glycosoaminoglycans, thrombospondin, vibronectin and von Willebrand's factor (vWF)(177). The roles of some of these molecules are presented in Table 3.I.

The subendothelial matrix provides structural integrity, mechanical strength and elasticity to the vessel wall. It can be mentioned that heparan sulfate, a proteoglycan with anticoagulant properties mediated by potentiation of antithrombin III, is less prominent in both the media and internal elastic lamina of veins, compared with arteries (40).

Table 3.I. Subendothelial molecules (with data from the text)

Molecule	Synthesis by EC	Functions
Collagens	+	• increased proliferation/inhibition of cell growth
Laminin	+	• involved in angiogenesis (induces tubes formation) • supports the adhesion of EC • necessary for EC growth
Fibronectin	+	• binds to fibrin, fibrinogen, collagen, and thrombospondin • binds to integrins • inhibits EC attachment, induces EC detachment
Thrombo-spondin	+	• mediates the adhesion of EC • inhibits EC attachment and induces EC detachment • binds to fibrin, fibrinogen, collagen and fibronectin
Glycosoamino-glycans	+ (heparan sulphate)	• initiate EC attachment • convey anticoagulant activity to the EC
Vibronectin		• supports attachment and spreading of EC • necessary for the activity of plasminogen activator inhibitors
von Willebrandt Factor	+	• stimulates platelet adhesion to the subendothelium • serves as carrier protein for factor VIII

Legend: EC = endothelial cells

Due to its high content of collagen, the basal lamina can be digested by collagenase. After treatment with collagenase, endothelial cells from various vessels (human umbilical vein, animal arteries, veins and microvessels) can be isolated and grown in tissue culture for in vitro studies (177).

The endothelium is a slowly renewing population of cells that rarely divide, the venous endothelial cells having a greater mitotic potential than those of arteries. The normal lifespan of a human endothelial cell is approximately 30 years (191).

3.1.2. The Roles of Venous Endothelium

The endothelium, including the venous one, plays a key role in cardiovascular homeostasis through its diverse influences on blood vessel structure and function.

3.1.2.1. The Role of Endothelium in Regulation of Vascular Tone

Endothelial cells influence vascular hemodynamics in physiologic state by releasing vasodilators such as nitric oxide (NO) and prostacyclin (PGI_2), as well as vasoconstrictor agents, including endothelin (ET), thromboxane A_2 and angiotensin II. These factors are not stored in intracellular granules; their activity is regulated by the location of specific receptors on vascular cells, through their rapid metabolism, or at the level of gene transcription (142, 175).

Generally, seven families of compounds have been associated with endothelium mediated vasomotor responses: prostanoids, nitric oxide, endothelins, angiotensins, hyperpolarizing factors, reactive oxygen species and other uncharacterized endothelium derived constrictors (41, 175). Aspects regarding the synthesis and actions of all these compounds are detailed in chapter 4.

Principal regulatory factors synthesized by the endothelium, their effects on the vasculature and other actions are presented in Tables 3.II and 3.III.

- *Eicosanoids*

  Similar to other vascular tissues, venous tissue synthesizes different prostanoids with known vasoactivity. The contribution of different layers of the venous wall to this production is still unclear. There are studies that suggest that both endothelium and venous smooth muscle cells take part in the production of both prostacyclin and thromboxane (137, 13). In vitro release of PGI_2 (in the form of its stable metabolite, 6-keto-$PGF_{1\alpha}$) was confirmed for several human veins, such as umbilical, saphenous, pulmonary, mesenteric veins (26, 27, 28, 78). The production of thromboxane (in the form of its stable metabolite, TxB_2) was proved for human umbilical veins, saphenous and pulmonary veins (120, 26). In vivo measurements of 6-keto-$PGF_{1\alpha}$ and TxB_2 were also performed in human hand veins (75). There are contradictory data concerning the amount of prostanoids produced by the venous tissue compared to the arterial one. Most publications reported that prostacyclin production of veins is lower than that in arteries, but there are authors that have found a similar or even a higher venous production (28, 26). Generally, prostacyclin relaxes and thromboxane contracts vascular smooth muscle; prostanoid receptors and the effects of these compounds on venous smooth muscle are presented in chapter 4.

- *Nitric oxide (NO)*
  The properties of EDRF from intact arteries and veins suggest that arterial and venous EDRF are similar: NO (85, 86). Endothelium-derived NO, which is synthesized from L-arginine activates cytoplasmic guanylate cyclase and thereby stimulates intracellular cGMP accumulation in vascular smooth muscle (130, 136, 87). NO-dependent relaxations were confirmed in several human venous preparations, such as human dorsal hand vein (in response to bradykinin and acetylcholine)(18), and human saphenous vein (in response to acetylcholine and calcium ionophore A23187)(167, 107). Several studies showed that venous relaxation to vasoactive agents via NO is generally smaller than that of arteries. For instance, NO mediates endothelium-dependent relaxations of both human internal mammary artery and saphenous vein, but the artery released more NO than the vein (206, 208).

Table 3.II. Relaxing factors produced by EC (with data from 130, 136, 87, 79, 175)

Substance	Secretion	Other effects
NO	• constitutive and • induced by thrombin, ADP, muscarinic agonists, bradykinin, substance P, shear stress, cytokines	• maintaining of vessel basal tone • inhibition of leukocyte adhesion • inhibition of platelet functions (adhesion, activation, secretion and aggregation) • inhibition of smooth muscle cell migration and proliferation
EDHF (identity)	Induced by muscarinic agonists	
PG I_2	induced at sites of vascular perturbation (is not constitutively produced and does not regulate basal systemic vascular tone)	• retardation of platelet aggregation and deposition

- *Hyperpolarizing factors*

  Evidence indicates that under specific conditions not all endothelium dependent relaxation can be fully explained by the release of NO and/or PGI_2. The factor or factors responsible for such an effect is/are called endothelium-derived hyperpolarizing factor/factors (EDHF). Although the nature of EDHF is unclear, it has been suggested that it may be epoxy-eicosatrienoic acids (short-lived metabolites of arachidonic acid produced by EC through the cytochrome P450-dependent pathway), K^+ or other substances (carbon monoxide, hydroxyl radicals, hydrogen peroxide)(96, 83, 52, 128); in some species, NO and prostacyclin also induced hyperpolarizations (36). The contribution of EDHF to endothelium-dependent relaxation varies along the vascular tree. There are just a few studies concerning EDHF in human venous tissue. For example, Yang and He (1997) noted that EDHF plays a role in the human saphenous vein (203), while Liu et al. (2000) reported that NO may be responsible for nearly 60% of the endothelium-dependent hyperpolarization induced by acetylcholine and bradykinin in the human saphenous vein (105).

- *Endothelin-1*
  Endothelin-1 is a 21 amino acid endothelium-derived peptide that produces sustained contractions of arterial and smooth muscle in vitro, being approximately 100 times more potent than angiotensin II (118). In contrast to NO, veins seem to be more sensitive to this peptide than arteries (142). For instance, endothelin-1 produced a greater contraction in the human saphenous vein than in the gastroepiploic artery or internal mammary artery and the constrictor effect of ET was rapidly reversed in arteries, but only to a lesser extent in veins (38). Other experiments showed that human mammary veins exhibited an enhanced sensitivity to ET-1 as compared to internal mammary artery and saphenous vein (206, 109).

- *Angiotensin II*
  The major components of the renin-angiotensin system (renin, angiotensin-converting enzyme, angiotensin, and angiotensin receptors) have been also identified in vascular tissue. Endothelial cells are considered to be the major source of angiotensin-converting enzyme (ACE) in the vascular tissue and they also contain the mRNA for angiotensinogen (51, 69). There are data concerning local generation and release of angiotensin II even in human veins, such as hand (11), saphenous (155, 19) and umbilical veins (125). Biological effects of Ang II are mediated by AT_1 (involved in vasoconstriction and stimulation of SMC proliferation) and AT_2 receptors (involved in fetal development) (187). The dominant venoactive effect of angiotensin II is constriction, demonstrated in the following human preparations: chorionic plate vein, hand veins, and saphenous veins (111, 11, 152). In addition to the direct constrictor action, angiotensin II augments the venoconstrictor response to sympathetic nerve stimulation via an increased release of norepinephrine from the nerve terminals (197, 126). The importance of the local renin-angiotensin system is underlined by the fact that local ACE inhibition in the wall of large veins along with the large arteries and resistance vessels contributes to the beneficial therapeutic effects of ACE inhibitors in hypertension and congestive heart failure (47). ACE inhibitors also decrease the magnitude of venous graft thickening, being useful in preventing late venous graft disease (19).

- *Reactive oxygen species (ROS)*
  Both endothelial cells and vascular smooth muscle cells are capable of producing ROS from a variety of enzymatic sources. In disease states, vascular production of these reactive oxygen metabolites can increase substantially. Low generation of ROS by cultures EC in response to different stimuli (cytokines, bradykinin, calcium ionophores, and phorbol esters) is widely reported (174, 4, 21). Potential sources of free radicals in EC cultures are numerous, including xantine-oxidase, mitocondrial enzymes, citochrome P-450, cyclooxygenases, lipooxygenases, NADPH-oxidase, and NADH-dependent oxidase (73). Increasing evidence indicates that under increased oxidative stress superoxide anions can contribute to endothelium-dependent contractions. Superoxide anions can participate in the formation of other ROS, such as hydrogen peroxide or hydroxyl radicals and can influence vascular tone by inactivation of NO (via a facile radical/radical reaction that occurs more rapidly than the reaction of superoxide anion with superoxide dismutase) and by inhibition of PGI_2 synthesis in endothelial cells (93, 80). Our studies (Siska et al., unpublished data) showed that in vitro administration of hydrogen peroxide induces both constriction and dilation of human saphenous vein smooth muscle, these two effects being dose-dependent (venodilation occurred just when high doses, such as 10^{-3} M, were used).

Table 3.III. Vasoconstrictors produced by EC (with data from 130, 136, 87, 79, 175)

Substance	**Secretion**	**Other effects**
Endothelin-1	induced	• stimulation of smooth muscle cells proliferation • increases platelet aggregation • stimulates interleukin expression in monocytes
Angiotensins	induced	• Ang I stimulates prostaglandin release in cultured EC
Thromboxane A_2	induced	• stimulation of platelet aggregation and deposition
Platelet-activating factor	induced	• promotion of leukocyte adhesion at cell surface

3.1.2.2. The Role of Endothelium in Coagulation and Fibrinolysis

Endothelial cells participate in hemostasis by producing both procoagulant and anticoagulant substances. In normal conditions, the anticoagulant activity prevails. As detected with peroxidase-conjugated antibodies, small vessels show more plasminogen activator than do large vessels, and veins show more than do arteries (177). Beside this, the thromboembolic reactions of the venules are of markedly shorter duration compared with the arterioles (one-sixth of the arteriolar reaction time), and these changes cannot be explained only by local hemodynamic factors (41).

The Role of endothelium in coagulation

Endothelial cells play a primary role in the regulation of blood clotting by two separate, but related mechanisms: participation to procoagulant pathways and inhibition of procoagulant proteins (17)(Fig. 3.1).

I. Anticoagulant activity

Endothelial cells produce and express on their extracellular surfaces small amounts of heparan sulfate, which localizes and increases the intrinsic activity of antithrombin III (ATIII); only 1% of plasma antithrombin III is bound to the endothelium, but this bound form is at least 1000 times more reactive than the unbound pool (41).

Endothelial cells also present thrombomodulin, an integral membrane glycoprotein on the luminal surface, which can remove thrombin from the blood by forming complexes with it, facilitating its internalization and subsequent degradation. When thrombin binds to thrombomodulin, it loses its procoagulant activity and the complex becomes a potent activator of protein C, an anticoagulant produced by the liver. Activated protein C binds to a specific receptor on EC and inhibits coagulation by degradation of factor Va and VIIIa. The anticoagulant properties of activated protein C are enhanced by protein S, synthesized in the liver, but also in endothelial cells; protein S increases the proteolytic activity of protein C, promoting its interaction with factor Va and VIIIa, and also facilitates endothelial cell and platelet binding (117, 108).

In addition to the production of Tissue factor, endothelial cells can generate specific inhibitors of Tissue factor, known as tissue factor pathway inhibitor (TFPI) and tissue factor pathway inhibitor-2 (TFPI-2). TFPI is present both in plasma and on the endothelial cells surface (17).

Another aspect of the anticoagulant activity of endothelium consists of the endothelial synthesis of factors which influence platelet functions: PGI_2, NO and ADP-ase. In platelets, PGI_2-mediated increases in cAMP concentration inhibit adhesion and the release of vasoconstrictors and proaggregatory compounds, such as thromboxane A_2, serotonin and ADP. Nitric oxide shares many of the properties of prostacyclin in that it can relax vascular smooth muscle and inhibit platelet aggregation (49, 142). The endothelial surface ectonucleotidases that metabolize ADP prevent platelet recruitment and form adenosine, which in turn elevates platelet cAMP levels and further inhibit platelet reactivity (67).

COAGULATION

ANTICOAGULANT FUNCTIONS	PROCOAGULANT FUNCTIONS
Coagulation protein binding sites expressed by EC •GAGs/ATIII •TFPI •Thrombomodulin	**Coagulation protein binding sites expressed by EC** •Binding sites for IX-IXa; X-Xa; XII; kallikrein •TF •PAR1 (thrombin receptor) •Receptor for protein C
Factors secreted/stored by EC that influence platelet function •PG I_2 •NO •ADP-ase	**Factors secreted/stored by EC that influence platelet function** •vWf •PAF •f I (fibrinogen) •fV •fXI •Tx A_2

Figure 3.1. Regulation of coagulation by endothelium (with data from the text)

II. Procoagulant activity

The main reaction of clot formation is the conversion of fibrinogen into fibrin, which is catalyzed by thrombin (115). Endothelium participates to this phenomenon by producing a number of factors, including high molecular weight kininogen (HMWK), Factor V, Factor VIII and Tissue factor (TF). Basal endothelial secretion of TF is low, but if stimulated or injured, the endothelial cells can increase its production by 10- to 40 fold (41). EC are also the main source of von Willebrandt Factor (vWF), which binds Factor VIII, and protect it against proteolysis mediated by activated protein C or Factor Xa; vWF also stimulates platelet adhesion to the subendothelial structures and serves as carrier protein for Factor VIII (194).

Furthermore, EC present binding sites for HMWK, and for factors VIII, IX-IXa, and X-Xa; activated protein C (APC); thrombin; fibrin (41, 64, 201, 143). The best-characterized EC binding site for a coagulation protein is the thrombin receptor, also known as protease-activated receptor-1 (PAR-1). After thrombin binding to PAR-1, which is a high-affinity G-protein-coupled protein, a wide array of changes in expression of both prothrombotic and antithrombotic molecules (TF, PAI-1, NO, PAF, ET, PGI_2) was noted (92). EC also express several receptors for fibrin and specific fibrin degradation products; binding of fibrin promotes the following processes: endothelial cells adhesion, spreading, proliferation, and migration, and also clot retraction, and inhibition of PGI_2 synthesis (143).

Endothelial cells can also regulate platelet function by production and release of platelet-activating factor (PAF)(Negro-Alvarez et al, 1997, quoted by 185).

The Role of endothelium in fibrinolysis

EC seem to express more antifibrinolytic activity than profibrinolytic activity, but contribution of EC to this mechanism needs to be clarified by further studies (30). The contribution of EC to the profibrinolytic-antifibrinolytic balance (Fig.3.2.) is influenced by numerous factors: metabolic status, vascular derivation, and the concentration of other hemostatically active molecules in the local plasma medium.

I. Antifibrinolytic activity

In cultured EC, an increased production of plasminogen activator inhibitors (PAIs) was noted.

- *PAI-1.* Quiescent EC express little or no PAI-1, but after exposure to inflammatory stimuli, EC in virtually every tissue express PAI-1 (163).

Its synthesis in EC is stimulated by numerous factors, such as thrombin, endotoxin, various cytokines, and oxidized LDL (106).

- *PAI-2.* PAI-2 is found normally in plasma only during pregnancy and is not synthesized by EC to an appreciable extent (6).

There are no data concerning endothelial production of PAI-3, but PAI-3 can bind to heparan sulfate proteoglycan on the luminal surface of endothelial cells, increasing its activity (66).

Another component of the antifibrinolytic activity of EC is thrombin-activatable fibrinolysis inhibitor (TAFI). TAFI is a procarboxy-peptidase-B-like molecule that, when activated by thrombin, cleaves carboxyterminal residues of fibrin and other proteins. The result of this process is a loss of plasminogen/plasmin and t-PA binding sites on fibrin, such that fibrinolysis is retarded (7).

FIBRINOLYSIS

ANTIFIBRINOLYTIC ACTIVITY	PROFIBRINOLYTIC ACTIVITY
Factors produced by EC •PAI-1 (after exposure to inflammatory stimuli) •PAI-2 (reduced)	**Factors produced by EC** •t-PA (microvasculature EC) •u-PA (EC involved in wound repair or angiogenesis
TAFI activation	**PA receptors expressed by EC** •u-PAR (EC involved in angiogenesis) •Annexin II (receptor for t-PA) •Plasminogen binding sites

Figure 3.2. Regulation of fibrinolysis by endothelium (with data from the text)

II. Profibrinolytic activity

The production and secretion of tissue plasminogen activators (t-PA) are a property of endothelial cells, but not from all type of vessels. For example, it seems that t-PA is associated only with a distinct subpopulation of the microvasculature, in both quiescent and activated cells (103). Humans exhibit higher plasma level after exercise or venous compression, but the source of this increase has not been established (102). Studies of deep veins of the lower limbs indicate the lowest fibrinolytic activity in the soleus sinuses, while the popliteal and the femoral vein endothelium had significantly higher levels of plasminogen activator.

u-PA (urokinase-type plasminogen activator) appears not to be expressed by quiescent EC, but is also important for vascular homeostasis (mice lacking u-PA develop inflammation-induced trombi)(200, 23)

EC also present receptors for t-PA (such as annexin II) and for u-PA (77, 10). The binding of t-PA to EC promotes its fibrinolytic activity and stimulates cell proliferation. After binding to u-PAR, single chain u-PA (the form found in plasma) exhibits increased plasminogen, activating efficiency and is relatively protected from inhibition by PAI-1 and PAI-2 (114, 81).

Endothelial cells express diverse binding sites for plasminogen, the identity of these sites being uncertain (147).

Pathological aspects

There are studies that demonstrated an increased fibrinolytic activity in both normal and varicose saphenous veins at the groin versus the ankle position. These differences could be explained by changes in the plasminogen system (tPA, uPA and PAI-1)(176). The levels of PAI-1 were comparable between normal and varicose specimens in the two regions. Levels of tPA were higher at the groin versus the ankle position in VV and tended to go in that direction with NV. Levels of uPA in the varicose saphenous veins were significantly higher than in normal veins, at both the groin and ankle positions, suggesting a role for uPA in the pathogenesis of varicose veins.

Venous thromboembolic disease is an important clinical entity, in which both acquired and genetic risk factors play a causative role. Genetic factors which increase thrombotic risk consist of rare heterogeneous loss-of-function mutations in coagulation-inhibitory factors, such as antithrombin, protein S and C, and more common, but unique, gain-of-function mutations in coagulation factors V and II, so-called factor V-Leiden and prothrombin gene variant G20210A. Elevated factor VIII levels, and deficiencies of thrombomodulin were also noted. The inherited deficiencies of antithrombin III, protein C and protein S occur in 10% of patients suffering from venous thrombosis, whereas factor V Leiden is present in as many as 20 to 60%. Less well-characterized disorders include elevated factor IX, X, and XI levels. (154, 22). Recently, polymorphisms of thrombin activatable fibrinolysis inhibitor (TAFI)' promoter, were suggested to contribute to an increased thrombotic risk (61). Beside this, low levels of heparin-releasable tissue factor pathway inhibitor (TFPI) were associated with deep venous thrombosis, indicating TFPI level as a possible risk factor, but there was no link between deep venous thrombosis and mutations in the nine exons of the TFPI gene (3).

3.1.2.3. The Role of endothelium in inflammation and interactions with blood cells

Circulating leukocytes and platelets may adhere to specific areas of the endothelium, to exposed subendothelial components, or to each other during the process of immune surveillance as well as in response to tissue injury or infection.

I. Endothelial-leukocyte interactions

Both EC and leukocytes express adhesion molecules that control leukocyte adhesion within circulation and migration into perivascular tissue. Endothelial cells express selectins (E and P-selectins) and adhesion proteins belonging to the immunoglobulin family (ICAM-1,2, VCAM-1, PECAM-1) whereas adhesion molecules on leukocytes comprise the selectins and the integrins. Expression of adhesion molecules changes rapidly with the activation status of both leukocytes and endothelial cells. Adhesion molecules may also be shed from the cells and their circulating level may be a measure of excessive or inappropriate endothelial or leukocyte activation (39, 185).

The endothelial adhesion molecules involved in endothelial-leukocyte interactions and their major roles are presented in Table 3.IV.

Table 3.IV. Main roles of endothelial adhesion molecules (with data from 112, 39)

Endothelial adhesion molecules	Main functions
P-selectin (CD62P) (induced)	Leukocyte rolling/early adhesion (N, E, B, Mo, memory T cells)
E-selectin (CD62E) (induced)	Leukocyte rolling/early adhesion (N, Mo, Ly)
ICAM-1 (CD54)(induced)	Leukocyte rolling/early adhesion (N, Mo, Ly)
ICAM-2 (CD102)	Leukocyte adhesion, stable arrest, and transmigration (all subsets)
VCAM-1 (CD106)(induced)	Leukocyte adhesion and transmigration (E, B, Mo, Ly)
CD44	Leukocyte adhesion, lymphocyte homing, endothelial cell binding of chemokines
CD40	Leukocyte adhesion, stimulation of endothelial cell activation induction of adhesion molecule expression
PECAM-1 (CD31)	Leukocyte transmigration (N, Mo, Ly), integrin activation
LFA-3 (induced)	Lymphocyte adhesion and costimulation
VAP-1	Lymphocyte adhesion
L-VAP-2	Lymphocyte adhesion
GlyCAM-1	Lymphocyte homing
MadCAM-1	Lymphocyte homing
CD34	Lymphocyte homing

Legend:
N = neutrophils; E = eosinophils; B = basophils; Mo = monocytes; Ly = lymphocytes

Leukocytes usually attach to endothelium under low shear stress, such as EC in the lining postcapillary venules. The fraction of leukocytes, which normally adhere to the endothelium, is considered as a specific dynamic leukocyte pool. During inflammation, leukocytes tether to and roll on the endothelial surface. Leukocyte rolling is mediated by adhesion molecules of the selectin family, such as P-selectin and E-selectin, depending on the type of stimuli (histamine or thrombin, and TNF or IL-1 respectively). The cells then arrest, spread, and finally migrate between EC to the underlying tissue. Adhesion molecules of the immunoglobulin superfamily, such as ICAM-1, ICAM-2, ICAM-3, and VCAM-1 or PECAM-1, mediate the firm adhesion of leukocytes to the vascular endothelium. The three ICAM-s are closely related and they bind to the same leukocyte integrin receptors, CD18/CD11.The best known inducers of these molecules include: for ICAM-1: TNF, IL-1, IFN-γ, linoleic acid, LPS, and for ICAM-2: TNF, IL-1, LPS. IL-1, oxidized LDL can induce the expression of VCAM-1. Phosphorilation of PECAM-1 may be involved in the reactive oxygen species-induced transendothelial migration of monocytes (112, 39, 185, 30).

Recent data proved that HUVEC and human intestinal endothelial cells could produce a wide spectrum of cytokines, including IL-3, IL-7, IL-8, IL-11, IL-14, IL-15, TNF, TGF-β and GM-CSF (140). Cytokines, which are inducible in endothelial cells, belong to the inflammatory family of inflammatory cytokines and their expression is regulated by NF-kB. However, the main sources of inflammatory cytokines in vasculature are monocytes and macrophages (185).

Pathological aspects

In 1987, Moyses et al. noticed that leukocyte sequestration occurred in normal subjects when the lower limb was subjected to venous hypertension for a 40 minutes period (135). Thomas et al. (1988) also observed a difference in white cell trapping between patients with chronic venous insufficiency (CVI) and control subjects with normal lower limb veins (186). Patients trapped 30% of white cells after 60 minutes of sitting, while controls trapped only 7%. After return to the lying position white cells began to leave the limb. Moreover, Coleridge-Smith et al. (1988) showed using video microscopy that the number of visible capillaries fell during a period of venous hypertension, suggesting that increased venous pressure reduced the capillary perfusion pressure and hence the capillary flow rate (31).

On the basis of these three observations, the hypothesis of white cell trapping was proposed (31). This hypothesis suggested that the "trapped" leukocytes were responsible for endothelial injury, which over a long period of time (months or years), resulted in damage to the microcirculation and leg ulceration. The standing position induces a rise in venous pressure and a decrease of blood flow to the lower limb, favoring adhesion of leukocytes to the microcirculatory endothelium. The reduced blood flow and the dilation of capillaries during ambulatory venous hypertension are responsible for the reduction of the shear rate in the microcirculation, an important factor influencing leukocyte adhesion. The reduction in shear rate favors neutrophil adhesion, which probably occurs in the post-capillary venules. In control subjects, the leukocyte adhesion is probably a physiological phenomenon that does not normally persist for any length of time, but in patients with CVI sustained venous hypertension occurs, so the leukocyte trapping may be more persistent. The trapped leukocytes become activated releasing free radicals and proteolytic enzymes (levels of lactoferrin and elastase were higher in patients with CVI than in controls)(172, 173). Endothelial adhesion of leukocytes during venous hypertension results in damage to the endothelium, as assessed by release of soluble adhesion molecules into the blood.

Immunohistochemical investigations have shown that the endothelium is perturbed, expressing increased amounts of factor VIII related antigen and adhesion molecules, especially intercellular adhesion molecule-1 (ICAM-1) (199, 192). Endothelial-leukocyte adhesion molecule-1 (ELAM-1/E-selectin) may be slightly upregulated, but vascular cell adhesion molecule (VCAM) appears to be normal in patients without venous ulceration. Damaged endothelium seems to more likely to attract the adhesion of leukocytes. A strong leukocyte infiltration has been measured in patients with venous disease and these cells were macrophages and T-lymphocytes (168). Saharay et al. (1998) measured the plasma levels of ELAM-1, ICAM-1, VCAM-1 before and after short-term venous hypertension in normal controls and in patients with chronic venous insufficiency subjected to short-term venous hypertension. In both the controls and the patients, the white/red cell ratio fell significantly in response to venous hypertension, confirming the sequestration of leukocytes. Basal levels of all three adhesion molecules (ELAM-1/E-selectin, ICAM-1, VCAM-1) were significantly higher in patients compared to controls. There was no significant change noted in either group in response to experimental venous hypertension. Increased levels of adhesion molecules suggest that endothelial activation is a feature of chronic venous insufficiency. Such increase, presumably due to endothelial damage in the skin, is supported by histological evidence, and is probably due to free radical and proteolytic enzyme release from activated leukocytes (161).

Ono et al. (1998) considered that venous valve damage in refluxing saphenous veins is associated with a monocyte-macrophage infiltrate. They noted a significant monocyte adherence on the valve leaflet and the vein wall, with a greater number in the valve sinus compared to the valve cusp and distal vein wall. Destruction of collagen in valve leaflets by monocyte-expressed collagenase may lead to the shrinking and shortening of valves that have been observed grossly and angioscopically (146).

Michiels et al. (1995) explained the alterations observed in the pathological vein as consequences of hypoxia resulting from venous stasis (122). Both *in vitro* studies on isolated human umbilical vein endothelial cells and experiments performed on human saphenous veins incubated in normoxic or hypoxic conditions proved that many neutrophils adhered to the hypoxic venous endothelium (CD18/CD11b - ICAM-1). Their experimental data show that hypoxia is able to activate endothelial cells, which release inflammatory mediators (PAF) and become adhesive for neutrophils. These adherent neutrophils were activated, releasing high amounts of superoxide anion and of B_4 leukotrienes. Free radicals and proteases release by activated neutrophils are able to degrade the extracellular matrix, the varicose saphenous vein losing as much as 60% of the collagen in its wall (153). In addition, hypoxia-activated endothelial cells secrete growth factors (bFGF, $PGF_{2\alpha}$), which will trigger smooth muscle cell proliferation and the synthesis of extracellular matrix components. Altogether and because they are frequently repeated, these processes could explain the alterations of the vascular wall in varicose veins. (121, 122, 123, 124).

II. Endothelial-platelets interactions

Normally, circulating platelets do not interact with the endothelial surface, because of the release of NO, PGI_2 and CD39 (ecto-ADP-ase)(164). Interestingly, platelet distribution differs substantially between venules and arterioles; near the vessel wall, platelet density is significantly lower in venules compared with arterioles (156).

During hemorrhage, platelets adhere to the exposed subendothelium and become activated. Platelet adhesion is more efficient under high shear stress, accounting for the greater number of platelets in fibrin clots within arteries compared with those within veins (156). In case of high shear stress (within arteries) platelet glycoprotein Ib-IX-V complex attaches to immobilized vWF (160). Under lower shear stresses (veins), unactivated platelets use the integrin $\alpha_{IIb}\beta_3$ to attach to and immediately arrest on immobilized fibrinogen; platelets also use integrins and other molecules to attach to subendothelial matrix components, such as fibronectin, laminin, and thrombospondin (97).

After adhesion to either vWF or fibrinogen, platelets become activated by secreted products (e,g, ADP) or by surface molecules (e.g. collagen), and adhere more avidly to subendothelium (through binding of activated $\alpha_{IIb}\beta_3$ to fibrinogen or to a distinct site of vWF)(160). As thrombin is generated, converting fibrinogen to fibrin, the aggregated platelets contract to strengthen the clot.

Pathological aspects

One of the three distinct processes of the saphenous vein graft disease is thrombosis. Thrombosis, intimal hyperplasia and atherosclerosis are interlinked pathophysiologically in the evolution of vein graft disease, being more or less temporally distinct. During the first month after bypass surgery, between 3% and 12% of saphenous vein grafts occlude, because of thrombosis. Graft thrombosis is caused by a association of factors: alterations in the vessel wall, modified properties and reactivity of venous grafts, changes in blood rheology, and altered flow dynamics (40, 134).

- *Alterations in vessel wall* are due to harvesting of venous conduits, frequently associated with endothelial loss and damage of the media.

Endothelial loss has several consequences (193, 158):

- accumulation of fibrin on the luminal surface,
- adhesion of platelets and neutrophils,
- decrease of tPA production,
- activation of extrinsic coagulation cascade by TF (constitutively expressed and also induced by inflammatory cytokines on the surface of EC).

Moreover, vein harvesting reduces the activity of thrombomodulin by up to 30%, while arterial flow downregulates its expression with a subsequent procoagulant effect (34, 72)

- Additionally, the *antithrombotic properties of veins are weak compared to the arterial ones*:
    - heparan sulfate is less extended in venous internal elastic lamina as compared to the arteries (40),
    - NO and PG I_2 synthesis is lower in veins than in arteries; low fluid shear stress in grafted venous conduits reduces the shear-dependent release of t-PA, NO and PG I_2 (110, 1).
    - the endothelial production of NO is stimulated by platelet derived-ADP and ATP in arterial conduits (internal mammary arteries), but not in venous grafts (saphenous vein); this might lead to the disaggregation of evolving platelet clot and antagonism of platelet-derived serotonin and thromboxane A_2-induced contraction, while in human saphenous vein this mechanism is poorly developed (Yang et al, 1991, quoted by 204).

- Another factor, which amplifies graft thrombosis, is represented by the *high sensitivity of denuded saphenous veins to circulating vasoactive agents.* For example, endothelin-1-induced contraction of venous conduit may attenuate flow and promotes stasis (134). Moreover, thrombin, a endothelium-dependent dilator in arteries, induces the constriction of saphenous veins (205).
  In human saphenous vein rings obtained during coronary bypass surgery contracted in response to noradrenaline, aggregating platelets induced a further increase in tension, while in rings of internal mammary artery precontracted with noradrenaline, aggregating platelets induced endothelium-dependent relaxation which was prevented by apyrase (with ADPase activity) and L-NG-monomethylarginine (NOS inhibitor). In quiescent veins, the platelet-induced contraction was greater than in arteries and facilitated by endothelium. Preincubation of platelets with aspirin (10 mmol/l) reduced the contraction, but contraction was abolished only in the presence of both the thromboxane receptor antagonist SQ-30741 and the serotoninergic $5HT_2$ receptor antagonist ketanserin, suggesting that thromboxane A_2 and serotonin mediate platelet-induced contraction in human saphenous vein (207, 204). Furthermore, platelet-derived growth factor is a potent mitogen for SV but not IMA smooth muscle proliferation, contributing to the low patency of SV compared to IMA grafts (204).
- *The circulating levels of some factors influencing hemostasis are also elevated, favoring the prothrombotic response.* The alterations of hemostatic parameters may persist for up to 30 days after surgery. Among these are increased plasma fibrinogen level and thrombin-antithrombin complexes. Patients with vein graft occlusion also showed lower basal preoperative tPA activity and factor VIII concentration (134).

All these data underline the importance of an effective antithrombotic therapy. In addition to classic antithrombotic therapy (aspirin, antiplatelet agents such as thienopyridines) new strategies are to be developed in prevention of saphenous vein graft disease: gene therapy, and modulation of platelet activation. A marked increase in venous NO endothelial production was obtained in cultured human saphenous veins transfected with an adenoviral vector encoding bovine eNOS. S-nitrosogluthatione, which is a platelet-selective NO donor that significantly inhibits platelet activation in venous grafts, may have a future role in improving early graft patency (134).

3.1.2.4. Venous Endothelium and Vascular Remodeling

Although all the vascular cells may participate in the vascular remodeling process, the endothelium is particularly suited to play a prominent part.

Endothelial cells are constantly exposed to physical forces, humoral factors, and inflammatory mediators, serving as sensory cells. Moreover, endothelial cells regulate smooth muscle cell growth by producing both growth promoting (PDGF, some FGF, TGF-α, oxygen free radicals, endothelin, and angiotensin II) and growth inhibiting factors (NO, PG I_2, some FGF, TGF-β, IGF-1, heparan sulfate and thrombospondin)(41).

However, under physiological conditions, growth inhibitors prevail, explaining why the blood vessel wall normally remains quiescent and does not proliferate (142).

Endothelial cells also present receptors for growth factors (24), such as:

- receptors for vascular endothelial growth factor (VEGF), which interacts with cellular receptors FLK1 (VEGF receptor-2) and FLT1 (VEGF receptor-2), promoting blood vessel formation, mainly EC proliferation, migration and survival;
- receptors for fibroblast growth factors (FGF); in vitro studies showed that FGF, especially FGF2, stimulates endothelial cell formation (migration, proliferation, release of proteolytic enzymes and capillary tubes formation);
- receptors for transforming growth factor-β1 (TGF-β1), which are serine/threonine kinases type I and II; TGF-β1 inhibits macrovascular endothelial cell proliferation, induces apoptosis, impairs endothelial cell migration and reduces their proteolytic activity in vitro. TGF-β1 may exert bimodal effects, depending on its concentration, on the type and density of endothelial cells, and on the interaction with other growth factors. Both in vitro and in vivo, TGF-β1 was also shown to have angiogenic properties.
- receptors for platelet-derived growth factor, involved in angiogenesis, with different effects in macro- and microvascular endothelial cells.
- receptors tyrosine kinases, TIE1 (tyrosine kinase with immunoglobulin and epidermal growth factor homology domains) and TIE2/TEK. TIE1 is involved in endothelial cell function (is required for structural integrity of microvascular EC, the control of fluid across capillaries, and hemodynamic stress resistance during blood vessels maturation), whereas

TIE2, which is the receptor for angiopoietin, seems to be implicated in blood vessel formation by acting on periendothelial cells. A mutation in the kinase domain at position 849 of TIE2 receptor has been related to the development of venous malformations (vessels with large lumina and increased number of EC compared to smooth muscle cells).

In addition, extracellular matrix composition can be influenced by the mixture of proteinases and proteinase inhibitors secreted by EC (24).

Table 3.V. The major roles of extracellular matrix proteinases (with data from 24, 32, 46)

PROTEINASES	**ROLES**
Plasminogen system:	
1. plasminogen	proenzyme
2. plasminogen activator (PA) • tissue-type PA (t-PA) • urokinase-type PA (u-PA)	• clot dissolution • pericellular proteolysis during cell migration and tissue remodeling during angiogenesis, atherosclerosis and restenosis
3. plasmin	• degradation of fibrin and extracellular matrix proteins • activation/release of growth factors from extracellular matrix (TGF-β1, FGF2, VEGF-A)
Matrix metalloproteinases	**(MMPs)**
MMP-2 (gelattinase A) MMP-9 (gellatinase B)	degradation of collagen type IV, V, VII and X, ellastin, denaturated collagens
MMP-13 (collagenase)	primary collagenase
MMP 3, 7, 10	degradation of proteoglycan core proteins, laminin, fibronectin, elastin, gelatin, non-helical collagens
MMP-12	degradation of insoluble ellastin, collagen IV, laminin, fibronectin, enatctin, proteoglycans
MT1-MMP, MT2-MMP (membrane-type MMPs)	activation of gellatinase A

- Proteinases include the plasminogen system (PA) and matrix metalloproteinases (MMPs).
- Proteinase inhibitors are represented by plasminogen activator inhibitors (PAIs), α_2-antiplasmin, and tissue inhibitors of MMPs (TIMPs: TIMP-1 and TIMP-2).

The roles of extracellular matrix proteinases are summarized in Table 3.V.

Quiescent endothelial cells express t-PA, MMP-2 and minimal MMP-1, the proteolysis being inhibited by PAI-1, TIMP-1, and TIMP-2, which are expressed in the same time. The expression of both proteinases and proteinase inhibitors is influenced by a variety of cytokines and growth factors (32).

Pathological aspects

Intimal hyperplasia in venous graft disease

Intimal hyperplasia is a major disease process in venous grafts between one month and one year after implantation; nearly all veins implanted into the arterial circulation develop intimal thickening within 4 to 6 weeks, which may reduce the lumen by up to 25%. This process represents the basis for later development of graft atheroma. Intimal hyperplasia begins with the proliferation of medial smooth muscle cells in response to a number of growth factors and cytokines released from endothelial cells, platelets, and macrophages. The following step is represented by migration of smooth muscle cells into the intima, with subsequent further proliferation. Later, progressive increase in intimal fibrosis and reduction of cellularity occurs, due to synthesis and deposition of extracellular matrix by activated smooth muscle cells. In contrast to arterial injury model, in the venous graft the major component of intimal hyperplasia occurs after neoendothelial formation (40, 1, 134). Several factors are involved in promotion of venous graft hyperplasia:

- reduced endothelial production of endothelial antiproliferative substances (NO, PGI_2, and adenosine), and increased superoxide generation, that directly stimulates smooth muscle cell proliferation; these phenomena occur as a consequence of transient ischemia incurred on explantation, followed by reperfusion after grafting (84, 150).
- platelets adhesion at sites of endothelial damage, followed by release of growth factors, such as PDGF and TGF-β1; PDGF is a very potent mitogen in human saphenous vein smooth muscle with a half-maximal effect at concentration in nanomolar range, while TGF-β1 inhibits PDGF and stretch-induced proliferation (76).

- pronounced proliferation of smooth muscle cells in saphenous veins induced by thrombin (in vitro data)(205)
- differentiation of perivascular fibroblasts into myofibroblasts after translocation through the media of newly placed vein grafts (171)
- increased wall stress incurred by saphenous veins on exposure to arterial pressures, which upregulates vein graft intimal receptors for bFGF released from damaged endothelial cells (138)
- reduction in shear stress because of vein distension under arterial pressure changes the profile of growth factors: increases the production of several growth factors (PDGF, bFGF, endothelin-1) and diminishes the generation of some growth inhibitors (TGFβ, NO)(40, 1)
- phenotypic modulation of a subpopulation of the circumferential medial VSMC to a synthetic phenotype, induced by surgical preparative injury (91)
- increased activity of matrix-degrading metalloproteinases (increased expression of pro-MMP-1 associated with a reduced expression of tissue-inhibitor of MMP, TIMP-2) due to surgical preparation of venous grafts (91).

A number of new approaches to prevent intimal hyperplasia have been studied. One strategy presumes the use of antisense nucleotides to block the expression of genes encoding cell cycle regulatory proteins in smooth muscle cells (116). Another possibility is represented by modulation of growth factors: inhibition of bFGF activity, local delivery of VEGF, with subsequent reduction of neointimal hyperplasia (studies in arterial injury animal models)(5). External stenting before graft implantation also decreases intimal and medial hyperplasia (porcine model)(88). There are studies investigating the role of ET-1 in isolated human saphenous vein smooth muscle cells and in an organ culture of the human saphenous vein. These studies demonstrated that ET-1 is a mediator of intimal hyperplasia in human saphenous vein in vitro, therefore endothelin receptor antagonists may be of therapeutic value in the modulation of vein graft intimal hyperplasia (119).

Varicose veins(VV)

Vascular remodeling was also described in varicose veins (95). Varicose vein walls differed from the normal saphenous veins by the presence of hypertrophic smooth muscle cells as well as disorganized elastin patterns, with a correlation between the hypertrophic SMC and an abnormal elastin pattern. Ultrastructurally, the SMC presented prominent microherniations and vesicles that bud from the cell, with microfilaments and microtubuli. The elastin fibers were disrupted from the hypertrophic SMC. The diameter of the smooth muscle cells in the varicose vein was significantly higher than that in the normal saphenous vein. The cellular hypertrophy of the SMC and the microherniations could be the basis for disruption of the elastin fibers connected to the SMC in varicose veins. Disrupted connections between SMC and elastin fibers could be responsible for the weakness of the venous wall observed in varicose vein disease.

Moreover, aging induces a continuous change in the bFGF/PDGF ratio (both growth factors decline, but bFGF decreased faster than PDGF), which may alter the composition of the extracellular matrix of the vein wall during aging and thus its susceptibility to varicose disease (48).

3.1.3. Heterogenity of Endothelial Function within Circulation

There are clear **differences between arterial and venous vessels** with respect to many endothelial functions. The same stimulus can elicit quantitatively or qualitatively different responses from arterial as compared to the venous endothelium in both macro- and microvascular beds.

At the *macrovascular level*, venous endothelium seems to have a lower capacity for production of relaxing factors, such as NO and prostaglandin I_2 (63). For instance, in humans, there is evidence of a continuous basal NO in arterial vessels of human forearm, while the endothelium of dorsal hand veins did not released NO in absence of stimuli (acetylcholine, bradykinin)(190, 33). Nevertheless, recent studies performed by Blackman et al. (2000) showed that human forerm capacitance veins exhibit both stimulated and basal NO activity, suggesting that NO also contributes to resting venous tone in healthy human subjects (14). Endothelial cells derived from saphenous vein have been reported to synthesize less PGI_2 than those from the internal mammary artery, a finding that may explain the rapidity with which pathogenic changes may develop in venous bypass grafts placed under arterial pressure (182).

Furthermore, mechanical forces such as pulsatile stretch and PDGF are potent mitogens for saphenous grafts, but not for internal mammary arteries (204).

At the *microvascular level*, there is histochemical evidence that less NO synthase is present in venular endothelium than in the arteriolar one (139). Moreover, there are studies that revealed arteriolar-venular differences in the capacity for releasing other endothelium-derived factors. In some arteriolar preparations, acetylcholine or shear stress elicited the co-release of endothelial NO and another unidentified relaxing factor, whereas in their paired venules they induced only NO release (15, 16).

Distinct subsets of endothelial cells often exist within a single organ. In situ studies of adult human liver showed two distinct types of sinusoidal endothelial phenotypes: hepatic periportal vessels express PECAM-1 and CD34, whereas sinusoidal intrahepatic endothelium does not (131).

Endothelial cells from diverse tissue are also **heterogenous with respect to their surface phenotype and protein expression**. Microvascular EC, express CD36, its expression being absent on human large vessels endothelium (umbilical vein), therefore CD36 may be considered a useful marker for EC of microvascular origin (184). Moreover, von Willebrandt factor, used commonly as an endothelial marker, is not expressed uniformly on cells from all types of vessels (98).

Endothelial cells also exhibit **heterogeneity with respect to hemostatic functions**. For example, it may be noted that microvascular endothelial cells show a more acute (brisk) ICAM-1 response to cytokines than do human umbilical endothelial cells (183).

The underlying causes of this heterogeneity remain largely unexplored, but they are probably multifactorial in origin. This diversity arises in part from the intrinsic molecular and biochemical differences that exist among some endothelial populations, on which other factors [differences in cell microenvironment, such as direct interactions with the adjacent cells, the activity of autocrine, paracrine and circulating factors, the influence of shear stress and pressure, the contact with circulating and tissue-based cells (eg, smooth muscle cells, perycites) and with microbes and their soluble products] are superimposed (30).

3.1.4. Pharmacological Aspects

Numerous types of ***receptors*** have been identified on the membrane of endothelial cells:

1. Specific receptors for blood-born factors, cotransmitters and autacoids which induce the NO release from the endothelial cells, such as: H_2 for

histamine, M_2 for acetylcholine, 5-HT_{1D} for serotonin, B_2 for bradykinin, receptor P_{2y} for ATP, and receptors for insulin (37,129). It is now widely accepted that α_2-and β-receptors exist on endothelial cells and contribute to the regulation of vasomotor tone, but the roles these receptors play are still debatable questions. Experimental data showed that α_2-adrenoceptor agonists do indeed have the capability of modulating vascular responsiveness via stimulation of the release of NO in large arteries and microcirculation. Moreover, removal of endothelium decreased the relaxations caused by β-adrenoceptor agonists in several isolated vessels from different species including humans, suggesting the existence of endothelial β-adrenoceptors (74). The presence of these receptors was confirmed by autoradiography in the endothelium of human saphenous vein (127) and by biochemical data in cultured human umbilical vein endothelial cells (57). This latter study, together with an in vivo study performed on forearm circulation (42) indicated that endothelial β-adrenoceptors were mostly of the β_2-subtype.

2. Endothelin receptors. The ET_B receptor, which is equally sensitive for the three endothelin isoforms, is present on both endothelium (subtype 1), where releases NO and prostacyclin, resulting in vasodilation, and on VSMC (subtype 2), where mediates vasoconstriction together with ET_A receptor (157).

3. Receptors for angiotensin, AT_1 (Saralasine>Ang II>Ang III), AT_2 (in smaller amounts) and AT_4 (Ang IV>Ang III). By stimulation of endothelial AT_1 receptors, Ang II induces production of endothelin, while activation of AT_2 receptors inhibits endothelial cell proliferation. Stimulation of AT_4 receptors is responsible for the vasodilator effect of Ang IV and III (185, 189).

Some of the receptors located on venous endothelial cells are depicted in figure 3.3.

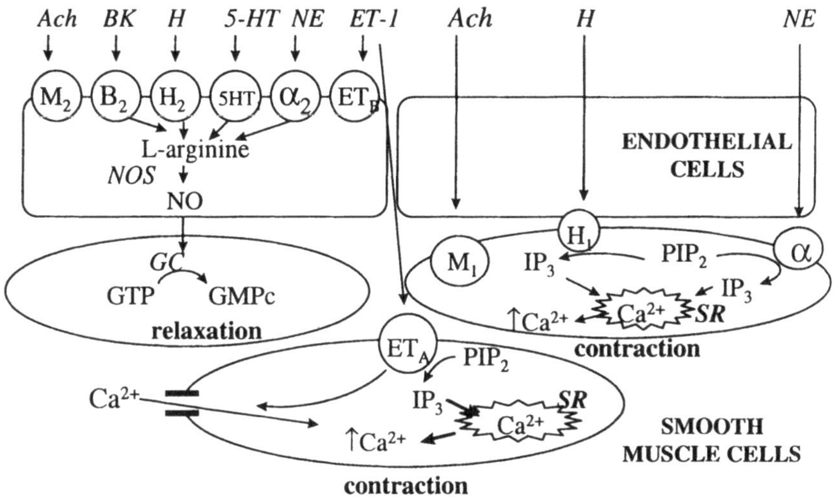

Figure 3.3. Receptors for several vasoactive agents are located on both venous endothelial and smooth muscle cells, being involved in either relaxation, either contraction of the smooth muscle cells.

Another important biological function of the endothelium is the ***conversion of inactive peptides to potent vasoactive agents***.

For instance:

- The conversion of decapeptide angiotensin I, to the potent vasoconstrictor octapeptide, angiotensin II, is accomplished by proteolytic cleavage of a Hys-Leu residue from the carboxy-terminal end catalyzed by angiotensin converting enzyme. In addition, ACE inactivates the peptide bradykinin, which as a potent stimulant for the NO production, acts as an indirect vasodilator. Blockade of ACE by ACE inhibitors provides an effective mean to treat hypertension; the antihypertensive action of the ACE inhibitors results from the inhibition of both the formation of the vasoconstrictor angiotensin II, and of the inactivation of bradykinin (55, 29).
- Endothelin is converted into its active form via two precursors, preproendothelin and proendothelin, also called "big-endothelin". The conversion from proendothelin to endothelin is controlled by a protease termed endothelin-converting enzyme (ECE)(159). Two different ECE isoforms with different expression sites have been identified: ECE-1, a membrane-bound enzyme with an extracellular domain, and ECE-2, an

enzyme with intracellular expression (166, 165, 53). The regulation of ECE expression remains to be clarified. There are data which suggest alternative promotors directing isoform-specific expression of human ECE-1 mRNA in cultured endothelial cells.

Endothelium also participates in the ***metabolic degradation*** of catecholamines, serotonin, and bradikynin (metabolized by cathecol-O-methyltransferase and monoamine oxidase) and of adenosine, taken up by the endothelial cells, and metabolized by adenosine deaminase (177). Recent experimental data demonstrated the existence of essential elements of the cholinergic system (choline acetyltransferase, vesicular acetylcholine transporter , acetylcholine) in the human endothelium (HUVEC, EC of dermal blood vessels). The biological functions of ACh synthesized by endothelial cells are to be clarified (94).

EC also ***produce several regulatory substances that can either be growth promoting*** (PDGF, bFGF, IGF-1, endothelin, angiotensin II) or ***growth inhibiting*** (collagen type V, glycosoaminoglycans, TGF-β, NO, PG I_2)(50, 68).

3.1.5. Hemodynamic Forces and the Endothelium

Venous EC are influenced by two major hemodynamic forces:

1. transmural pressure gradients, which influence the vessel wall distention and development of wall tension (Laplace's law)

$T = \Delta P \times r$

T = wall tension, ΔP = transmural pressure gradient, r = vessel radius

Because wall tension rises with increasing vessel radius, for any given transmural pressure gradient, tension is greatest in highly distensible vessels, like veins. The stretch due to ΔP occurs in all directions, deforming all vessel wall components (8).

2. wall'shear stress, generated by blood flowing over their apical surfaces. The shear stress depends upon mean fluid flow rate, blood viscosity and the physical dimensions of blood vessels. The stretch due to shear stress acts in one direction, and only EC are exposed to this force. Mean shear stress is lowest in the large veins (1 dyne/cm^2), increases in small venules (20-40 dynes/cm^2), and is the highest in small arterioles (60-80 dynes/cm^2) (8).

Shear stress is a very important factor in cell signaling. Endothelial cell shear stress mechanosensors include membrane receptor kinases, intergrins, G proteins, ion channels, intercellular junction proteins, membrane lipids and the cytoskeleton. These sensors are linked to signaling cascades, inducing various responses due to the level and pattern of shear stress (58).

Acute shear stress occurs in vivo when blood flow is reestablished after a temporary occlusion. In endothelial cells, acute shear stress induces the following responses:

- rapid reorganization of the cytoskeleton (the cells will align in the direction of flow), due to actin depolymerization followed by repolymerization, both processes being dependent upon intracellular calcium concentration (198, 133)
- activation of ion channels (activates endothelial stretch-responsive Ca^{2+} channels and calcium activated K^+ channels)(35, 170)
- stimulation of PLC and PKC, leading to rapid generation of IP_3 and DAG, these events being related to intracellular calcium mobilization (148, 209)
- activation PLA_2, with release of arachidonic acid from membrane phospholipids (12)
- stimulation of NO and prostacyclin secretion by EC (141, 62)
- activates gene transcription (PDGF-B, COX II, eNOS, manganese SOD, tissue factor, C-type natriuretic peptide, TGF-β1)(151, 188, 104, 144,145) and c-fos and c-jun (149).
- acute shear stress activates ET-1 gene transcription (132, 113).
- rapid downregulation of thrombomodulin (in human saphenous vein exposed to arterial flow for 45-90 minutes); this response was sufficient to limit protein C activation, and seemed to be induced by the increased shear stress (72).

In case of **chronic shear stress**, modifications in endothelial cell structure and function were also reported (8):

- cell' arrangement in the direction of flow and flattening;
- structural reorganization (cell hypertrophy, increased density of actin microfilaments and focal adhesions, increased density of Weibel-Palade bodies);
- enhanced cell adhesion;
- marked down-regulation of ET-1 gene expression;
- profound down-regulation of PDGF-B transcription.

In endothelial cells, various patterns of flow and shear stress may induce different responses (58):

- sustained laminar shear stress induces a transient activation of Ras-mitogen-activated protein kinase kinase (MEKK)-c-Jun aminoterminal kinase (JNK) pathway with transient monocyte chemotactic protein-1 (MCP-1) expression, followed by its downregulation.
- in case of complex flow patterns, such as those seen at the branch points, MCP-1 downregulation was not observed.

All of these findings show that endothelium, including the venous one, plays an important role in the regulation of vasomotor tone. Furthermore, these cellular responses might explain the effects of reduced shear stress associated with thrombotic occlusion and of increased shear stress associated with hypertension.

3.2. VENOUS SMOOTH MUSCLE

3.2.1. Microscopic Aspects

Smooth muscle cells represent the prevailing component of the venous media. The media of small veins contains two to four layers of smooth muscle fibers interspersed between a thin network of elastic and collagen fibers (177).

In medium-size veins, the media is thinner than in arteries of same caliber: two to four circular layers of smooth muscle, separated by bundles of longitudinal collagen fibers interspersed with a delicate network of elastic fibers and a few fibroblasts. The circumferential distensibility of the veins is due to the circular-helical arrangement of muscle fibers, while the changes in length are facilitated by the longitudinal orientation of some smooth muscle, elastic and collagen fibers. The elastica externa is poorly defined (177).

The media of large veins is thin, with a few layers of smooth muscle fibers. Rare processes of endothelial cells penetrate the elastica interna to establish myoendothelial junctions. Elastica externa is poorly defined or missing. In the largest vessels of the venous system, such as the venae cavae, the smooth muscle fibers are disposed longitudinally rather than in a circular fashion (177).

Functional adaptations have introduced augmentation or reduction of structural elements especially in the muscular composition of some veins. An increased number of longitudinally oriented muscle bundles may be encountered in all the three tunics. For instance, there are veins rich in smooth muscle in the intima: (internal jugular vein, saphenous, femoral, and popliteal veins, veins of forearm), or in the media (limbs and umbilical veins), and in the adventitia (veins of abdominal cavity). Veins devoid of smooth also were also identified (veins of retina and bone, maternal placenta, meningeal and dural sinuses)(177).

Vascular smooth muscle cells are smaller (25 - 80 μm) than the smooth muscle cells in other locations, with surface vesicles (caveolae), which increase the surface membrane area by about 25%. They are organized in characteristic longitudinal rows with vesicle-free regions in between. The cells are embedded in connective tissue, which contributes to the distribution of forces developed by the smooth muscle. Smooth muscle cells touch one another through gap-junctions, regions of close apposition between the outer leaflets of the plasma membranes of neighboring cells. Gap junctions are dynamic structures, generally less frequent in large veins than in arterioles and small arteries. These structures are clusters of transmembrane hydrophilic channels (connexons), which allow direct exchange of ions and small molecules between adjacent cells (electric and metabolic coupling)(178).

Contractile apparatus

Most of the data concerning the contractile apparatus and the contraction mechanism of VSMC were obtained using arterial muscle cells, and no significant differences between arterial and venous SMC were reported

The organization of filaments in vascular smooth muscles is less apparent than in striated muscles. Three types of filaments can be observed: thick, thin and intermediate.

The thick myosin filament is composed of two heavy chains (MW 200,000 and 204,000 Da) and two sets of light-chain subunits: LC_{20} (MW 20,000 Da, regulatory) and LC_{17} (MW 17,000 Da, alkali). Serine-19 of LC_{20} is phosphorilated by myosin light chain kinase (MLCK), which is activated by calcium and calcium-binding protein, calmodulin (CaM). In vascular smooth muscle, MLCK (MW 160,000 Da) binds 1 mol calmodulin/mol enzyme. Threonine 18 is phosphorylated rarely by MLCK; beside MLCK, PKC also phosphorylates LC (serine 1, serine2, and threonine9 sites). The phosphorilation of LC_{20} is the signal that activates the cycling of cross-bridges and initiates contraction. The state of phosphorilation of myosin is also regulated by the opposing action of myosin light chain phosphatase (MLCP) and by modulation of MLCK activity (e.g. phosphorilation of serine-512 of LC_{20} by cAMP-protein kinase and Ca^{2+}/calmodulin-dependent protein-kinase II reduces the affinity of MLCK for calmodulin)(178, 9).

In vascular smooth muscle, thin filaments comprise actin, the main constituent, and other proteins: tropomyosin, caldesmon and calponin (179, 2, 196, 162).

Filamentous actin is a two-stranded helix made up of actin monomers of 42,500 Da and bind tropomyosin that lies in the groove on either side of the actin filament. The weight ratio of actin:myosin in smooth muscle is 1.5 to 3:1, and the ratio of action to myosin filaments is approximately 13:1. The actin: myosin ratio is somewhat higher in (at least in some) arterial than in venous smooth muscles. Actin filaments provide strength, connections to other cells and the extracellular matrix, paths for intracellular transport and a scaffold for generating force (179). Recently, a number of signal transduction pathways have been identified that regulate actin polymerization and contractility. GTP-binding proteins, protein kinases, phosphoinositide kinases, and protein phosphatases all play important roles in determining the location and extent of actin polymerization and contractility of actin/myosin filaments. These pathways allow cells to respond to extracellular signals to regulate movement and the tone of vascular smooth muscle cells (25).

Caldesmon (CaD)(87 kDa) is a long, flexible protein, containing binding sites for myosin, actin, tropomyosin and Ca^{2+}-calmodulin. Caldesmon inhibits actomyosin ATP-ase activity. In tonic vascular muscles, the ratio caldesmon: actin is 1:205. Caldesmon is phosphorylated in vitro by Ca^{2+}-calmodulin protein-kinase II (CaMK II), PKC, casein kinase II and MAP kinase, the phosphorilation within the appropriate domain lowering the affinity of the molecule for actin or myosin. Caldesmon seem to be implicated in the regulation of crossbridge cycling, inhibiting actomyosin ATP-ase activity and the movement of actin filaments over phosphorylated myosin (in vitro motility assay)(101, 2, 196).

Calponin (CaP)(MW 34 kDa) is a protein containing binding sites for actin tropomyosin, and Ca^{2+}-calmodulin, which is located peripherally along the long-pitch actin helix. Calponin inhibits actomyosin ATP-ase activity by up to 80% and this inhibition is reversed by calcium and calmodulin as well as by the phosphorilation of the protein by protein-kinase C or CaMK II and restored following dephosphorylation of calponin by a type 2A protein phosphatase. In vascular smooth muscle cells, calponin is present at the same molar concentration as tropomyosin (1 calponin:1 tropomyosin:7 actins)(82, 2, 196, 90).

Within the cytoplasm, thin filaments insert into fusiform dense bodies, which are functionally analogous to Z-lines of striated muscle. Intermediate filaments form a "citoskeleton" linking the dense bodies throughout the cell, maintaining its shape. These filaments are composed of proteins, desmin and/or vimentin (178).

The tone generating capacity of vascular smooth muscle is dependent on interaction between two major contractile proteins, actin and myosin.

In vascular smooth muscle, which is devoid of troponin C, the regulation of actin-myosin interaction is predominantly regulated by a myosin-linked system, which includes calmodulin and MLCK. When calcium rises in the cytosol, it binds to calmodulin and the resulting Ca^{2+}-calmodulin complex then binds to hydrophobic sites of the MLCK. Calmodulin is a 17 kDa protein with four Ca^{2+}-binding sites: two Ca^{2+}-binding sites in the N-terminal region and the other two at the C-terminal region with the Ca^{2+}-binding sites connected by seven fold rotated α-helical structures. Calmodulin binds calcium with different affinities: the two Ca^{2+}-binding sites located in the C domain strongly bind to Ca^{2+}, whereas the other two Ca^{2+}-binding sites in the N-domain bind weakly. Calmodulin regulates the second messenger system through several mechanisms: activation of protein kinases (MLCK, phosphorylase kinase, protein kinase II and others) and protein phosphatases and by regulation of second messenger levels (enhances the activities of guanilate cyclase, cyclic phosphodiesterase and IP_3 kinase, which converts IP_3 to IP_4)(2, 196, 9).

3.2.2. Contraction-Relaxation Cycle

Neural or hormonal stimulation of vascular smooth muscle cells results in an increase of intracellular calcium concentration, from approximately 140 nM in the resting cell to 500-700 nM. Ca^{2+} enters the sarcoplasm via voltage -gated or receptor operated Ca^{2+}-channels, or from the sarcoplasmic reticulum via IP_3 receptor/Ca^{2+} release channels or ryanodine receptor/Ca^{2+}-release channels. As a consequence, Ca^{2+} binds to CaM (4 ions per molecule of CaM) inducing a conformational change that exposes hydrophobic sites of interaction with MLCK. The resulting ternary complex $(Ca^{2+})_4$-CaM-MLCK, representing the active form of MLCK, catalysis the transfer of the terminal phosphoryl group of ATP to Ser19 on each of the two 20kDa light chains of myosin. This phosphorylation triggers the cycling of myosin crossbridges along the actin filaments, with development of force and contraction of the muscle. In addition to MLCK, calmodulin kinase II can also phosphorylate Ser19 of MLC_{20}, but only at very slow rate (1/20 of the Vmax of MLCK), which is unlikely to contribute to the physiological initiation of contraction (179, 2, 196, 9, 162).

Relaxation of vascular smooth muscle follows the restoration of resting intracellular calcium, by extrusion of Ca^{2+} from the cell by a sarcolemal pump or a Na^{+}-Ca^{2+} exchanger, or pumping of Ca^{2+} into the sarcoplasmic reticulum by a calcium pump in the SR membrane. MLCK is rapidly inactivated by the dissociation of CaM, and myosin is dephosphorylated by MLCP. The rate and extent of Ca^{2+} pumping into SR is sufficient to cause relaxation, but plasma membrane Ca^{2+}-ATP-ase and, to a lesser extent the Na^{+}-Ca^{2+} exchanger, contribute to the maintenance of the steady-state levels of total cell calcium. Inhibition of Ca^{2+} influx, through hyperpolarization or by Ca^{2+}-entry blockers, can also reduce $[Ca^{2+}]i$ and cause relaxation (179, 2, 196, 9, 162).

3.2.3. Regulation of Smooth Muscle Contraction

The intracellular level of Ca^{2+} provides the link between excitation and contraction, being considered the primary regulator of the contractile state of vascular smooth muscle, since it dictates the level of myosin phosphorylation. Mechanisms of regulation of intracellular calcium level can be divided into two types: electromechanical and pharmacomechanical coupling mechanisms (Fig. 3.4).

Electromechanical coupling mechanism

Electromechanical coupling operates through changes in surface membrane potential.

The resting membrane potential of smooth muscle is negative, ranging between -40 and -70 mV (depending on cell type: smooth muscles which show spontaneous, rhythmic electrical activity, such as the portal vein smooth muscle have a less negative membrane potential).

Excitatory drugs and neurotransmitters induce depolarization of the sarcolemma, which activates L-type Ca^{2+} channels, resulting in Ca^{2+} entry to the sarcoplasm from the extracellular space down its concentration gradient (1.5-2 mM extracellular and 120-270 nM intracellular). Opening of the calcium channels results in a rather modest increase in calcium intracellular level to 500-700 nM, but this is sufficient to trigger myosin phosphorilation and contraction of the muscle. The Ca^{2+} current carried by the action potential releases additional Ca^{2+} through calcium-induced calcium release (CICR) from the sarcoplasmic reticulum (179, 2, 196, 9, 162).

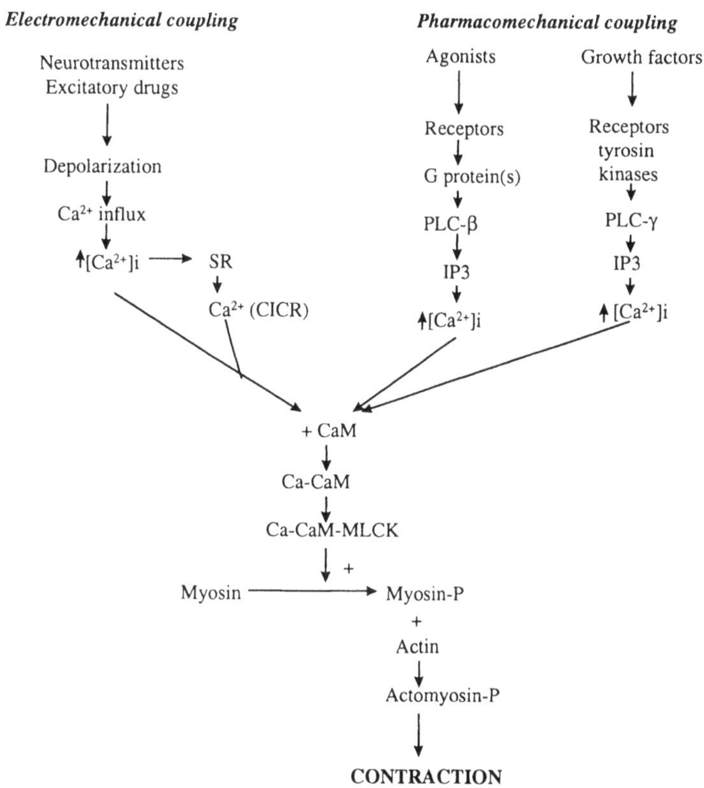

Figure 3.4. Pathways of excitation-contraction coupling (with data from 179, 2, 196).

Pharmacomechanical coupling mechanism

Mechanisms whereby $[Ca^{2+}]i$ is regulated without a change in membrane potential are referred to as pharmacomechanical coupling.

Various extracellular signals alter $[Ca^{2+}]i$ without affecting the membrane potential (179, 2, 196, 162):

- acetylcholine, angiotensin, vasopressin, bradikinin, histamine, thromboxane A_2 and even catecholamines (through α_1-adrenoceptors) binding to their specific membrane receptors, induces the activation of phospholipase C (specifically PLC β isoenzymes) activation with subsequent generation of IP_3, which triggers contraction via the release of Ca^{2+} from sarcoplasmic reticulum. This signal transduction pathway involves members of the Gq subfamily of heterotrimeric GTP-binding proteins (G_q and G_{11}). A distinct sarcoplasmic reticulum Ca^{2+} release channel, the ryanodine receptor, is activated by an increase in $[Ca^{2+}]i$; this process is commonly referred as Ca^{2+}-induced Ca^{2+}-release; this receptor has been suggested to be involved in amplification of an agonist-induced calcium signal, initiation of sarcoplasmic Ca^{2+} oscillations and propagation of calcium waves;
- growth factors, such as PDGF and EGF, acting via receptors that contain a tyrosine kinase catalytic site, activate PLC-γ isoenzymes, resulting in IP_3 production and Ca^{2+} release from SR. This signal transduction pathway does not involve a GTP-binding protein.
- other signals activate calcium entry into the smooth muscle cell via L-type Ca^{2+} channels or receptor-operated Ca^{2+} channels.

Phamacomechanical coupling mechanisms can also contract or relax vascular smooth muscle without a change in $[Ca^{2+}]i$, via Ca^{2+} sensitization and desensitization (Fig.3.5)(179, 2, 196, 162).

Ca^{2+} sensitization.

Ca^{2+} sensitization include the contractions induced at constant $[Ca^{2+}]i$ by certain agonists, and caused by MLCP inhibition, with subsequent increased LC phosphorylation and contraction. MLCP, also known as SMPP-1M, consists of a 110-130 kDa regulatory subunit ($M_{110-130}$), a 37 kDa catalitic subunit (PP-1C), and a 20kDa subunit with identified function (180, 181).

Three pathways that inhibit MLCP activity were identified:

- activation of Rho-kinase by RhoA-GTP, enzyme which phosphorylates the $M_{110-130}$ regulatory subunit and inhibits the catalytic activity of MLCP. Depending on the receptors and cell types involved, several trimeric G-proteins, including $G\alpha_q$, $G\alpha_{12,13}$ and $G\alpha_{1-2}$, can activate RhoA. Phosphorylation of $M_{110-130}$ in its C-terminal half may be also induced by other kinases (70, 181, 56)

RhoA is a monomeric G-protein, which is active when contains GTP and inactive when the bound nucleotide is GDP. MLCP inhibition requires the translocation of RhoA•GTP to the plasma membrane. In resting smooth muscle the inactive RhoA forms are present in the cytosol, where are complexed with RhoGDI, forming RhoA•RhoGDI. Cytosolic RhoA•RhoGDI is activated by Rho-GEFs, which stimulate the replacement of GDP with GTP, followed by dissociation and translocation of RhoA•GTP to the plasma membrane (71, 181)

The Rho-kinase inhibitors, such as C3 and Y-27632, were shown to inhibit thrombin-stimulated migration of vascular smooth muscle cells and endothelial contraction, suggesting that the Rho-/Rho-kinase pathway may be involved in the formation of atheromatous plaques and post-angioplasty re-stenosis (169, 54).

- activation of Rho-kinase by arachidonic acid increase due to a variety of stimuli; arachidonic acid also inhibits the activity of MLCP by dissociating $M_{110-130}$ subunit from the catalytic one (181)
- phosphorylation of CPI-17 by protein kinase C (PKC), CPI-17P inducing a direct inhibition of the catalytic subunit PP-1C. PKCs may be constitutively active, and can also be activated by phorbol esters or diacylglycerol (195, 181).

These mechanisms seem to operate in parallel with and independently of the activation of MLCK by calcium release from sarcoplasmic reticulum by IP_3 or by Ca^{2+} influx (181).

Ca^{2+} desensitization

Ca^{2+} desensitization can be mediated by inhibition of MLCK and/or activation of SMPP-1M:

- phosphorylation of site A of MLCK by calmodulin-dependent protein kinase II (in vivo) and several kinases (in vitro) is followed by a decrease of its affinity to Ca^{2+}-calmodulin. If the smooth muscle cell is exposed to high $[Ca^{2+}]i$, the Ca^{2+}-calmodulin-dependent protein kinase II (CaMK II) becomes activated. CaMK II phosphorylates MLCK, lowering its affinity for calcium-calmodulin, thereby inhibiting MLCK activity and favoring smooth muscle relaxation owing to myosin dephosphorylation by MLCP (65). In permeabilized smooth muscle of the rabbit portal vein, Kureishi et al. (2000) showed the existence of other kinases, distinct from Rho-associated kinase, myosin light chain kinase, and protein kinase C, which phosphorylate myosin light chain at serine-19 and induce Ca^{2+}-independent smooth muscle contraction (99).

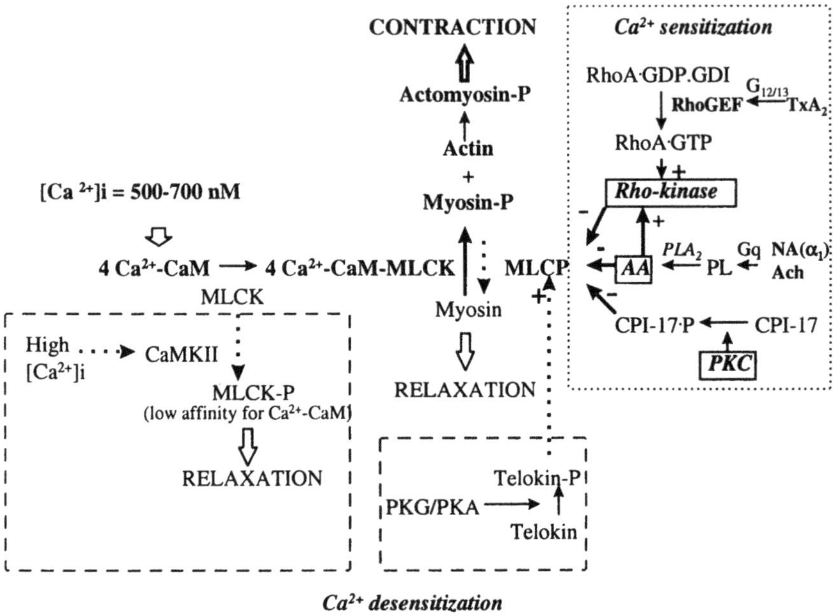

Figure 3.5. Mechanism of the vascular smooth muscle contraction-relaxation. (with data from 179, 2, 196, 99, 202)

PKG and/or PKA and telokin cooperate in the Ca^{2+} desensitizing mechanism mediated by enhancement of MLC_{20} dephosphorylation. Telokin, also known as kinase-related protein, has a structure identical to the COOH terminus of smooth muscle MLCK, and presents a characteristic immunoglobulin fold. The roles of telokin include: binding to the S1/S2 region of unphosphorylated smooth muscle myosin, stabilization of myosin filaments, modulation of MLCK oligomerization (in vitro) and inhibition of myosin phosphorylation by MLCK, through competitive inhibition for the MLCK site. Experimental studies showed that the major in situ effect of telokin is desensitization to $[Ca^{2+}]i$ through a mechanism that accelerates the dephosphorylation of LC20, acting sinergistically with the effect of 8-Br-cGMP-activated kinase. The effect of telokin was enhanced by its phosphorylation by PKG and PKA (202).

Direct regulation of crossbridge cycling

A direct regulation of crossbridge cycling is also possible and involves the two regulatory proteins associated to the actin filament: caldesmon and calponin (Fig.3.6.)(179, 2, 196, 90):

- Caldesmon may interact with actin, myosin and tropomyosin in a Ca^{2+}-independent manner, and with calmodulin in a Ca^{2+}-dependent manner. The physiological roles of caldesmon include the ability to cross-link actin and myosin filaments (structural role) and the ability to inhibit actomyosin ATP-ase activity and thus, the crossbridge cycling rate. These functions of caldesmon may be regulated by phosphorylation, which affect the interactions of caldesmon with both actin and myosin filaments. Briefly, activation of PKC by phorbol esters results in the conversion of Ras from the inactive GDP-bound form to its active GTP-bound form. Activated Ras converts Raf , a serine-treonine kinase, to an active state, thereby triggering the phosphorylation of MAP kinase kinase (MAPKK) and MAP kinase (MAPK). The latter phosphorylates caldesmon, alleviating its inhibition of the actomyosin ATP-ase, thereby triggering contraction.

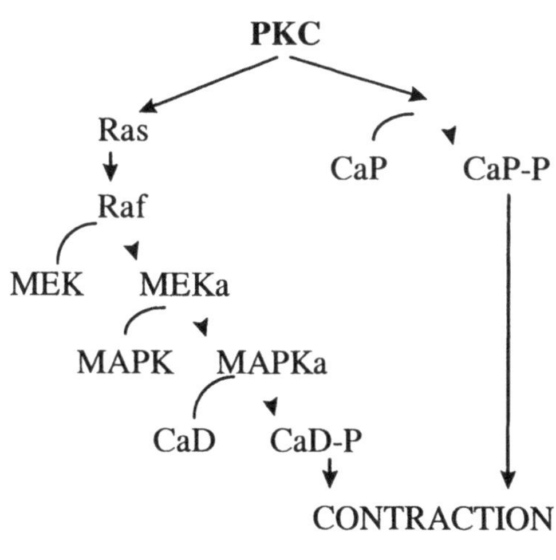

Figure 3.6. Direct regulation of crossbridge cycling involving caldesmon and calponin (with data from 179, 2, 196, 162)

- Calponin (*cal*modulin-binding, tro*ponin* T-like protein) inhibits actomyosin ATP-ase activity, this inhibition being reversed by calcium and calmodulin, but also by its phosphorylation by PKC or CaMK II. The proposed mechanism of calponin physiological role in the regulation of cross-bridge cycling rate in smooth muscle can be summarized as follows: In the resting state, at low intracellular calcium levels, calponin associated to with the actin filament serves to inhibit the cross-bridge cycling rate, and the muscle is relaxed. After stimulation, $[Ca^{2+}]i$ rises, triggering MLCK activation by Ca^{2+}-CaM. But phosphorylated myosin presents a low ATP-ase activity, which will be enhanced in the presence of actin. However, as long as calponin remains attached to the actin filament, the crossbridge cycling rate is inhibited. This inhibition is released by phosphorylation of calponin by PKC or CaMK II and/or by binding of calponin to Ca^{2+}-caltropin (a calcium-binding protein), with consecutive dissociation of calponin from actin.

Finally, we can say that vascular smooth muscle tone is regulated primarily by $[Ca^{2+}]i$, which stimulates myosin phosphorylation and activates myosin ATP-ase by actin. The regulation of vascular smooth muscle tone involves mechanisms of regulation of intracellular calcium level, but also other mechanisms like Ca^{2+}-independent contraction and regulation of crossbridge cycling by thin filament-associated proteins. Almost all studies concerning the mechanism of vascular smooth muscle contraction-relaxation were performed on arterial smooth muscles, but there are no data underlining important differences between venous and arterial smooth muscle activity.

3.3. VENOUS ADVENTITIA

Small veins have an adventitia with longitudinally oriented elastic fibers and delicate bundles of collagen.

The adventitia of medium-size veins is thicker than the media and is composed of loose connective tissue with collagen fibers, and smooth muscle cells frequently oriented longitudinally; vasa vasorum, lymphatics, and unmyelinated nerves are consistently present.

The adventitia represents the greatest part of the large veins walls and is continuous with the surrounding connective tissue. It contains the loose connective tissue with thick bundles of elastic and collagen fibers longitudinally oriented and smooth muscle fibers with similar arrangement.

The connective tissue cells of the vascular wall represent a pluripotential system, being involved in the production, storage and secretion of local vasoactive mediators (mast cells frequently located along the pericytic venules release histamine and serotonin), phagocytosis (performed by macrophages), immune reactions (involving plasma cells and eosinophils) and secretion of connective tissue fibers (performed mostly by fibroblasts). Differences concerning the ratio between collagen and elastin in arteries and veins were noted. For instance, in humans, vena cava contains about seven times more collagen (types I, III and IV) than elastin, while in aorta collagen (type III prevalent) and elastin, each represent 20% of the dry weight (177).

The venous wall adventitia is provided with its own nutrient vessels, called vasa vasorum, while the rest of the wall is nourished by diffusion. Vasa vasorum of veins are more abundant and penetrate much closer to the intima than do those of arteries. A rich nervous plexus is also encountered (177).

Venous wall undergoes changes and transformations with increasing age, but in a less stereotyped way that the corresponding arteries. For instance, human saphenous veins from elderly subjects present the following characteristics: various degrees of intimal thickening, fibrosis of the three tunics, with gradual increase in collagens I, II and especially IV in the circular layers of the media, and overall decrease in the elastic network (20).

REFERENCES

1. Allaire E, Clowes AW. Endothelial cell injury in cardiovascular surgery: the intimal hyperplastic response. Ann Thorac Surg 1997; 63: 582-591
2. Allen BG, Walsh MP. The biochemical basis of the regulation of smooth-muscle contraction. TIBS 1994; 19: 362-367
3. Amini-Nekoo A, Futers TS, Moia M, Mannucci PM, Grant PJ, Ariens RA. Analysis of the tissue factor pathway inhibitor gene and antigen levels in relation to venous thrombosis, Br J Haematol 2001; 113: 537-543.
4. Arnal JF, Tack I, Besombes JP, Pipy B, Negre-Salvayre A. Nitric oxide and superoxide anion production during endothelial cell proliferation. Am J Physiol 1996; 271: C1521-1526
5. Asahara T T, Bauters C, Pastore C, Kearney M, Rossow S, Bunting S, Ferrara N, Symes JF, Isner JM. Local delivery of vascular endothelial growth factor accelerates

re-endothelialization and attenuates intimal hyperplasia in baloon-injured rat carotid artery. Circulation 1995; 91: 2793-2801

6. Astedt B, Hagerstrandt I, Lecander I. Cellular localization in placenta of placental type plasminogen activator inhibitor. Thromb Haemost 1986; 56: 63-65
7. Bajzar L, Morser J, Nesheim M. TAFI, or plasma procarboxy-peptidase B, couples the coagulation and fybrinolytic cascades through the thrombin-thrombomodulin complex. J Biol Chem 1996; 271: 16603-16608
8. Ballermann BJ, Dardik A, Eng E, Liu A. Shear stress and the endothelium. Kidney International 1998; 54: 100-108
9. Barany M, Barany K. Protein phosphrylation during contraction and relaxation. In Biochemistry of Smooth Muscle Contraction. Ed. M Barany, Academic Press, 1996; 321-339
10. Barnathan ES, Kuo A, Rosenfeld L, Kariko K, Leski M, Robbiati F, Nolli ML, Henkin J, Cines DB. Interaction of single chain urokinase type plasminogen activator with human endothelial cells. J Biol Chem 1990; 265: 2865-2872
11. Belz GG, Berrmann J, Schloos J, KleinBloesem CH. The effect of oral clazapril and prazosin on the constrictor effects of locally infused angiotensin I and noradrenaline in human hand veins. Br J Clin Pharmacol 1989; 28: 608-611
12. Bhagyalakshmi A, Berthiaume F, Reich KM, Frangos JA. Fluid shear stress stimulates membrane phospholipid metabolism in cultured human endothelial cells. J Vasc Res 1992; 29: 443-449
13. Bishop-Bailey D, Pepper JR, Larkin SW, Mitchell JA, Differential induction of cyclooxigenase-2 in human arterial and venous smooth muscle. Role of endogenous prostanoids, Arterioscler Thromb Vasc Biol 1998; 18: 1655-1661
14. Blackman DJ, Morris-Thurgood JA, Atherton JJ, Ellis GR, Anderson RA, Cockcroft JR, Frenneaux MP, Endothelium-derived nitric oxide contributes to the regulation of venous tone in humans, Circulation 2000; 101: 165-170
15. Boegehold MA. Flow-dependent arteriolar dilation in normotensive rats fed low- or high-salt diets. Am J Physiol 1995; 269: H1407-1414
16. Boegehold MA. Shear-dependent release of venular nitric oxide: effect on arteriolar tone in rat striated muscle. Am J Physiol 1996; 271: H387-395
17. Bombeli T, Meller M, Haeberli A. Anticoagulant properties of the vascular endothelium. Thromb Haemost 1997; 77: 408-423
18. Bonner G, Preis S, Schunk U, Wagmann M, Chrosch R, Toussaint C. Effect of bradykinin on arteries and veins in systemic and pulmonary circulation. J Cardiovasc Pharmacol 1992; 20(suppl.9): S21-S27
19. Borland JA, Chester AH, Crabbe S, Parkerson JB, Catravas JD, Yacoub MH. Differential action of angiotensin II and activity of angiotensin-converting enzyme in human bypass grafts. J Thorac Cardiovasc Surg 1998; 116: 206-212
20. Bouissou H, Julian M, Pieraggi, MTh, Louge L. Vein morphology. Phlebology 1988; 3 (supL1.): 1-11
21. Brandes RP, Barton M, Philippens KM, Schweitzer G, Mugge A. Endothelial-derived superoxide anions in pig coconary arteries: evidence from lucigenin chemiluminiscence and histochemical techniques. J Physiol 1997; 500: 331-342
22. Caprini JA, Arcelus JI, Reyna JJ. Effective risk stratification of surgical and nonsurgical patients for venous thromboembolic disease. Semin Hematol 2001; 38(Suppl 5): 12-19

23. Carmeliet P, Schoonjans L, Kiekens L, Ream B, Degan J, Bronson R, De Vos R, van den Oord JJ, Collen D, Mulligan RC. Physiological consequence of loss of plasminogen activator gene function in mice. Nature 1994; 369: 419-424
24. Carmeliet P, Collen D. Vascular development and disorders: Molecular analysis and pathogenic insights. Kidney International 1998; 53: 1519-1549
25. Carpenter CL. Actin cytoskeleton and cell signaling, Crit Care Med 2000; 28(4 Suppl): N94-9
26. Carter AJ, Bevan JA, Hanley SP, Morgan WE, Turner DR. A comparison of human pulmonary arterial and venous prostacyclin and thromboxane synthesis. Effect of a thromboxane synthase inhibitor. Thromb Haemostasis 1984; 51:257-260
27. Carter AJ, Eisert WG, Muller TH. Thrombin stimulates inositol phosphate accumulation and prostacyclin synthesis in human ednothelial cells from umbilical vein but not from omentum. Thromb Haemostasis 1989; 61: 122-126
28. Chaikouni A, Crawford FA, Kochel PJ, Olanoff LS, Haluschka PV. Human internal mammary artery produces more prostacyclin than saphenous vein. J Thorac Cardiovasc Surg 1986; 92: 88-91
29. Chappel MC, Pirro NT, Sykes A, Ferrario CM. Metabolism of angiotensin-(1-7) by angiotensin converting enzyme. Hypertension 1998; 31: 362-367
30. Cines DB, Pollak ES, Buck CA, Loscalzo j, Zimmerman GA, McEver RP, Pober JS, Wick TM, Konkle BA, Schwartz BS, Barnathan ES, McCrae KR, Hug BA, Schmidt A-M, Stern DM. Endothelial cells in physiology and in the pathophysiology of vascular disorders. Blood 1998; 91: 3527-3561
31. Coleridge Smith PD, Thomas P, Scurr JH, Dormandy JA. Causes of venous ulceration: a new hypothesis. Br Med J 1988; 296: 1726-1728
32. Collen D, Lijnen HR. Basic and clinical aspects of fibrinolysis and thrombolysis. Blood 1991; 78: 3114-3124
33. Collier J, Vallance P. L-NMMA increase arteriolar but not venous tone in humans: The mechansim appears to be independent of sympathetic tone. J Cardiovasc Pharmacol 1991; 17(Suppl.3): S182-S185
34. Cook JM, Cook CD, Marlar R, Solis MM, Fink L, Eidt JF. Thrombomodulin activity in human sapgenous grafts prepared for coronary artery bypass. J Vasc Surg 1991; 14: 147-151
35. Cooke JP, Rossitch E jr., Andon NA, Loscalzo J, Dzau VJ. Flow activates an endothelial potassium channel to release an endogenous nitrovasodilator. J Clin Invest 1991; 88: 1663-1671
36. Corriu C, Feletou M, Canet E, Vanhoutte PM. Endothelium-derived factors and hypepolarizations of isolated carotid artery of the guinea pig. Br J Pharmacol 1996; 119: 959-964
37. Cosentino F, Lüscher TF. Maintenance of vascular integrity: role of nitric oxide and other bradikinin mediators, Eur Heart J 1995; 16: K4-12
38. Costello KB, Stewart DJ, Baffour R. Endothelin is a potent constrictor of human vessels used in coronary revascularization surgery. Eur J Pharmacol 1990; 186: 311-314
39. Cotran RS, Mayadas-Norton T. Endothelial adhesion molecules in health and disease. Path Biol 1998; 46: 164-170
40. Cox JL, Chiasson DA, Gotlieb AI. Stranger in a strange land: the pathogenesis of saphenous graft stenosis with emphasis on structural and functional difference between veins and arteries. Prog Cardiovasc Dis 1991; 34: 45-68
41. Davies MG, Hagen PO. The vascular endothelium. A new horizon. Ann Surg 1993;

218: 593-609

42. Dawes M, Chowienczyk PJ, Ritter JM. Effects of inhibition of the L-arginine/nitric oxide pathway on vasodilation caused by β-adrenergic agonists in human forearm. Circulation 1997; 95: 2293-2297
43. Dejana E, Corada M, Lampugnani MG. Endothelial cell-to-cell junctions. FASEB J 1995; 9: 910-918
44. Dejana E, Lostaglio S. Endothelial cell-to-cell junctions and their role in angiogenesis. Forum 1996; 6: 380-389
45. Dejana E, Valiron O, Navarro P, Lampugnani MG. Intercellular junctions in the endothelium and the control of vascular permeability. Ann N Y Acad Sci 1997; 811: 36-43
46. Dollery CM, McEwan JR, Henney AM. Matrix metalloproteinases and cardiovascular disease. Circ Res 1995; 77: 863-868
47. Drexler H, Hornig B. Endothelial dysfunction in human disease. J Moll Cell Cardiol 1999; 31: 51-60
48. Drubaix I, Giakoumakis A, Robert L, Robert AM. Preliminary data on the age-dependent decrease in basic fibroblast growth factor and platelet-derived growth factor in the human vein wall and in their influence on cell proliferation. Gerontology 1998; 44: 9-14
49. Dusting GJ, Fennessy P, Yin ZL, Gurevich V. Nitric oxide in atherosclerotis: vascular protector or villain? Clin Exp Pharmacol Physiol 1998; 25: S34-S41
50. Dzau VJ, Gibbons GH. "The role of the endothelium in vascular remodelling." In *Cardiovascular significance of endothelium-derived vasoactive factors*, Rubanyi GM, ed. Futura Publishing Co.Inc, Mount Kisco, NY, 1991; 281-290
51. Dzau VJ. Cell biology and genetics of angiotensin in cardiovascular disease. J Hypertens 1994; Suppl 12: S3-10
52. Edwards G, Dora KA, Gardener MJ, Garland CJ, Weston AH. K^+ is an endothelium-derived hyperpolarizing factor in rat arteries. Nature 1998; 396: 269-272
53. Emoto N, Yanagisawa M. Endothelin-converting enzyme-2 is a membrane bound, phosphoramidon-sensitive metalloprotease with acidic pH optimum. J Biol Chem 1995; 270: 15262-15268
54. Essler M, Retzer M, Bauer M, Heemskerk JW, Aepfelbacher M, Siess W. Mildly oxidized low density lipoprotein induces contraction of human ednothelial cells through activation of rho/Rhokinase and inhibition of myosin light chain phosphatase. J Biol Chem 1999; 274: 30361-30363
55. Falkenhahn M, Gohlke P, Paul MSA. The renin-angiotensin system in the heart and vascular wall: new therapeutic aspects. J Cardiovasc Pharm 1994; 24(suppl.2): S6-13
56. Feng J, Ito M, Kureishi Y, Ichikawa K, Amano M, Isaka N, Okawa K, Iwamatsu A, Kaibuchi K, Hartshorne D J, Nakano. Rho-associated kinase of chicken gizzard smooth muscle. J Biol Chem 1999; 274: 3744-3752
57. Ferro A, Queen LR, Priest RM, Xu B, Ritter JM, Poston L, Ward JPT. Activation of the nitric oxide synthase by β_2-adrenoceptors in human umbilical vein endothelium in vitro. Br J Pharmacol 1999; 126: 1872-1880
58. Fisher AB, Chien S, Barakat AI, Nerem RM. Endothelial cellular response to altered shear stress. Am J Physiol Lung Cell Mol Physiol 2001; 281: L529-533
59. Fishman AP. Endothelium: A distributed organ of diverse capabilities. Ann NY Acad Sci 1982; 401: 1-8
60. Florey L. The endothelial cell. Br Med J 1966; 2: 487-490

61. Franco RF, Fagundes MG, Meijers JC, Reitsma PH, Lourenco D, Morelli V, Maffei FH, Ferrari IC, Piccinato CE, Silva WA Jr, Zago MA. Identification of polymorphisms in the 5'-untranslated region of the TAFI gene: relationship with plasma TAFI levels and risk of venous thrombosis. Haematologica 2001; 86:510-517
62. Frangos JA, Eskin SG, McIntire LV, Ives CL. Flow effects on prostacyclin production by cultured human endothelial cells. Science 1985; 227: 1477-1479
63. Fukaya Y, Ohhashi T. Acetylcholine- and flow-induced production and release of nitric oxide in arterial and venous endothelial cells. Am J Physiol 1996; 270: H99-H106
64. Fukudome K, Kurosawa S, Stearns-Kurosawa D-J, He X, Rezaie AR, Esmon CT. The endothelial cell protein C receptor. Cell surface expression and direct ligand binding by the soluble receptor. J Biol Chem 1996; 271: 17491-17498
65. Gallagher PJ, Herring BP, Stull JT. Myosin light chain kinases. J Muscle Res Cell Motil 1997; 18: 1-16
66. Geiger M, Prilinger U, Griffin JH, Binder BR. Urinary protein C inhibitor. Glycosaminoglycans synthetized by the epithelial cell line TC1-598 enhance its interaction with urokinase. J Biol Chem 1991; 266: 11851-11857
67. Gertler JP, Abbott WM. Prothrombotic and fibrinolytic function of normal and perturbed endothelium. J Surg Res 1992; 52: 89-92
68. Gibbons GH, Dzau VJ. The emerging concept of vascular remodeling. N Engl J Med 1994; 330: 1431-1438
69. Gibbons GH. Endothelial function as a determinant of vascular function and structure: a new therapeutic target. Am J Cardiol 1997; 79: 3-8
70. Gohla A, Schultz G, Offermanns S. Role for G_{12}/G_{13} in agonist-induced vascular smooth muscle cells contraction. *Circ Res* 2000; 87: 221-227
71. Gong MC, Fujihara H, Somlyo AV, Somlyo AP. Translocation of rhoA associated with Ca^{2+}-sensitization of smooth muscle. J Biol Chem 1997; 272: 10704-10709
72. Gosling M, Golledge J, Turner RJ, Powell JT. Arterial flow conditions downregulate thrombomodulin on saphenous vein endothelium. Circulation 1999; 99: 1047-1053
73. Griendling KK, Sorescu D, Lassegue B, Ushio-Fukai M. Modulation of Protein-kinase activity and gene expression by reactive oxygen species and their role in vascular physiology and pathophysiology, Arteriscler Thromb Vasc Biol 2000; 20: 2175-2183
74. Guimaraes S, de Moura D. Vascular Adrenoceptors: An Update, Phamacol Rev 2001; 53: 319-356
75. Haastrup A, Gadegbeku CA, Zhang D, Mukhin YV, Greene EL, Jaffa AA, Egan BM. Lipids stimulate the production of 6-keto-prostaglandin F1α in human dorsal hand veins. Hypertension 2001; 38: 858-863
76. Hafizi S, Nobin R, Allen SP, Chester AH, Yacoub MH. Contrasting effects of platelet-derived growth factor (PDGF) isomers on mitogenesis, contraction and intracellular calcium concentration in human vascular smooth muscle. Acta Physiol Scand 1998; 164: 191-199
77. Hajjar KA, Jacovina AT, Checko J. An endothelial cell receptor for plasminogen/tissue plasminogen activator. J Biol Chem 1994; 269: 21191-21194
78. Hanley SP, Bevan J. Inhibition by aspirin of human arterial and venous prostacyclin synthesis. Prostaglandin Leukotriene Med 1985; 20: 141-149
79. Harrison DG, Sayegh H, Ohara Y, Inoue N, Venema RC. Regulation of expression of the endothelial cell nitric oxide synthase. Clin Exp Pharmacol Physiol 1996; 23: 251-255
80. Harrison DG. Endothelial function and oxidant stress. Clin Cardiol 1997; 20: II11-17

81. Higazi AA-R, Mazar A, Wang J, Reilly R, Henkin J, Kniss D, Cines D. Single chain urokinase-type plasminogen activator bound to its receptor is relatively resistant to plasminogen activator inhibitor type I. Blood 1996; 269: 3545-3549
82. Hodgkinson JL, El-Mezgueldi M, Craig R, Vibert P, Marston SB, Lehman W. 3-D image reconstruction of reconstituted smooth muscle thin filaments containing calponin: visualization of interactions between F-actin and calponin. J Mol Biol 1997; 273: 159-169
83. Hoebel BG, Steyrer E, Graier WF. Origin and function of epoxyeicosatrienoic acids in vascular endothelial cells: more than just endothelium-derived hyperpolarizing factor? Clin Exp Pharmacol Physiol 1998; 25: 826-830
84. Holt CM, Francis SE, Newby AC, Rogers S, Gadson PA, Taylot T, Angelini GD. Comparison of response to injury in organ culture of human saphenous vein and internal mammary artery. Ann Thorac Surg 1993; 55: 1522-1528
85. Ignarro LJ. Biological actions and properties of endothelium-derived nitric oxide formed and released from artery and vein. Circ Res 1982; 65: 1-21
86. Ignarro LJ, Buga GM, Chaudhuri G. EDRF generation and release from perfused bovine pulmonary artery and vein. Eur J Pharmacol 1988; 149: 79-88
87. Ignarro LJ, Heme-dependent activation of guanilate-cyclase by nitric oxide: a novel signal transduction mechanism, Blood Vessels 1991; 28: 67-73
88. Izzat MB, Mehta D, Bryan AJ, reeves B, Newby AC, Angelini GD. Influence of external stent size on early medial and neointimal thickening in a pig model of saphenous vein bypass grafting. Circulation 1996; 94: 1741-1745
89. Jaffe EA. Culture of human endothelial cells from umbilical cord vein: identification by morphologic and immunologic criteria. J Clin Invest 1973; 52: 2745-2756
90. Jin JP; Walsh MP; Sutherland C; Chen W. A role for serine-175 in modulating the molecular conformation of calponin, Biochem J 2000; 350: 579-88
91. Johnson JL, van Eys GJJM, Angelini GD, George SJ. Injury induces dedifferentiation of smooth muscle cells and increased matrix-0degrading metalloproteinase activity in human saphenous vein. Arterioscl Thromb Vasc Biol 2001; 21: 1146-1152
92. Kanthou C, Benzakour O. Cellular effects of thrombin and their signaling pathways. 1995; 2: 293-298
93. Katusic ZS, Vanhoutte PM. Superoxide anion is an endothelium-derived contracting factor. Am J Physiol 1989; 257: H33-37
94. Kirkpatrick CJ, Bittinger F, Unger RE, Kriegsmann J, Kilbinger H, Wessler I. The non-neuronal cholinergic system in the endothelium: evidence and possible pathobiological significance. Jpn J Pharmacol 2001; 85: 24-28 (abstract)
95. Kockx MM, Knaapen MW, Bortier HE, Cromheeke KM, Boutherin-Falson O, Finet M. Vascular remodeling in varicose veins. Angiology 1998; 49:871-877
96. Komori K, Vanhoutte PM. Endothelium-derived hyperpolarizing factor. Blood Vessels 1990; 27: 238-245
97. Kroll MH, Hellums JD, McIntire LV, Schafer AI, Moake JL. Platelets and shear stress. Blood 1996; 88: 1525-1541
98. Kumar S, West DC, Ager A. Heterogeneity in endothelial cells from large vessels and microvessels. Differentiation 1987; 36: 57-70
99. Kureishi Y, Ito M, Feng J, Okinaka T, Isaka N, Nakano T. Regulation of Ca^{2+}-independent smooth muscle contraction by alternative staurosporine-sensitive kinase, Eur J Pharmacol 1999; 376: 315-320
100. Lampugnani MG, Dejana E. Interendothelial junctions: structure, signaling and functional roles. Curr Opin Cell Biol 1997; 9: 674-682

101. Lehman W, Vibert P, Craig R. Vizualization of caldesmon on smooth muscle thin filaments. J Mol Biol 1997; 274: 310-317
102. Levin EG, Santell L. Thrombin- and histamine-induced signal transduction in human endothelial cells. Stimulation and agonist-dependent desensitization of protein phosphorylation. J Biol Chem 1991; 266: 174-181
103. Levin EG, Osborn KG. The expression of endothelial cell tissue plasminogen activator in vivo: A function defined by vessel size and anatomic location. J Cell Sci 1997; 11: 139-148
104. Lin MC, Almusjacobs F, Chen HH, Parry GCN, Mackman N, Shyy JYJ. Atherosclerosis, thrombosis, gene expression, hemodynamics, signal transduction: Shear stress induction of the tissue factor gene. J Clin Invest 1997; 99: 737-744
105. Liu ZG; Ge ZD; He GW. Difference in endothelium-derived hyperpolarizing factor-mediated hyperpolarization and nitric oxide release between human internal mammary artery and saphenous vein. Circulation 2000; 102: III296-301
106. Loskutoff DJ, Sawdy M, Mimuro J. "Type 1 plasminogen activator inhibitor." In *Progress in Hemostasis and Thrombosis*. Coller BS, ed. Saunders 1989: 87-99
107. Lowell RC, Gloviczki P, Miller VM, In vitro evaluation of endothelial and smooth muscle function of primary varicose veins, J Vasc Surg 1992; 16: 679-86
108. Lu D, Kalafatis M, Mann KG, Long GL. Comparison of activated protein C/protein S-mediated inactivation of human factor VIII and factor V. Blood 1996; 87: 4708-4717
109. Lüscher TF, Yang Z, Tschudi M, von Segesser L, Stulz P, Boulanger C, Siebenmann R, Turina M, Bühler FR. Interaction between endothelin-1 and endothelium-derived relaxing factor in human arteries and veins, Circ Res 1990; 66:1088-1094
110. Lüscher TF. Vascular biology of coronary bypass grafts. Coronary Artery Disease 1992; 3: 157-165
111. Maigaard S, Forman A, Andersson KE. Differential effects of angiotensin, vasopressin, and oxytocin on various smooth muscle tissues within the human uteroplacental unit. Acta Physiol Scand 1986; 128: 23-31
112. Malik AB, Lo SK. Vascular endothelial adhesion molecules and tissue inflammation. Pharm Rev 1996; 48: 213-233
113. Malek AM, Greene AL, Izumo S. Regulation of endothelin 1 gene by fluid shear stress is transcriptionally mediated and independent of protein kinase C and cAMP. Proc Natl Acad Sci U S A. 1993; 90: 5999-6003
114. Manchanda N, Schwartz BS. Single chain urokinase. Augmentation of enzymatic activity upon binding to monocytes. J Biol Chem 1991; 266:14580-14584.
115. Mann KG. Thrombosis: theoretical considerations. Am J Clin Nutr 1997; 65(suppl. 5): 1675S-1664S
116. Mann MJ, Gibbons GH, Kernoff RS, Diet FP, Tsao PS, Cooke JP, Kaneda Y, Dzau VJ. Genetic engineering of vein grafts resistant to atherosclerosis. Proc Natl Acad Sci USA. 1995; 92: 4502-4506
117. Maruyama I. Thrombomodulin, an endothelial anticoagulant: its structure, function and expression. Jpn Circ J 1992; 56: 187-191
118. Masaki T. Possible role of endothelin in endothelial regulation of vascular tone. Annu Rev Pharmacol Toxicol 1995; 35: 235-255
119. Masood I, Porter KE, London NJ. Endothelin-1 is a mediator of intimal hyperplasia in organ culture of human saphenous vein. Br J Surg 1997; 84: 499-503
120. Mehta J, Roberts A. Human vascular tissue produce thromboxane as well as prostacyclin. Am J Physiol 1983; 244: R839-844

121. Michiels C, Arnould T, Remacle J. Role de l'hypoxie et des cellules endotheliales dans le developpement des veines variqueuses. Med Sci 1994; 10:845-853
122. Michiels C, Arnould T, Janssens D, Bajou K, Geron I, Remacle J. Interactions entre les cellules musculaires lisses apres activation par l'hypoxie. Une etiologie possible de la maladie veineuse. Phlebologie 1995; 48: 141-149
123. Michiels C, Arnould T, Janssens D, Bajou K, Geron I, Remacle J. Interactions between endothelial cells and smooth muscle cells after their activation by hypoxia. A possible etiology for venous disease. Int Angiol 1996; 15:124-30
124. Michiels C, Arnould T, Thibaut-Vercruyssen R, Bouaziz N, Janssens D, Remacle J. Perfused human saphenous veins for the study of the origin of varicose veins: role of the endothelium and of hypoxia. Int Angiol 1997; 16:134-141
125. Mizuno K, Niimura S, Tani SM, Haga H, Inagami T, Fukuchii S. Direct proof for local generation and release of angiotensin II in peripheral human vascular tissue. Am J Hypertens 1991; 4 (suppl): 67S-72S
126. Molderings GJ, Likungu J, Hentrich F, Gothert M. Facilitatory presynaptic angiotensin receptors on the sympathetic nerves of the human saphenous vein and pulmonary artery. Potential involvement in beta-adrenoceptor-mediated facilitation of noradrenaline release. Naunyn Schmiedebergs Arch Pharmacol 1988; 338: 228-233
127. Molenaar P, Malta E, Jones CR, Buxton BF, Summers RJ. Autoradiographic localization and function of beta-adrenoceptors on the human internal mammary artery and saphenous vein. Br J Pharmacol 1988; 95:225-233
128. Mombouli J-V, Vanhoutte PM. Endothelium-dependent hyperpolarizing factor(s): updating the unknown. Trends Pharmacol Sci 1997; 18: 252-256
129. Mombouli J-V, Vanhoutte PM. Endothelial dysfunction: from physiology to therapy. J Moll Cell Cardiol 1999; 31: 61-74
130. Moncada S, Higgs A. The L-arginine-nitric oxide pathway. N Engl J Med 1993; 329: 2002-2012
131. Morin O, Patry P, Lafleur L. Heterogeneuty of endothelial cells of adult liver rat as resolved by sedimentation velocity and flowcitometry. J Cell Physiol 1984; 119: 327-331
132. Morita T, Kurihara H, Maemura K, Yoshizumi M, Yazaki Y. Disruption of cytoskeletal structures mediates shear stress-induced endothelin-1 gene expression in cultured porcine aortic endothelial cells. J Clin Invest 1993; 92: 1706-1712
133. Morita T, Kurihara H, Maemura K, Yoshizumi M, Nagai R, Yazaki Y. Role of Ca^{2+} and protein kinase C in shear stress-induced actin depolymerization and endothelin 1 gene expression, Circ Res 1994; 75: 630-636
134. Motwani JG, Topol EJ. Aortocoronary saphenous vein graft disease. Pathogenesis, predisposition, and prevention. Circulation 1998; 97: 916-931
135. Moyses C, Cederholm-William SA, Michel CC. Haemoconcentration and accumulation of white cells in the feet during venous stasis. Int J Microcirc Clin Exp 1987; 5: 311-320
136. Murad E, Waldman S, Molina C, Bennett B, Leitman D. Regulation and role of guanylate cyclase-cyclic GMP in vascular relaxation. Prog Clin Biol Res 1987; 249: 65-76
137. Nadasy GL, Szekacs B, Juhasz I, Feher J, Kowach AGB, Monos E., Role of endothelium, oxygen and ionic milieu in the prostacyclin and thromboxane production of rat aortic tissue slices, Acta Physiol Hung 1991; 78: 77-87

138. Nguyen HC, Grossi EA, LeBoutellier M, Steinberg BM, Rifkin DB, Baumann FG, Colvin SB, Galloway AC. Mammary artery versus saphenous vein grafts: assessment of basic fibroblast growth factor receptors. Ann Thorac Surg 1994; 58: 308-311
139. Nichols K, Staines W, Rubin S, Krantis A. Distribution of nitric oxide synthase activity in arterioles and venules of rat and human intestine. Am J Physiol 1994; 267: G270-275
140. Nilsen EM, Johansen FE, Jahnsen FL, Landin KE, Scholtz T, Brandtzaeg P, Haraldsen G. Cytokine profiles of cultured microvascular endothelial cells from the human intestine. Gut 1998; 42: 635-642
141. Nishida K, Harrison DG, Navas JP, Fisher AA, Dockery SP, Uematsu M, Nerem RM, Alexander RW, Murphy TJ. Molecular cloning and characterization of the constitutive bovine aortic endothelial cell nitric oxide synthase. J Clin Invest 1992; 90: 1092-2096
142. Noll G, Luscher TF. The endothelium in acute coronary syndromes. Eur Heart J 1998; 19(suppl. C): C30-C38
143. Odriljn TM, Francis CW, Sporn LA, Bunce LA, Marder VJ, Simpson-Haidaris PJ. Heparin-binding domain of fibrin mediates its binding to endothelial cells. Arterisocl Thromb Vasc Biol 1996; 16: 1544-1551
144. Okahara K, Kambayshi J, Ohnishi T, Fujiwara Y, Monden M. Shear stress induces expression of CNP gene in human endothelial cells. FEBS Lett 1995; 373: 108-110
145. Onho M, Cooke JP, Dzau VJ, Gibbons GH. Fluid shear stress induced endothelial transforming growth factor beta-1 transcription and production: Modulation by potassium channel blockade. J Clin Invest 1995; 95: 1363-1369
146. Ono T, Bergan JJ, Schmid-Schonbein GW, Takase S. Monocyte infiltration into venous valves. J Vasc Surg 1998; 27: 158-166
147. Ploplis VA, Carmeliet P, Vazirzadeh S, van Vlaenderen I, Moons L, Plow EF, Collen D. Effects of disruption of the plasminogen gene on thrombosis, growth, and health in mice. Circulation 1995; 92: 2585-2593
148. Prasad AR, Logan SA, Nerem RM, Schwartz CJ, Sprague EA. Flow-related responses of intracellular inositol phosphate levels in cultured aortic endothelial cells. Circ Res 1993; 72: 822-836
149. Ranjan V, Waterbury R, Xiao ZH, Diamond SL. Fluid shear stress induction of the transcriptional activator c-fos in human and bovine endothelial cells, HeLa, and Chinese hamster ovary cells. Biotech Bioeng 1996; 49: 383-390
150. Rao GN, Berk BC. Active oxygen species stimulate vascular smooth muscle cell growth and proto-oncogene expression. Circ Res 1992; 70: 593-599
151. Resnick N, Collins T, Atkinson W, Bonthron DT, Dewey CF jr., Gimbrone MAjr. Platelet-derived growth factor B chain promoter contains a cis-acting fluid shear stress-responsive element. Proc Natl Acd Sci USA 1993; 90: 4591-4595
152. Rizzi A, Quaglio D, Vasquez G, Mascoli F, Amadesi S, Calo G, Regoli D, Zamboni P. Effects of vasoactive agents in healthy and diseased human saphenous veins. J Vasc Surg 1998; 28:855-861
153. Robert A. Extracellular matrix and vascular pathologies. Role of proteases and oxygenated free radicals. Ann Cardiol Angeiol 1992; 24:A18-23
154. Robetorye RS, Rodgers GM. Update on selected inherited venous thrombotic disorders. Am J Hematol 2001; 68: 256-268
155. Rogerson FM, Chai SY, Schlawe I, Murray WK, Marley PD, Mendelsohn FA. Presence of angiotensin converting enzyme in the adventitia of large blood vessels. J Hypertens 1992; 10: 615-620

156. Roth GJ. Platelets and blood vessels: The adhesion event. Immunol Today 1992; 13: 100-105
157. Rothermund L, Paul M. The role of endothelin in hypertension. Curr Opin Nephrol Hypertens 1998; 7: 451-456
158. Roubos N, Rosenfeldt FL, Richards SM, Conyers RAJ, Davis BB. Improved preservation of saphneous grafts by the use of glyceril trinitrate - verapamil solution during harvesting. Circulation 1995; 92(suppl. II): II31-II36
159. Rubanyi GM, Polokoff MA. Endothelins: Molecular Biology, Biochemistry, Pharmacology, Physiology, and Pathophysiology. Pharm Rev 1994; 46: 328-394
160. Ruggeri Z, Ware J. von Willebrandt factor. FASEB J 1993: 7: 308-312
161. Saharay M, Shields DA, Georgiannos SN, Porter JB, Scurr JH, Coleridge Smith PD. Endothelial activation in patients with chronic venous disease. Eur J Vasc Endovasc Surg 1998; 15: 342-349
162. Savineau JP, Marthan R. Modulation of the calcium sensitivity of the smooth muscle contractile apparatus: molecular mechanisms, pharmacological and pathophysiological implications, Fundam Clin Pharmacol 1997; 11: 289-299
163. Sawdy MS, Loskutoff DJ. Regulation of murine type 1 plasminogen activator inhibitor gene in vivo. Tissue specificity and induction by lypopolysaccharide, tumor necrosis factor-α, and transforming growth factor-β. J Clin Invest 1991; 88: 1346-1342
164. Schafer AI. Vascular endothelium: In defense of blood fluidity. J Clin Invest 1997; 99: 1143-1152
165. Schimada K, Matsushita Y, Wakabayashi K, Takahashi M, Matsubara A, Iijima A, Tanzawa K. Cloning and functional expression of endothelin-converting enzyme cDNA. Biochem Biophys Res Commun 1995; 207: 807-812
166. Schmidt M, Kroger B, Jacob E., Seulberger H, Subkowski T, Otter R, Meyer T, Schmalzing G, Hillen H. Molecular characterization of human and bovine endothelin-converting enzyme (ECE-1). FEBS Lett, 1994; 356: 238-243
167. Schwartz LB, Radic ZS, O'Donohoe MK, Mikat EM, McCann RL, Hagen PO. Saphenous vein endothelium-dependent relaxation in patients with peripheral vascular disease. Ann Vasc Surg 1996; 6:425-432
168. Scott HJ, McMullin GM, Coleridge Smith PD, Scurr JH. A histological study into white blood cells and their association with lipodermatosclerosis and ulceration. Br J Surg 1990; 78: 210-211
169. Seasholtz TM, Majumdar M, Kaplan DD, Brown JH. Rho and Rho kinase mediate thrombin-stimulated vascular smooth muscle cell DNA synthesis and migration. Circ Res 1999; 84: 1186-1193
170. Shen J, Luscinskas FW, Conolly A, Dewey CF jr., Gimbrone MA jr. Fluid shear stress modulates cytosolic free calcium in vascular endothelial cells. Am J Physiol 1992; 262: C384-390
171. Shi Y, O'Brien JE Jr, Mannion JD, Morrison RC, Chung W, Fard A, Zalewski A. Remodeling of autologous saphenous vein grafts: the role of perivascular myofibroblasts. Circulation 1997; 95: 2684-2693
172. Shields DA, Andaz S, Abeysinghe RD, Porter JB, Scurr JH, Coleridge Smith PD. Plasma lactoferrin as a marker of white cell degranulation in venous disease. Phlebology 1994; 9:55-58
173. Shields DA, Andaz SK, Sarin S, Scurr JH, Coleridge Smith PD. Plasma elastase in venous disease. Br J Surg 1994; 81:1496-1499.

174. Shimizu S, Ishii M, Yamamoto T, Kawanishi T, Momose K, Kuroiwa Y. Bradykinin induces generation of reactive oxygen species in bovine aortic endothelial cells. Res Commun Chem Pathol Pharmacol 1994; 84: 301-314
175. Shimokawa H. Primary Endothelial Dysfunction: Atherosclerosis. J Mol Cell Cardiol 1999; 31: 23-37
176. Shireman PK, McCarthy WJ, Pearce WH, Shively VP, Cipollone M, Kwaan HC, Yao JST. Plasminogen activator levels are influenced by location and varicosity in greater saphenous vein. J Vasc Surg 1996; 24: 719-724
177. Simionescu N, Simionescu M. "The cardiovascular system." In *Cell and Tissue. A Textbook of Histology*, 6th edition. Weiss L., ed. Urban and Schwartzenberg, Baltimore and Münich, 1988; 353-401
178. Somlyo AP, Somlyo AV. "Smooth Muscle Structure and Function." In *The Heart and Cardiovascular System. Scientific Foundations*, 2nd edition. Fozzard HA, Haber E, Jennings RB, Katz AM, Morgan HE, ed. Raven Press New York, 1991; 845-864
179. Somlyo AP, Somlyo AV. Signal transduction and regulation in smooth muscle, Nature 1994; 372: 231-236
180. Somlyo AP. Kinases, myosin phosphatases and Rho proteins: curioser and curioser. J Physiol 1999; 516: 630
181. Somlyo AP, Somlyo AV. Signal transduction by G-proteins, Rho-kinase and protein phosphatase to smooth muscle and non-muscle myosin II. J Physiol 2000; 522: 177-185
182. Subramanian VA, Hernandez Ym Tack-Goldman K, Grabowski EF, Weksler BB. Prostacyclin production by internal mammary artery as a factor in coronary artery bypass grafts. Surgery 1986; 100: 376-380
183. Swerlick RA, Garcia-Gonzalez E, Kubota Y, Xu Y, Lawley TJ. Studies of the modulation of MHC antigen and cell adhesion molecule expression on human dermal microvascular endothelial cells. J Invest Dermatol 1991; 97: 190-196
184. Swerlick RA, Lee KH, Wick TM, Lawley TJ. Human dermal microvascular endothelial but not human umbilical vein endothelial cells express CD36 in vivo and in vitro. J Immunol 1992; 148: 78-83
185. Taborek M, Kaiser S. Endothelial cells functions. Relationship to atherogenesis. Basic Res Cardiol 1999; 94: 295-314
186. Thomas PR, Nash GB, Dormandy JA. White cell accumulation in dependent legs of patients with venous hypertension: a possible mechanism for trophic changes in the skin. Br Med J 1988; 27: 1693-1695
187. Timmermanns PB, Wong PC, Chiu AT, Herblin WF, Benfield P, Carini DJ, Lee RJ, Wexler RR, Saye JA, Smith RD. Angiotensin II receptors and angiotensin II receptor antagonists. Pharmacol Rev 1993; 45: 205-251
188. Topper JN, Cai J, Falb D, Gimbrone MA jr. Identification of vascular endothelial genes differentially responsive to fluid mechanical stimuli: cyclooxygenase-2, manganese superoxide dismutase, endothelial cell nitric oxide synthase are selectively up-regulated by steady laminar shear stress. Proc Natl Acad Sci USA 1996; 93: 10417-10422
189. Touyz RM, Schiffrin EL. Signal transduction mechanisms mediating the physiological and pathophysiological actions of angiotensin II in vascular smooth muscle cells. Pharmacol Rev 2000; 52: 639-672
190. Vallance P, Collier J, Moncada S. Nitric oxide synthesized from L-arginine mediates endothelium dependent dilation in human veins in vivo. Cardiovasc Res 1989, 23: 1053-1057
191. Vanhoutte PM. Endothelial dysfunction and atherosclerosis. Eur Heart J. 1997; 18:

E19-29
192. Veraart JC, Verhaegh ME, Neumann HA, Hulsmans RF, Arends JW. Adhesion molecule expression in venous leg ulcers. Vasa 1993; 22: 213-218.
193. Verrier ED, Boyle E. Endothelial cell injury in cardiovascular surgery. Ann Thorac Surg 1996; 62: 915-922
194. Vlot AJ, Koppelman SJ, Bouma BN, Sixma JJ. Factor VIII and von Willebrandt factor. Thromb Haemost 1998; 79: 456-465
195. Walker LA, Gailly P, Jensen PE, Somlyo AV, Somlyo AP. The unimportance of being (protein kinase C) epsilon. FASEB J 1998; 12: 813-821
196. Walsh MP. Regulation of vascular smooth muscle tone. Can J Physiol Pharmacol 1994; 72: 919-936
197. Webb DJ, Benjamin N, Cockcroft JR, Collier JG. Augmentation of sympathetic venoconstriction by angiotensin II in human dorsal hand veins. Am J Hypertens 1989; 2: 721-723
198. Wechezak AR, Wight TN, Viggers RF, Sauvage LR. Endothelial adherence under shear stress is dependent upon microfilament reorganization. J Cell Physiol 1989; 139: 136-146
199. Wilkinson LS, Bunker C, Edwards JC, Scurr JH; Coleridge Smith PD. Leukocytes: their role in the etiopathogenesis of skin damage in venous disease. J Vasc Surg. 1993; 17: 669-675.
200. Wojta J, Hoover RL, Daniel TO. Vascular origin determinates plasminogen activator expression in human endothelial cells. Renal endothelial cells produce large amounts of single chain urokinase type plasminogen activator. J Biol Chem 1989; 264: 2846-2852
201. Woolkanis MJ, De Melfi TN jr., Blanchard N, Hoxie JA, Brass LF. Regulation of thrombin receptors on HUVECs. J Biol Chem 1995; 270: 9686-9692
202. Wu X, Haystead TAJ, Nakamoto HK, Somlyo AV, Somlyo AP. Acceleration of myosin light chain dephosphorylation and relaxation of smooth muscle by telokin. J Biol Chem 1998; 273: 11362-11369
203. Yang JA, He GW. Surgical preparation abolishes endothelium-derived hyperpolarizing factor-mediated hyperpolarization in the human saphenous vein. Ann Thorac Surg 1997; 63: 429-433
204. Yang Z, Lüscher TF. Basic cellular mechanisms of coronary bypass graft disease. Eur Heart J 1993; 14(suppl I): 193-197
205. Yang Z, Ruschitzka F, Rabelink TJ, Noll G, Julmy F, Joch H, Gafner V, Aleksic I, Althaus U, Luscher TF. Different effects of thrombin receptor activation on endothelium and smooth muscle cells of human coronary bypass vessels: implications for venous bypass graft failure. Circulation 1997; 95: 1870-1876
206. Yang ZH, Diederich D, Schneider K, Siebenmann R, Stulz P, von Segesser L, Turina M, Bühler FR, Lüscher TF. Endothelium-derived relaxing factor and protection against contractions induced by histamine and serotonin in the human internal mammary artery and in the saphenous vein. Circulation 1989; 80:1041-1048
207. Yang ZH, Stulz P, von Segesser L., Bauer E, Turina M, Lüscher TF. Different interactions of platelets with arterial and venous coronary bypass vessels. Lancet 1991; 337: 939-943
208. Yang ZH, von Segesser L., Bauer E, Stulz P, Turina M, Lüscher TF. Different activation of the endothelial L-arginine and cyclooxygenase pathway in the human internal mammary artery and saphenous vein, Circ Res 1991; 68:52-60 (abstract)
209. Ziegelstein RC, Cheng L., Capogrossi MC. Flow-dependent cytosolic acidification of vascular endothelial cells. Science 1992; 258: 656-659

CHAPTER 4

REGULATION OF THE VENOUS TONE

TAKE HOME MESSAGES

- **Neural control** of the venous tone is provided by the adrenergic innervation. In some venous territories, a cholinergic innervation, and/or a non-adrenergic non-cholinergic one were identified.
- **Hormones** are also involved in the control of venous tone.

-catecholamines and angiotensin II are most important venoconstrictors.
-the relaxing action of estrogen and progesterone was studied just in some venous territories.
-vasopressin, somatostatin, insulin, and thyroid hormones have actions just in pathophysiologic states.

- **Local control** of venous tone includes: *metabolic regulation*; *humoral control* (which involves vasoconstrictor substances, vasodilator factors and factors with both constrictor and relaxing actions); *ions*; *endothelium-dependent regulation* (venous endothelial cells produce vasodilators – NO, PGI_2 and EDHF – and also vasoconstrictors – ET-1, TxA_2 and PGH_2; veins exhibit a less pronounced endothelium-dependent control and a different response profile to endogenous vasoactive substances than arteries); *other factors* (reactive oxygen species, cytokines, fibrinogen, thrombin, oxidized LDL and vasostatins).
- **Myogenic control** of veins is less important than arterial one.
- Pharmacological agents can modulate venous tone.

4.1. NEURAL CONTROL

4.1.1. Sympathetic Control

The control of venous smooth muscle tone and venous function is dominated by the sympathetic nervous system, its activity being coordinated in the vasomotor center in the brainstem. The degree of adrenergic innervation of the veins varies widely; cutaneous and splachnic veins are most densely innervated, while large conduit veins and the deep limb veins receive only scarce adrenergic innervation (396).

The adrenergic nerve terminals in the venous wall, when activated, release norepinephrine (which in turn binds to the specific adrenergic receptors (predominant α-adrenoceptors) of the venous smooth muscles, causing contraction. The function of the adrenergic nerve terminals in the vein wall is not different from that of sympathetic endings in other vascular tissue. Many adrenergic axons ramify over the adventitial surface of veins and arteries; the terminal axons of these regions present varicosities of 1μm diameter and 2 μm length. The terminal branch of each nervous fiber contain several hundred varicosities, which contain norepinephrine (NE), and cotransmitters, such as ATP, VIP (vasoactive intestinal peptide), CGRP (calcitonin-gene-related peptide) (164, 314), and neuropeptide Y (NPY) (322, 210). In vascular smooth muscle tissues, two synaptic vesicles types were identified: small dense-cores vesicles, which contain NE and ATP and large dense-cored vesicles that contain NE, ATP and neuropeptide (320, 210)

The nerve impulse is propagated along to the terminal at 0.5 m/sec., invades the varicosities, and activates voltage-dependent N-type calcium channels. At the terminal, the impulse speed is about 0.5 μm/sec. and release of neurotransmitter requires Ca^{2+} (210).

4.1.1.1. Neurotransmitters Released by the Sympathetic Nervous Fibers (norepinephrine, ATP, neuropeptide Y, CGRP)

Norepinephrine (NE)

Varicosities contain the enzymatic apparatus necessary for NE biosynthesis, storage and release. NE is synthesized through hydroxylation of tyrosine to desoxyphenylalanine (DOPA), followed by DOPA decarboxylation to dopamine. The final step involves the β-hydroxylation of dopamine to norepinephrine by dopamine β-hydroxylase, present in storage vesicles in adrenergic varicosities. The rate-limiting enzyme in NE synthesis is tyrosine hydroxylase.

NE released from the adrenergic nerve varicosities enters the synaptic cleft and activates the adrenoceptors on the vascular cells.

Finally, several processes remove NE:

- uptake in the nerve endings where part of it is enzymatically degraded by the intraneuronal monoamine oxidase (MAO) to 3,4 dihydroxyphenylglycol (DOPEG), but most of it is recycled to the storage vesicles;
- diffusion to the capillaries;
- uptake by the effector cells and enzymatic degradation by monoamine oxidase (MAO) and catechol-O-methyltransferase (COMT) to inactive metabolites, monohydroxyphenylglycol (MOPEG) and methoxy-4-hydroxymandelic acid (VMA)(396, 415).

The human saphenous vein metabolizes exogenous noradrenaline following a pattern different from that shown to occur in various animal blood vessels. These veins had a relatively low content of noradrenaline, but a high content of deaminated metabolites (DOPEG and dihydroxymandelic acid). In saphenous vein segments incubated with 3H-noradrenaline, the oxidative deamination pathway predominated over the O-methylating one. The deamination process occurred both at neuronal and extraneuronal level. DOPEG was considered a good index of intraneuronal deamination, whereas dihydroxymandelic acid and O-methylated and deaminated metabolites were formed mainly extraneuronally (62).

The adrenergic nerve endings in the venous wall are endowed with presynaptic receptors capable of modulating norepinephrine release:

1. receptors which inhibit NE release (Fig. 4.1.)
   - α_{2A}-adrenergic receptors [human saphenous vein (265)];
   - histamine receptors, H_2 şi H_3 [human saphenous vein, (263)];
   - muscarinic receptors, M_2 [rat portal vein, (325); human saphenous vein (333); human cutaneous veins (395)];
   - receptors for serotonin, 5-HT_{1B} [rat vena cava (162)] and 5-HT_{1D} [human and canine saphenous vein (262)];
   - purinergic receptors [rat portal vein (128, 129)];
   - receptors for NPY (Y_2)[human mesenteric veins, Pernow et al., 1987, quoted by 321];
   - EP_3 receptors for PG E_2 [human saphenous vein (264)];
   - receptors for dopamine (DA)[rat portal vein (283)]

Hydrogen, potassium ions, and increased osmolarity also inhibit norepinephrine release when sympathetic nerves are stimulated (396).

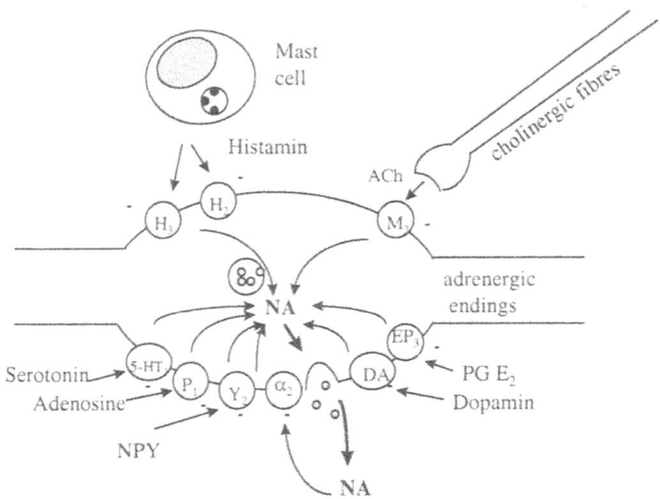

Figure 4.1. Prejunctional receptors, which inhibit noradrenaline (NA) release (with data from the text)

2. receptors which facilitate NE release (Fig. 4.2.):
- β_2 adrenergic receptors [human saphenous vein (395, 401)]
- receptors for angiotensin II [human saphenous vein (261)]

These data concerning the presynaptic receptors involved in the modulation of NE release indicate regional and species-related differences in their distribution.

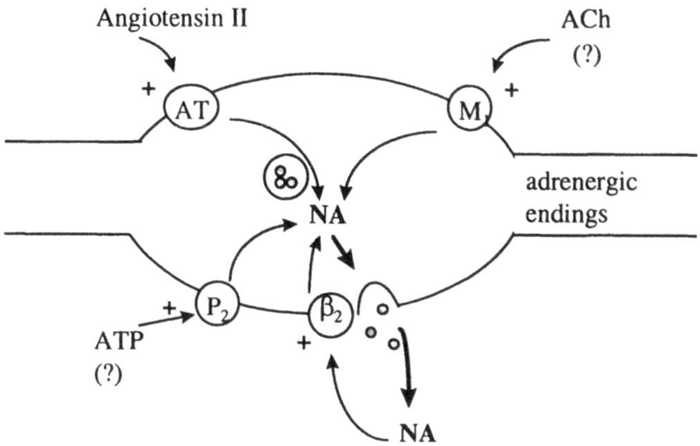

Figure 4.2. Prejunctional receptors, which facilitate noradrenaline (NA) release (with data from the text)

Under physiologic conditions, the depolarization of the membrane induced by a single excitatory junction potential evoked by perivascular nerve stimulation is small and is not always enough to activate voltage-dependent calcium channels. Repetitive excitation of perivascular fibers leads to summation of EXPS, followed by release of neurotransmitters, in amounts that depend on the frequency and number of stimuli. The spike potential evoked by EJPS produces calcium influx and also enables propagation of excitation from one cell to another, because vascular smooth muscle cells are present a functional syncytial structure. (Stjarne et al., 1989, 1990, quoted by 210).

Finally, NE activates post-junctional receptors, mainly α_1 and α_2-adrenergic receptors in vascular smooth muscle cells. Both α-adrenoceptors are important for the control of vascular tone, but neither α_1- nor α_2-adrenoceptors constitute homogeneous groups. Each α-adrenoceptor type can be subdivided into different subtypes.

The present classification of α_1-adrenoceptors stands as follows (79):

- α_{1A}-adrenoceptor subtype (cloned α_{1c} and redesignated $\alpha_{1a/c}$);
- α_{1B}-adrenoceptor subtype (cloned α_{1b});
- α_{1D}-adrenoceptor subtype (cloned α_{1d} and redesignated $\alpha_{1a/d}$).

It seems that the α_{1A}-adrenoceptor subtype is more implicated in the maintenance of vascular basal tone and of arterial blood pressure in conscious animals, and the α_{1B}-adrenoceptor subtype participates more in responses to exogenous agonists (79).

The present classification of α_2-adrenoceptors stands as follows (79):

- $\alpha_{2A/D}$-adrenoceptor subtype (today it is accepted that the α_{2A}-adrenoceptor subtype and the α_{2D} adrenoceptor subtype are the same receptor but they were identified in different species: the α_{2A} in human and the α_{2D} in rat);
- α_{2B}-adrenoceptor subtype (cloned α_{2b});
- α_{2C}-adrenoceptor subtype (cloned α_{2c}).

The $\alpha_{2A/D}$- and α_{2B}-adrenoceptor subtypes are involved in the control of arterial contraction, and that the α_{2C}-adrenoceptor subtype is responsible above all for venous vasoconstriction (79).

Despite the validity of the above-mentioned classification of the α_1- and α_2-adrenoceptors, it seems clear that the contractions of a large number of tissues including human venous smooth muscle are mediated by more than one α-adrenoceptor subtype. The following paragraphs present the subtypes of adrenoceptors identified in several human veins.

There are data indicating that the human saphenous vein possesses both α_1- and α_2-adrenoceptors postjunctionally and, that both contribute to contractile responses (416, 173, 257), but α_2-adrenoceptors are the predominant receptors mediating contraction (117). The α_1-adrenoceptor involved in the vasomotor activity of human saphenous vein has tentatively been associated with the α_{1B} adrenoceptor family subtype (318), but RNA expression for α_{1A}, α_{1B} (337, 166) and α_{1C}-adrenoceptors (114) was found (337, 166). Postjunctional α_2-adrenoceptor of human saphenous vein resembled a α_{2B}-ligand binding site more than a α_{2A}-ligand binding site (363), but recent studies (156) concluded that the functional postjunctional α_2-adrenoceptor mediating contractions of the human saphenous vein closely resembled the human recombinant α_{2C}-adrenoceptor ligand-binding site.

In cutaneous veins, the NE released from adrenergic fibers appears to activate preferentially the post-junctional α_2-adrenoceptors (166).

In human pulmonary vein, in terms of level of mRNA expression for α_1-adrenoceptor subtypes, the ranking order was: $\alpha_{1A}>\alpha_{1B}>\alpha_{1D}$ (337).

Some venous territories also contain post-junctional β-receptors, mediating venodilation: human facial vein (250) and human saphenous vein (β_1,β_2)(140).

ATP

There are studies which proved that ATP is a sympathetic cotransmitter in human veins, such as ovarian or saphenous veins (372, 339). The ATP released from the vesicles in the sympathetic nerve terminals acts locally and probably only post-junctional, being rapidly hydrolyzed by ecto-ATP-ase (life-time less than 100 msec). ATP induces a transient inward current via ligand-gated channels, which produces excitatory junctional potentials, action potentials and a phasic contraction of the effector tissue. It has been assumed that this ATPase activity is due to membrane bound ecto-ATPases on the surface of the effector tissue, however, the recently identified soluble ATPase released during nerve stimulation could also be involved in inactivation of ATP. The relative importance of ecto-ATPase and the releasable ATPase is yet to be determined (364).

ATP induces both vasoconstriction and vasodilation in the vessels from many arterial and venous branches.

Neuronally released ATP is involved in the contractile response of cutaneous vein exposure to cold (144) and has been shown to exert a trophic action on venous myocytes (4). The P_{2X} receptors are responsible for the vasoconstrictor response produced as a consequence of the release of ATP from sympathetic perivascular nerves, while P_{2Y}-purinoceptors may be implicated in mediating the relaxing response to ATP after its release as a cotransmitter with norepinephrine. The subclassification of P_2 receptors has advanced dramatically in the past few years due to the use of molecular biology methods allowing the cloning and expression of 14 different subclasses of P_2 receptors, seven P_{2X} and seven P_{2Y} (364). Various purinoceptors subtypes were identified in human venous preparations.

For instance, Cario-Toumaniantz et al (1998) showed that in human saphenous vein myocytes both hP_{2X1} and hP_{2X7} receptors are expressed as 2 separated populations of channels and are involved in ATP-induced tension. Moreover, cell lysis consequent to hP_{2X7} receptor-induced pore formation might contribute to the disorganization and decrease in the amount of contractile myocytes in the media of varicose veins (72).

Racchi et al. (1999) investigated human saphenous veins in order to assess the cooperative participation of ATP, NPY, and noradrenaline in the vasomotor responses elicited following electrical depolarization of the perivascular nerve terminals. Their results supported the physiological role of ATP in sympathetic neurotransmission and the involvement of human sympathetic vasomotor reflexes in the coordinated motor action of ATP, NPY, and NE acting on vascular smooth muscle cells (318).

Neuropeptide Y (NPY)

The colocalization and corelease of NPY with NE was demonstrated in the sympathetic fibers from several venous territories, including human mesenteric, saphenous, and uterine veins (386, 228).

Receptors for NPY were classified into Y_1 and Y_2 subtypes (Michel, 1991 quoted by 210, 150). Y_1 receptor is located mainly post-junctional, being involved in vasoconstriction and potentiation of norepinephrine-induced contraction; Y_2 receptor was detected at pre- and post-junctional sites and it seems to mediate the pre-junctional inhibition of norepinephrine release. For instance, in human saphenous vein, NPY elicited a prolonged contraction, reaching its maximum plateau after 20 minutes after each dose (228).

Studies concerning the actions of NPY in relation to endothelium are controversial: endothelium removal was followed by an increase (315), a decrease of NPY-induced vasoconstriction (106) or was not influenced by this maneuver (308).

Moreover NPY seems to have a mitogenic effect, mediated by Y_1 receptors, and thus may be considered as a sympathetic trophic agent involved in vascular hypertrophy (438).

Calcitonin gene-related peptide (CGRP)

There are studies, which reported that CGRP is contained in both adrenergic and NANC fibers distributed to different components of the cardiovascular system. (314, 36). The actions exerted by CGRP were detailed in paragraph 4.3.

4.1.2. Cholinergic Innervation

Immunohistochemical, biochemical and functional studies have revealed two separate cholinergic systems in the vascular wall:

- *Endothelial cells* represent the ubiquitous *intrinsic, intimal system*; they contain the acetylcholine-synthesizing enzyme, choline acetyltransferase, release a choline ester, and contain functional muscarinic receptors. The intimal system serves as a general regulator of basal vascular tone and wall structure responding to local, luminal stimuli (209).
- *Perivascular autonomic nerve fibers* represent the *extrinsic, adventitial system.* These axons are not ubiquitous but show a highly selective distribution among and even within organs, and utilize co-mediators

(NO, neuropeptides) in an organ-specific pattern. The perivascular nerve fibers act on top of this basal tone by providing fine-tuning in response to reflex activation due to systemic demands (209).

Most vascular tissues are innervated mainly by adrenergic fibers, but there are studies that reported the existence of a cholinergic innervation of several arteries (199) and veins. Yoshioka et al. (1988) and Tsuru et al. (1994) demonstrated evidence for an excitatory cholinergic innervation in canine portal vein and in rabbit portal vein (431, 389). In vivo electrical stimulation of the greater splachnic nerves in the dog produced an elevation of the pressure in the vena cava that was completely blocked by atropine, suggesting the presence of a cholinergic innervation in this region (280).

More recently Walch et al. (1997) treated the pulmonary vessels with cholinesterase (ChE) inhibitors to determine the role of these enzymes in the regulation of vascular tone. In human pulmonary veins, the ChE activity was two fold greater than in arteries, but a role for ChE activity in the control of venous tone was difficult to observe, even though this tissue contained a greater amount of enzyme than the artery. Moreover, experimental data showed the absence of sufficient spontaneous release of ACh to modulate human pulmonary vessel basal tone (404).

Acetylcholine (ACh) can contract and relax vascular tissue, vasodilation being endothelium-dependent. Generally, muscarinic M_3 receptors mediate endothelium-dependent vasodilation (enhancing the release of NO, EDHF or other relaxing agents), whereas contraction is mediate via several subtypes. Vascular smooth muscle relaxation may also be mediated by endothelium-independent mechanisms, depending upon species and anatomical location of the vessel (123, 74). For instance, M_1 receptors are involved in the mediation of ACh-induced relaxation of human pulmonary veins (404). Acetylcholine-induced contraction is thought to involve coupling of the muscarinic receptor, via a G protein, to a phosphoinositide-specific PLC, inducing formation of IP_3 and DAG. Another mechanism, which might explain vascular smooth muscle contraction, involves inhibition of adenylyl cyclase activity, via a pertussis toxin-sensitive G protein (123).

Interesting aspects concerning ACh effects on pulmonary veins were reported. For instance, the ability of ACh to induce pulmonary vasoconstriction was found to be species dependent. In vessels derived from sheep lung, ACh induced contractions in veins but not in arteries whereas in human pulmonary vessels the reverse was observed (406). To characterize the muscarinic receptors on human pulmonary veins associated with the acetylcholine-induced relaxation, isolated venous preparations were pre-contracted with noradrenaline and were subsequently challenged with ACh in the absence or presence of selective muscarinic antagonists: pirenzepine (M_1), darifenacin (M_3), himbacine (M_2, M_4), methoctramine (M_2) and pFHHSiD (M_1, M_3). All agents inhibited ACh-induced relaxations in venous preparations, but the pK(B) values obtained for these antagonists were not those predicted for the involvement of $M_{2\text{-}5}$ receptors in the ACh-induced relaxation in human pulmonary veins, suggesting that the relaxations induced by ACh are due to the activation of M_1 receptors on endothelial cells in isolated human pulmonary veins.

4.1.3. Non-Adrenergic Non-Cholinergic Innervation (NANC)

Several studies reported a distribution of a non-adrenergic non-cholinergic innervation in vascular tissues, including veins. ATP, VIP, CGRP, and more recently NO were designed as neurotransmitters released by these NANC fibers (Table 4.I).

Table. 4.I. Human venous tissues in which NANC innervation was reported.

Human venous tissue	NANC neurotransmitters	References
cutaneous veins	ATP	72
pulmonary veins	ATP	437
deep dorsal penile vein	NPY, VIP, dopamine	102
cortical, cerebral veins	substance P	279
uterine veins	NO	384
inferior vena cava, renal veins, femoral veins	CGRP	36
saphenous vein	CGRP	182

A coarse network of VIP-immunoreactive nerve fibers was reported in some venous territories, including human veins. A great density of nerves supplying the deep dorsal penile vein and vasa vasorum were neuropeptide Y-immunoreactive nerves followed by vasoactive intestinal polypeptide- and dopamine beta-hydroxylase-immunoreactive nerves (102).

In human cutaneous veins where purinergic neurotransmission is more prominent compared with in deep vessels, physiological and pathological roles of nerve-released ATP have been described. Neuronally released ATP has been reported to act through activation of unidentified ionotropic P_{2X} receptors. In human saphenous vein smooth muscle, both hP_{2X1} and hP_{2X7} receptors are expressed as two separated populations of channels in human saphenous vein myocytes and are involved in ATP-induced tension (72).

Purinergic neurotransmission was also reported to take part in the regulation of pulmonary circulation. Semi-quantitation of the autoradiographs (performed by using [3H] alpha, beta-methylene ATP ([3H] alpha, beta-MeATP) as the radioligand) revealed significant differences in the densities of P_{2X}-purinoceptors among the pulmonary vessels studied, the veins being sparsely labeled and only in the media (437).

The use of monoclonal antibodies allowed the identification of NOS in perivascular nerve endings, forming the so-called "nitroxidergic innervation". An involvement of nitroxidergic nerves in the relaxation of dog and monkey temporal veins, was reported by Toda et al. (385). Human uterine veins are also innervated by vasodilator nerves from which NO is liberated as a vasodilator neurotransmitter (384).

An abundantly vasodilatory innervation releasing substance P was identified in the venous cerebral territory (cortical veins, deep cerebral veins, dural sinuses)(279). Substance P also dilated human pial veins, superficial hand veins and omental veins precontracted with either norepinephrine or prostaglandin $F_{2\alpha}$ (121, 244, 386).

CGRP-immunoreactive nerve fibers are distributed widely in the cardiovascular system and generally are more numerous around arteries and veins and human blood vessels display a lower density than those of other mammalian vascular territories. Varicose and smooth CGRP-immunoreactive nerve fibers were seen at the junction of the adventitia and the media, passing into the muscle layer. A high-density CGRP-innervation, occurring as a dense varicose mesh with occasional penetrating branches, was found in the inferior vena cava, and in renal and femoral veins (36). A peptidergic innervation mainly localized along the vasa vasorum and associated with immunoreactivity of substance P and CGRP was found which yields evidence for a mechanosensory innervation of human greater saphenous vein (182).

Vasorelaxation in response to CGRP was demonstrated in several human blood vessels in vitro, including veins: omental veins (121), pulmonary veins (243), intracerebral venules (122). CGRP was found to be a potent vasodilator of precontracted human epicardial coronary veins in vitro (343). The potency of the vasorelaxant effect of CGRP, and the requirement of this action of intact endothelium presents a marked regional variation. For instance, CGRP induced endothelium-independent vasodilation in human pulmonary arteries and veins (243) and in human saphenous veins (228). At present, there is no consensus regarding the involvement of NO and cGMP in the endothelium-dependent CGRP-induced vasodilation, but the synthesis and release of prostacyclin in response to CGRP was demonstrated in endothelial cells from human umbilical veins (101).

CGRP also promotes the proliferation of endothelial cells from human umbilical veins (168).

4.2. HORMONES AND VENOUS TONE

4.2.1. Catecholamines

Catecholamines, as circulating hormones, are synthesized and released from the chromaffin cells of the adrenal medulla in response to emotion or stress; the most important catecholamine secreted is epinephrine. The biosynthetic pathway is similar to that described in adrenergic nerve varicosities. Epinephrine contained within the secretory vesicles of pheochromocytes is released in response to acetylcholine liberated by preganglionic nerve fibers that terminate in the medulla; most of epinephrine is carried away acting upon distant target tissues or is metabolized by catechol-O-methyltransferase (396, 415).

In vascular tissues, α and β-adrenoceptors are not located close to each other, explaining the differences in case of stimulation by a high concentration of circulating adrenaline or in case of a noradrenaline release from the sympathetic nerve fibers. This contributes to the different sensitivity of various vessels to sympathomimetic amines; some of them being under control of circulating catecholamines, whereas others are not (166). In arteries, experimental data indicated that α_1-receptors are situated in the vicinity of sympathetic nerve terminals, strategically located to be activated by noradrenaline released by nerve endings, whereas α_2-adrenoceptors are placed extrajunctionally, being activated preferentially by circulating adrenaline. In contrast to arteries, veins seem to present α_2-adrenoceptors closer to sympathetic nerve terminals than α_1-adrenoceptors (211, 169, 145). Similar differences were noted for β-adrenoceptors: β_1-adrenoceptors, that are stimulated by noradrenaline are located near the nerve endings, while β_2-adrenoceptors that are insensitive to noradrenaline and function as receptors for circulating adrenaline are situated outside of neuronal influence. Results on veins, indicated that in these vessels, β_2 subtype are close to the nerve terminals and β_1-adrenoceptors are scarce or not present, since adrenaline caused relaxation, whereas noradrenaline did not (67, Guimaraes and Paiva, 1981, quoted by 166).

It is now widely accepted that α_2- and β-adrenoceptors exist on endothelial cells and contribute to the regulation of vasomotor tone. In several veins, adrenergic agonists caused relaxation that was inhibited by selective α_2-adrenoceptor antagonists and was eliminated by endothelium removal (256); it was demonstrated that activation of endothelial α_2-adrenoceptors stimulates the release of NO. However, in human hand veins, Haefeli et al. (1993) found no evidence for endothelial α_2-adrenoceptor-mediated release of EDRF/NO (167).

The presence of β-adrenoceptors was confirmed by autoradiography in the endothelium of human saphenous vein (266), and by biochemical analysis in cultured human umbilical vein endothelial cells (141). This latter study, together with an in vivo study performed on forearm circulation (111) showed that endothelial β-adrenoceptors is totally or at least predominantly of the β_2-subtype. Moreover, after L-NAME treatment or endothelium removal, propranolol had no influence on isoprenaline-induced vasodilation, suggesting that this effect was mediated by β_3- and/or low-affinity state of β_1-adrenoceptors, formerly proposed as putative β_4-adrenoceptors (63).

Vascular adrenergic mechanisms are influenced by aging and temperature. Docherty (1994) demonstrated an age-related decrease in α_2-adrenoceptor-mediated contractile responsiveness in the human saphenous vein (116).

Aging was also associated with a decline in beta-adrenergic responsiveness in human dorsal hand vein (isoprenaline-induced venodilation was significantly lower in elderly than in young subjects)(149). The decreased effect of beta-adrenoceptor agonists (such as, isoproterenol) in human hand vein might be caused by reduced production of cyclic AMP in elderly subjects (172). Cooling (from 37° C to 24° C) augmented saphenous vein reactivity to norepinephrine by an apparent increase in the responsiveness of α_2-adrenoceptors to agonists. The relationship between temperature and adrenoceptor responsiveness may be of pivotal importance in defining the mechanism of cold-induced vasospasm (173, 174). Another study (91) indicated that human saphenous vein contractility to a partial α_1-adrenoceptor agonist increased when the temperature was raised, a response that contrasted to that noted with full α_1- and α_2-adrenoceptor agonists. This observation could be of importance for the treatment of the symptoms of venous insufficiency, favored during warm days.

In some pathological states, veins seem more or less responsive to α-agonists. For instance:

- The saphenous vein from hypertensive patients is less distensible, slower to relax, and more reactive to norepinephrine, these differences being probably involved in the reduced patency of this graft (258).
- A significant reduction in norepinephrine-induced contractile activity was reported in varicose veins, extending previous observations regarding the impairment of smooth muscle contractility in primary chronic venous insufficiency (382, 222, 330, 257).
- Alterations in smooth muscle responsiveness to norepinephrine was also noted in human vein grafts explanted from the arterial circulation (mean duration between grafting and revision was 16 months): norepinephrine produced endothelium-independent and dose-dependent contractions in both human saphenous grafts and normal saphenous veins, but maximal contractions were significantly reduced in venous grafts compared to controls (305). These experimental data suggested that increased wall tension in grafted segments might be responsible for attenuation of venous smooth muscle contraction.

The possibility for genetic variability in venous responsiveness was also explored. Studies performed in twins showed that interindividual variability in venous responsiveness of superficial hand veins to locally infused norepinephrine was much smaller between monozygotic twins than between dizygotic twins or unrelated subjects (226, 227). Using dorsal hand vein technique, differences in venoreactivity of healthy White and Latin Americans were studied (391). A significant difference in venous responsiveness between two groups was noted. Latin Americans had less maximal venoconstrictive response to the α_1-adrenergic agonist, phenylephrine, and required a greater infusion rate of isoproterenol (β_2-

adrenergic agonist) to produce half maximal response. These results suggested that normotensive Latin Americans may have different peripheral vascular responsiveness to adrenergic agonists, explaining why factors that usually predispose to hypertension development in White subjects are not as predominate in the Latin American population (380). A similar study was performed by Eichler et al. (1990), who showed that responsiveness of superficial hand veins to phenylephrine was significantly greater in White normotensive subjects, compared to that of Black normotensive males (125).

4.2.2. Angiotensins

Traditionally, the renin-angiotensin system (RAS) has been viewed as an endocrine system, which plays an important role in the regulation of blood pressure and fluid homeostasis. According to the classical concept, liver-derived angiotensinogen is cleaved by renin produced by the kidneys, forming angiotensin I. Then, angiotensin I is converted by angiotensin-converting enzyme (ACE) in the lungs, to angiotensin II, one of the most potent vasoconstrictors and a stimulant of aldosterone release. Finally, angiotensin II is degraded by aminopeptidases to angiotensin III and IV (134).

All components of the RAS, except renin, were demonstrated to be produced in several tissues, including vessel wall (108):

- Angiotensinogen mRNA and protein was identified in vascular smooth muscle, endothelium, and perivascular fat;
- ACE was found in the adventitia, endothelial cells and vascular smooth muscle cells in culture.

These data indicate the existence of a so-called local or tissue renin-angiotensin system. Whereas the circulating renin-angiotensin system is considered to provide short-term cardiorenal homeostasis, the tissue system is believed to provide local tonic control of vascular resistance and influence tissue specific functions. For instance, in human forearm, in situ generation of angiotensin II seems more important for vasoconstriction than circulating angiotensin II (344).

In addition to ACE-dependent pathway, a chymase (chymotripsin-like serine protease) pathway was also demonstrated in human vascular tissue (58).

Angiotensin II, the principal effector of renin-angiotensin cascade exerts two types of effects: vasoconstriction and aldosterone release, which occur in seconds or minutes, and slower responses, which take days or weeks, and include vascular growth, ventricular hypertrophy, and the pressor effect at very low doses. These last effects are likely to be more important in the pathogenesis of some cardiovascular diseases (108, 120, 134, 159, 387).

The synthesis and actions of angiotensins in venous tissue are presented in chapter 4.3.2.

4.2.3. Estrogen and Progesterone

4.2.3.1. Estrogens

The beneficial actions of **estrogens** on vascular integrity include (148):

- decrease of vascular tone,
- cytoprotective action on the arterial wall,
- increase of HDL cholesterol, together with a decrease of LDL cholesterol
- inhibition of LDL-oxidation,
- decrease of plasminogen and fibrinogen levels.

Estrogen activates two types of receptors, named two types of nuclear receptors, named ERα and ERβ. The genes for these receptors are located on different chromosomes. Both receptors form homo- and heterodimers with each other, which have been shown to be active in experimental systems, considerably enhancing the variety and function al expression of estrogen. There are differences in tissue distribution of ERα and ERβ receptors, and also in binding affinities of the different estrogens to these two receptors (148).

Estrogens have quantitatively different vascular effects on different tissues, depending on species and experimental preparations, but its major effect is vasodilation. The relative roles of ERα and β in mediating relaxation of blood vessels are still to be clarified.

Some of the vasodilatory actions of estrogens in pharmacologic doses might be direct and rapid (non-genomic effects). The relaxing effect of estrogen might be caused by:

- increased synthesis of endothelium-dependent relaxing factors (NO, PGI_2, EDHF or others)(148). However, conjugated estrogens significantly reduced greater saphenous vein endothelial prostacyclin production in a group receiving four daily infusions of conjugated estrogens compared to control subjects (190). Recent studies showed that in human umbilical veins, 17β-estradiol activated MAP kinase as well as GMPc synthesis and NO release, and that these effects could be triggered with membrane-impermeant forms of 17β-estradiol; these actions could be blocked by ER antagonist ICI-182, 780 (341).

- decreased production of vasoconstrictor factors, such as endothelin (295) or superoxide anion (16).
- decreased calcium entry into vascular smooth muscle cells by activation of both receptor-operated and voltage-dependent calcium channels (89). Farhat et al (1996) suggested an involvement of membrane specific binding proteins, because 17β-estradiol rapidly increased cAMP level in pulmonary vascular smooth muscle cells (135).
- decreased α-adrenergic responsiveness in venous smooth muscle cells, thereby decreasing venous tone and contributing to the pathogenesis of varicosities. Nevertheless, an in vivo study performed by Jilma et al. (1994) showed that one administration of estradiol valerate had no significant effect on α-adrenergic responsiveness on the smooth muscle of human hand veins, assessed by venous compliance (197).

Calcagno et al. (1992) reported that the effects of estrogen on veins differs from those reported in arteries, and these differences were seen both in vitro in veins taken from their normal location and in vivo in veins placed in the arterial circulation. For instance, 17 beta-estradiol did not significantly alter thymidine uptake in vitro in segments from human saphenous veins (70).

An enhancement of venous compliance after ingestion of oral estrogen-containing contraceptives and occurrence of varicose veins as an adverse reaction to these contraceptives were also reported (160, 83).

Table 4.11. Human venous territories in which receptors for sex hormones were identified

Human veins	Receptors	References
Uterine veins	ER	39
Saphenous veins	ER	201
	ER, PR	311, 312, 239
Placental veins	PR	292

Legend: ER = estrogen receptors; PR = progesterone receptors

Pathophysiology

Varicose veins

Clinical and epidemiological observations regarding varicose veins, such as their predominance in women and the occurrence of venous stasis during sex-hormone therapy, the luteal phase of the menstrual cycle, and pregnancy, suggested a sex hormone-dependency of this venous pathology.

Bergqvist et al. (1993) showed low estrogen and progesterone receptor level in all arterial and vein samples with no statistical difference between fertile and post menopausal women. Estrogen receptors were found in all peripheral vein samples from fertile women but not in all samples from post-menopausal women and men. There were significant differences with higher levels of estrogen receptors in cytosol and nuclear fraction, in uterine veins from fertile women compared to peripheral veins from fertile women, post-menopausal women and men, respectively. These data suggested that the hormonal regulation of peripheral vein walls is different than that of uterine veins (39).

Several studies concerning the expression of estrogen receptors in human saphenous veins smooth muscle were performed:

- Karas et al. (1994, 1995) demonstrated that human saphenous vein vascular smooth muscle cells express estrogen-receptor mRNA and protein and that this receptor is capable of estrogen-dependent gene activation, suggesting a direct mechanism of estrogen on vascular smooth muscle cells. In addition to the classical estrogen receptor, human VSM cells also expressed an estrogen receptor isoform containing an in-frame deletion of Exon 4 (ER delta 4)(201, 202).
- Contrary results were reported in varicose veins. In varicose saphenous veins removed from both men and pre- or post-menopausal women no estrogen receptors (ER) or extremely low levels of ER were detected (by EIA and RT-PCR) (311, 312). By staining with anti-estrogen receptor antibodies, Mashiah et al. (1999) detected ER in the nuclear regions of the intima and media in females and males, while in the adventitia they were found only in nuclei of the vasa vasorum. Estrogen receptor levels were lower in non-varicose segments of varicose veins compared with normal veins. In varicose segments, estrogen receptors were more abundant than in the non-varicose parts of the same vein, especially in females, suggesting an involvement of estrogens in varicosis development. These differences could be ascribed to the different number of patients, their age, the pathological status of the veins, and also to culture conditions, which might have altered the phenotype of smooth muscle cells (239).

- Immunohistochemical, radioligand binding, Western immunoblotting and RT-PCR studies of isolated human umbilical vein endothelial and human umbilical vein smooth muscle cells failed to detect the classic estrogen receptor α and estrogen receptor β isoforms (23).

4.2.3.2. Progesterone

Physiological venous changes related to **progesterone** have been described on the basis of hormonal status, such as venous stasis during luteal phase or pregnancy. Consequently, these steroid hormones may directly modulate venous blood flow. For instance, the existence of PR staining in smooth muscle cells of spiral arteries in early pregnancy correlates with large increases in endometrial and myometrial blood flow that occur in order to support fetal growth and homeostasis (310).

Several studies reported the existence of progesterone receptors in various venous tissues and progesterone effects on venous tone:

- In human placental veins progesterone produced a dose-dependent relaxation. The relaxation was endothelium-independent and seemed to be mediated by a receptor-activated cAMP mechanism. The relaxing action of progesterone could be physiologically important in maintaining low resistance and adequate blood flow in the placental circulation (292).
- The presence of progesterone receptors was investigated in the walls of normal and varicose veins by various methods (immunoassay and immunocytochemistry). PR staining was observed in the cell nuclei of the tunica media and the subendothelial layer (neointima), with no significant variation in the PR content of different regions within the same saphenous vein. PR was also detected by RT-PCR in biopsy samples. This observation suggested that progesterone acts directly on these veins via a classic receptor-mediated pathway (311, 312). Progesterone receptor levels were higher in varicose segments compared to non-varicose portions of the same vein and in these non-varicose parts were higher in females (239). The presence of PR in the media of saphenous veins suggests that progesterone may influence venous structure and/or function. In vitro experimental studies showed that progesterone induced the decrease of noradrenaline and calcium-induced contractions in isolated human saphenous veins (309).

4.2.4. Other Hormones (vasopressin, somatostatin, insulin, thyroid hormones)

4.2.4.1. Vasopressin

The effects of vasopressin might attain significance in physiologic or pathophysiologic states characterized by an increased plasmatic level of the peptide, such as dehydration, exercise, and hypertension, and congestive heart failure.

Vasopressin induced vasoconstriction in some, but not all venous territories. The venoconstrictor effect was reported in human chorionic plate vein (231) and human saphenous vein (5). The constrictor action of vasopressin seems to be lower in veins, compared to arterial preparations, probably due to a low population or sensitivity of receptors sites for this peptide (238, 5). Collier et al. (1972) found no constrictor effect after the local infusion of vasopressin into superficial hand veins (85).

In human saphenous vein, the V_1 receptor seems to mediate the contractile response of this peptide; after V_1-receptor blockade, vasopressin produced an endothelium-dependent relaxation of venous preparations. The relaxing effect was independent of V_2-receptor stimulation of NO formation, but was inhibited by indomethacin, suggesting the release of vasodilator prostaglandins from the endothelial cells in response to vasopressin (5).

In vivo studies showed have shown that the effects of vasopressin on human forearm blood flow, as measured by venous occlusion pletismography, are biphasic. Lower doses of vasopressin caused vasoconstriction, while the administration of higher doses was followed by vasodilation (377).

4.2.4.2. Somatostatin

Somatostatin presents both venoconstrictor and venodilator actions.

- The contractile effect of somatostatin was noted in human preparations such as mesenteric veins (386), hand veins (304), and saphenous veins (228). In human hand veins, somatostatin also augmented the contractions induced by norepinephrine, epinephrine and dopamine (304).
- The dilator effect of somatostatin was reported in the venous portal tree. The decrease of portal venous inflow and portal pressure induced

somatostatin may be used in the pharmacological treatment of portal hypertension. A combination of somatostatin, vasopressin, and nitroglycerin seems to be very effective in patients with portal hypertension (329, 68).

The presence of somatostatin receptors in human blood vessels was also investigated. Human blood vessels, normal veins and arteries, expressed high levels of somatostatin receptor 1 (SSTR-1) with significantly lower levels of SSTR-2 and -4. Immunocytochemical studies demonstrated that SSTR-1 was present in endothelial but not vascular smooth muscle cells. The levels of SSTR-1 varied between individuals, indicating that a vascular disease process may have affected SSTR gene expression (105).

Human umbilical vein endothelial cells exposed to 10 nM somatostatin or 10 nM SSTR-1-specific agonist presented alterations of actin cytoskeleton, as characterized by a loss of actin stress fibers coupled with an increase in lamellipodia formation at the plasma membrane. These results might explain the lack of effectiveness of angiopeptin (a somatostatin analog) in inhibiting intimal hyperplasia in humans by the differential expression of SSTR-1 in human endothelial cells (105). Another somatostatin analog octreotide was an effective inhibitor of the proliferation of human umbilical vein endothelial cells (107).

The use of a range of somatostatin analogues allowed the characterization of the receptor-mediating contraction of the human saphenous vein. Their contractile responses suggested that in human saphenous vein the recombinant somatostatin receptor 2 (SST2) mediated somatostatin venoconstriction. The receptor transduction mechanism seemed to involve activation of L-type calcium channels and entry of extracellular calcium (115).

Somatostatin receptors were detected by quantitative receptor autoradiography in peritumoral veins of various human cancer tissue specimens (colonic adenocarcinomas, carcinoids, renal-cell carcinomas malignant lymphomas). In all cases, the somatostatin receptors were localized in the venous smooth-muscle cell layer, exhibiting specific and high-affinity binding of somatostatin-14, somatostatin-28 and octreotide, and suggesting a preferential expression of the SSTR2 receptor subtype. Since the vessels of normal non-neoplastic human tissues have few somatostatin receptors, the increased somatostatin receptor expression in peritumoral vessels suggested that somatostatin and somatostatin receptors may play a regulatory role for hemodynamic tumor-host interactions, possibly involving tumor stroma generation, tumor environment, angiogenesis and, particularly, vascular drainage of poorly differentiated neoplasms (326).

4.2.4.3. Insulin

Recent experimental studies indicate that insulin plays a role in the regulation of vascular tone in human vessels, including venous tone. It has been observed that insulin attenuates vasoconstrictor responses to pressor agonists and increases the vasorelaxing effect in precontracted arteries, this action being endothelium-dependent. Controversy persists about the mechanisms of insulin-induced vasodilation; among these possible mechanisms are:

- decreased vascular sensitivity to α-adrenergic agonists and an enhanced sensitivity to β-adrenoceptor agonists (100);
- stimulation of nitric oxide release from endothelial cells (371, 345);
- activation of ATP-dependent potassium channels (246, 196).

There are also proofs for long term insulin actions in vascular smooth muscle cells, such as increase of Na^+-K^+-ATP-ase and Na^+-Ca^{2+} exchanger (383; Smith and Smith, 1994, quoted by 300).

The presence of specific receptors for insulin on human arterial as well as human venous endothelial cells was reported; the concentration of insulin receptors varied among endothelial cells derived from different vascular sources, the number of binding sites in veins being lower than in arteries (25, 259).

In endothelial cells, the effect of insulin is not limited to the influence upon NO synthesis. Insulin also stimulated the production and secretion of ET-1 in cultured endothelial cells, but hyperinsulinemia was not associated with increased plasma ET-1 levels in healthy men in vivo (189, 251).

There are a few studies regarding the direct action of insulin on human venous smooth muscle as well as the influence of diabetes upon venous reactivity.

Insulin and insulin-like growth factor-I (IGF-I) are endogenous peptides with vasoactive activities. Their vasodilatory effects on human vessels (internal mammary artery and saphenous vein) taken from patients with and without noninsulin-dependent diabetes mellitus were studied. In both groups, insulin and IGF-I evoked greater relaxation in arterial rings than they did in saphenous-vein rings. The relaxing effect was not affected by the removal of the endothelium and by inhibition of the production of nitric oxide, but was completely abolished by KCl, and was attenuated by the nonspecific potassium-channel blocker tetraethylammonium. These data suggested that both insulin and IGF-I induced endothelial-independent, nitric oxide-independent vasorelaxation of human saphenous veins, through a mechanism involving activation of potassium channels, with no significant differences between vessels from patients with and without non-insulin-dependent diabetes mellitus (196). A high-affinity IGF-I binding sites in the wall of saphenous vein was also reported, indicating that insulin-like growth factor-I plays an important role in regulating the proliferation of venous wall cellular components, an essential step in the process of venous intimal hyperplasia (357).

In human hand veins, insulin caused a dose-dependent dilation of preconstricted veins, and this effect was impaired in hypertensive patients (137).

Several research teams reported the influence of diabetes upon venous reactivity:

- The effect of diabetes on the vasodilator responses and ultrastructure of saphenous vein harvested from patients undergoing infrainguinal bypass surgery for limb salvage and the development of stenosis within the vein grafts was studied by Hicks et al. (1997). Endothelium-dependent relaxation by NO pathways stimulated after bradykinin and thrombin addition was not different in vein rings from diabetic and nondiabetic patients, while fibrinogen-mediated vasorelaxation was negligible in vein from diabetic patients. These data suggested that diabetes is not a risk factor for early (12 months) infrainguinal vein graft stenosis (184).
- In non-insulin-dependent diabetes mellitus, a deficit in the vasorelaxant activity of endothelium, leading to an increase in contractility of human saphenous vein, was reported by Karasu et al. (1995)(203).
- In human placental arteries and veins, gestational diabetes produced an enhancement of hypoxia-induced relaxation and an increase of the contraction caused by reoxygenation or micromolar concentrations of hydrogen peroxide (143).
- Blochl-Daum et al. (1992) speculated that disease states like diabetes, that are associated with endothelium dysfunction, might facilitate the access of endothelin to vascular smooth muscle, causing increased vasoconstriction (50). However, their study, carried out in patients with type 2 diabetes found no such change. Other studies reported an increased response of human hand veins to noradrenaline in insulin-dependent diabetics with microalbuminuria, as well as in diabetic patients with autonomic neuropathy (54, 126).

4.2.4.4. Thyroid Hormones

Thyroid hormone (3,5,3'-triiodo-L-thyronine), which might be used as a positive inotrope and vasodilator for patients undergoing cardiac surgery, produced dose-dependent relaxation of human saphenous vein rings preconstricted with potassium or phenylephrine. The relaxing effect was noted only in case of supraphysiological and suprapharmacological concentrations, whereas triiodothyronine had no vasomotor effect in clinically relevant concentrations. In vivo, triiodothyronine administration had little direct effect on the tone of human vascular smooth muscle (208).

4.3. LOCAL CONTROL

The local control of veins has been much less extensively studied than that of arteries. In vitro studies have been performed mostly on large veins, the extrapolation of these data to venous microvessels remains to be confirmed. However, the contractility of large veins seems to be less sensitive to local metabolic factors compared with the smaller ones.

Some veins were more studied than others: hand veins, pulmonary veins, saphenous veins and umbilical veins. In addition, human umbilical vein endothelial cells (HUVEC) culture is one of the most used models in the research of endothelial functions and its interactions with leukocytes and platelets.

4.3.1. Metabolic Control

4.3.1.1. PO_2

PO_2 represents an important factor in local metabolic regulation of vascular tone, including venous one. The effects induced by PO_2 changes are conditioned by the degree and duration of the hypoxia or hyperoxia and depends on the equilibrium among several factors, which are worked out mainly in the vascular endothelial cell layer. Veins respond to PO_2 changes in different ways and the mechanisms of the observed effects of hypoxia on the vein wall are still uncertain:

- Chronic hypoxia impaired pulmonary venous smooth muscle contractility and reduced pulmonary venous reactivity and sensitivity to phenylephrine and angiotensin II, without changing the pulmonary venous contractile response to acute hypoxia (435). Hypoxic contraction of isolated pulmonary vessels was found to be Ca^{2+}-dependent (434) and seemed to be mediated by a reactive oxygen species (such as H_2O_2), which in turn could modulate the ratio of prostacyclin and thromboxane release or the sensitivity to these substances (346, 353). Anoxic constriction might be mediated by ET-1 release from the endothelial cells (398).
- Placental veins presented hypoxic relaxation and reoxygenation contraction, which were prevented by an inhibitor of cyclooxygenase pathway, indomethacin (142, 291).

4.3.1.2. PCO_2 and pH

There are just a few data concerning the influence of these two factors upon venous tone. In isolated veins, lowered pH and increased PCO_2 decreased smooth muscle contractility (394). For example, in isolated human hand veins, a pH shift from 7.6 to 6.9 inhibited the contractile response to norepinephrine, serotonin and $PGF_{2\alpha}$ (18).

4.3.1.3. Lactate

Lactate might be produced by the venous wall, even in normoxic conditions (aerobic glycolysis); in case of local hypoxia, lactate release is elevated, probably due to the fact that LDH subunit composition in venous tissue is better suited for transformation of pyruvate into lactate than the enzyme in arterial tissue (234). Relaxation to lactate was markedly inhibited in both placental arteries and veins of women with severe preeclampsia compared with vessels from uncomplicated term or preterm pregnancies, suggesting that in severe preeclampsia, absence of lactate-induced dilatation of placental vessels may contribute to the fetal complications associated with impaired blood flow and vasospasm (143).

4.3.1.4. Adenosine

Adenosine is well known for its powerful relaxing effects in many vascular beds, being considered one of the factors, which mediate the adjustment of resistance vessels to metabolic needs of the tissue. P_1-purinoceptors present an agonist potency: adenosine>AMP>ADP>ATP, are selectively antagonized by methylxantines and their activation induces changes in intracellular cAMP levels. P1-purinoceptors have been further subdivided into A_1 and A_2, which inhibit or activate adenylate cyclase (320). In case of venous tissue, data concerning adenosine are scarce and contrary. Adenosine relaxed human saphenous rings and human hand veins (in vivo) in a dose-dependent manner (342, 149) and induced dilation of placental veins (mediated by A_1 and A_2 receptors)(328).

4.3.1.5. ADP and ATP

ATP and ADP are components of blood-borne elements, such as platelets and erythrocytes, and can also be released from endothelial cells and smooth muscle cells (320).

Activation of specific P_2-purinoceptors located on the smooth muscle can produce either vasoconstriction or vasodilation, whereas endothelial P_2 receptors usually mediate relaxation via production of NO. Agonist potency for these receptors is: ATP>ADP>AMP>adenosine and they are not antagonized by methylxantines. P_2-purinoceptors have been subdivided into P_{2X}, P_{2Y} (320).

- ***The*** P_{2X}***-receptor*** located on vascular smooth muscle cells are responsible for the ***vasoconstrictor responses*** produced by the ATP released from sympathetic perivascular fibers.

The effects of exogenous ATP were studied using different preparations:

- In human saphenous vein freshly isolated myocytes, contractions were mediated only by activation of P_{2x} receptor channels. The ATP-induced $[Ca^{2+}]i$ rise was due to both Ca^{2+} entry and Ca^{2+} release activated by Ca^{2+} ions that enter the cell through P_{2x} receptor channels (221).
- In isolated umbilical arteries and veins from normal term pregnancy, with or without endothelium, both ATP and alpha, beta-methylene ATP caused concentration-dependent contractions. Immunohistochemical studies with specific polyclonal antibodies against P_{2X1-6} receptors showed that positive immunostaining was restricted to smooth muscle cells,

the strongest signals being produced by antibodies against P_{2X1} receptors. Therefore, P_{2X1}-purinoceptors seem to mediate ATP-induced contraction of umbilical vessels (51).

- ***P_{2Y}-receptor*** is located mainly on endothelial cells, although in some vessels it was present on the smooth muscle; these purinoceptors are involved in the ***relaxant response*** induced by ATP, ADP and other structural analogues (320).

In situations where the intimal smooth muscle is exposed to the blood, as in cases of endothelial cell injury, the purines may act at P_{2X}-purinoceptors to cause vasospasm. Endothelial ATP receptors activate rapid mobilization of intracellular calcium stores (through activation of PLC and PLD-based signal transduction pathways) and the increased cytosolic Ca^{2+} concentration is associated with the rapid release of several vasorelaxant agents, such as nitric oxide and prostacyclin (320, 119, 90).

ADP induced relaxation of vascular smooth muscle, including venous one, through a receptor-coupled mechanism, resulted in an increase of cAMP activity in both endothelial and smooth muscle cells. In patients undergoing vascular surgical procedures, the saphenous veins presented negligible relaxation in response to adenosine diphosphate (12.1±12.8% at $1x10^{-5}$ M)(352); similar results were reported by Yang and Lüscher (1989)(423). Lowell et al. (1992) showed that healthy and varicose human saphenous veins precontracted with norepinephrine presented no differences in maximal relaxations in response to ADP and PGI_2, and that ADP-induced venodilation was not altered by endothelium removal. This experimental data indicated that in lower limbs varicosities receptor-coupled activation of cAMP by prostacyclin and ADP was preserved (222).

4.3.2. Humoral Control

Local humoral control involves vasoconstrictor factors, vasodilator factors and factors with both constrictor and relaxing actions. Experimental data concerning the effects of various humoral factors upon human veins are summarized in Table 4.III and Table 4.IV.

Table 4.III. Humoral factors producing constriction of human veins

Humoral contracting factors	Human preparation	References
angiotensin II	hand veins	85, 37, 21, 167
	saphenous veins	29, 330, 58
	chorionic plate veins	231
$PGF_{2\alpha}$	saphenous vein	27, 222
	penile circumflex vein	205
ThromboxaneA_2	pulmonary vein	408
	hand vein	19
	saphenous vein	232, 369,154, 247, 388
	placental vein	104, 214
Bradykinin	umbilical vein	138, 323, 331
Histamine (H_1)	saphenous vein	76
	placental chorionic veins	103
	fetal umbilical vein	233
	pulmonary veins	255
Serotonin	pulmonary veins	399, 428, 27, 158
	placental chorionic veins	275, 327
	hand veins	292, 113

Table. 4.IV. Humoral factors producing relaxation of human veins

Humoral relaxing factors	Human preparation	References
ANP, BNP, CNP	saphenous veins	317, 433
ANP	hand veins	14
PGI_2	penile circumflex veins	205
	hand veins	17, 18
	saphenous veins	424
PGE_2	pulmonary vein	408
	hand vein	19
$PGF_{2\alpha}$	hand vein	20
Bradykinin	saphenous veins	185, 219, 380
	hand veins	55
Histamine (H_2)	saphenous veins	349, 290, 3
	placental chorionic veins	103
Substance P	saphenous vein	228
	superficial hand vein	244, 375
	omental vein	121, 53
	mesenteric vein	386

4.3.2.1. Angiotensins

The major components of the renin-angiotensin system have been demonstrated to exist in vascular tissue, including venous wall. For instance, local generation and release of angiotensin II was demonstrated in:

- isolated perfused human umbilical veins (260);
- human hand veins (37);
- human saphenous veins. Using RT-PCR, Paul et al. (1993) demonstrated that all components of the RAS were widely expressed in human organ samples, including human saphenous veins (0.02±0.01 pg renin/micrograms total RNA)(306).

Angiotensin-converting enzyme (ACE) activity was found in the endothelium, but also in the adventitia of large veins, such as human saphenous vein, explaining the persistence of ACE activity after endothelium removal and revealing another source of ACE distant from the luminal surface of the venous wall (332). More recently, Borland et al. (1998), using an immunohistochemical technique with streptavidin biotin peroxidase, localized ACE to both EC and SMC. Moreover, they demonstrated the existence of an alternative Ang I converting pathway to that of ACE, involving chymase, enzyme confined to mast cells in the adventitia of the vessel wall (58).

All angiotensins present venoactive actions.

The constrictor effect of **angiotensin I** (Ang I) was proved in both human hand veins and saphenous veins:

- Ang I caused a marked venoconstriction limited by rapid tachyphylaxis (dorsal hand vein compliance technique). At high doses, cilazaprilat and enalaprilat completely inhibited angiotensin I-induced venoconstriction, the process being reversible after 14-31 min, suggesting an inhibition of ACE associated with the vein wall (124).
- In human saphenous vein, the contractile response to angiotensin I was significantly inhibited by incubation with the AT_1 receptor antagonist losartan (57).

The constrictor effect of **angiotensin II** (Ang II) was proved in various human venous preparations, such as: hand veins (85, 37, 21), chorionic plate vein (231), saphenous veins (330, 58). In addition to its direct constrictor effect, angiotensin II potentiates the venoconstrictor response to sympathetic nerve stimulation via an increased release of NE from the nerve terminals, mechanism demonstrated in several human veins (hand veins and saphenous veins)(414, 261).

Elevated levels of Ang II and its degradation products **angiotensin III** (Ang III) **and angiotensin IV** (Ang IV) may contribute to the regulation of vascular tone under various clinical circumstances. Ang II, Ang III, and Ang IV produced concentration-dependent contractions in endothelium-denuded human saphenous vein preparations with comparable maximal responses. Ang III was 16 times less active than Ang II, whereas Ang IV was approximately 2,700-fold less potent than Ang II. The contractile responses to all three peptides were mediated via AT_1-receptors but not AT_2-receptors, because Ang II receptor antagonist losartan shifted all the concentration-response curves to the right in a parallel manner. Ang II showed strong tachyphylaxis, whereas Ang III and Ang IV did not. These results indicated that in endothelium-denuded human SV, Ang II, but also Ang III and Ang IV are efficacious vasoconstrictor agents (216).

There are data, which demonstrated the existence of important differences in angiotensin-converting enzyme activity and AT_1 receptor responses in veins compared to arteries. For example, human saphenous vein produced greater maximum responses to Ang II than did the internal thoracic artery, this effect being unchanged by inhibition of NOS, COX, or by an endothelin receptor antagonist in either vessel. Losartan inhibited the vasoconstrictor response in both blood vessels. Homogenates of saphenous vein displayed a threefold greater tissue ACE activity compared to internal thoracic artery. Both the contractile response to angiotensin II and the enzyme activity were retained in venous grafts removed up to 20 years after coronary bypass surgery. These findings may have important implications for vein graft patency, as well as for the use of ACE inhibitors and AT_1 receptor antagonists in the prevention and treatment of vein graft disease (58).

The influence exerted by angiotensin-converting enzyme inhibitor upon venous smooth muscle was also studied. The ACE inhibitor enalaprilat markedly augmented endothelium-dependent relaxations to bradykinin in saphenous vein and had no effect on endothelium-dependent relaxations to acetylcholine. These data indicated that in human saphenous vein ACE inactivates bradykinin and thereby blunts endothelium-dependent relaxations to the peptide and converts Ang I to Ang II (427).

In some pathological states, such as varicose veins, the reactivity of venous smooth muscle to angiotensin II is impaired. A significant and gradual reduction (progressively with the increasing severity of the disease) in Ang II, NE, and ET-1 contractile activities in the diseased veins as compared with the control tissues was demonstrated. The dramatic reduction of Ang II affinity appeared in an early stage of the disease, supporting the hypothesis that such an abnormality within the venous wall could play a role in the pathogenesis of primary varicose vein disease (330). Measurements of serum ACE, as a plasma marker of endothelial lesions, were considered useful in order to identify patients with high risk of deep vein thrombosis (118).

4.3.2.2. Natriuretic Peptides

Natriuretic peptides, ANP, BNP and CNP, are a family of peptides encoded by genes with similar overall structure. They exert their affects through interaction with one or more of three NP receptors, two of them stimulating guanylate cyclase, whereas the third appears mostly as a clearance receptor. In contrast to ANP (mainly synthesized within the atrial myocytes) and BNP (predominantly produced in atria and brain), CNP is predominantly secreted from the vascular endothelium. CNP released from endothelial cells acts in a paracrine manner, being involved in the control of vascular tone. CNP is a potent venodilator and a selective arterial relaxing agent (mediated via the ANPR-B receptor expressed in vascular smooth muscle), with minimal natriuretic and diuretic actions (155, 403, 24).

The vasoactive effects of natriuretic peptides were studied just in a few human veins such as hand veins and saphenous veins.

Locally infused ANP on superficial human hand veins, with or without preconstriction, induced only a small dilator effect, suggesting that at physiological doses, ANP did not produce a significant venorelaxing effect (413). However, in another study, performed in vivo, intraarterial administration of ANP was followed by venodilation (14).

The venodilator effects of human ANP, BNP, and CNP on human vascular tissue prepared from saphenous were also investigated. With regard to potency and magnitude of effect, all three natriuretic peptides exhibited just a weak venodilating action (317). However, another study showed that in segments of intact saphenous vein, C-type natriuretic peptide was significantly more effective than atrial natriuretic peptide (16-fold increase in cyclic GMP in response to 1 microM of C-type natriuretic peptide versus six-fold increase in cyclic GMP in response to 1 microM of atrial natriuretic peptide). In cultured smooth muscle cells from saphenous vein, the pattern of response to C-type natriuretic peptide and atrial natriuretic peptide was the same as in the intact vessels. Due to this observation, the authors suggested that increased concentrations of C-type natriuretic peptide could contribute to venous pooling in septic shock (433).

Human ANP and BNP might indirectly influence vascular tone. In HUVEC cultures, both natriuretic peptides inhibited ET-1 secretion, induced by angiotensin II or thrombin (206).

4.3.2.3. Eicosanoids

Prostanoids

Venous tissues are capable of producing eicosanoids, but the normal values for the vasoactive **prostanoid** production was difficult to characterize, because its dependence on the method used (274).

The production of prostacyclin and thromboxane A_2 (in vitro studies) was confirmed for different human venous tissues, such as umbilical veins (248, 249), pulmonary veins (73), mesenteric veins (171), and saphenous veins (248, 249).

The contribution of venous wall layers to prostanoid production was also investigated; it seems that both endothelium and smooth muscle take part in production of both prostacyclin and thromboxane (278).

- Human umbilical vein endothelial cells synthesize in normal conditions large amounts of PG, especially PGI_2 (1.42 ng/ml PGE_2, 1.00 ng/ml PGD_2, 7.69 ng/ml $PGF_{2\alpha}$, and 26.92 ng/ml PGI_2)(253).
- Bishop-Bailey et al (1998) noted that both venous (human saphenous vein) and arterial smooth muscle cells (internal mammary artery) in culture released low levels of cyclooxygenase (COX) metabolites in absence of cytokines, suggesting that smooth muscle cells do not normally express COX enzymes. After treatment with IL-1β, TNF-α, LPS, or cytokine mix, both arterial and venous smooth muscle cells released increased amounts of COX metabolites, PGE_2 being release preferentially, followed by PGI_2 and very low levels of PGI_2; venous cells release more PGE_2 than did arterial cells. Both arterial and venous tissue contain two forms of COX: the constitutive form COX-1, located in the endothelial layer, and a cytokine-inducible isoform, COX-2, which can be induced in vascular smooth muscle by IL-1β, TNF-α, bacterial LPS, growth factors, and phorbol esters; these authors demonstrated that human venous smooth muscle expressed higher amounts of COX-2 than the arterial one (47).
- There are other several investigators who reported that veins produce less (Chaikpuny et al, 1986 - saphenous vein versus internal mammary artery), more (Mehta and Roberts, 1983 - umbilical vein versus umbilical artery) or a similar amount (Carter et al., 1984 - venous versus

arterial pulmonary tissue) of prostacyclin, these differences being related to the investigated venous territory and/or species (75, 249, 73).

Generally speaking, prostacyclin relaxes and thromboxane contracts vascular smooth muscle, whereas the effects of PGE_2 and $PGF_{2\alpha}$ seem to be inconsistent, with contracting effects in some territories, and relaxing actions in other vascular beds. This general pattern was questioned by Sinzinger and Fitscha (1984), who found contraction in human saphenous veins in vitro; at high concentrations, $\geq 1\mu M$, PGI_2 became vasoconstrictor in both large arteries and veins (358); these actions were blocked by thromboxane-receptor antagonists, suggesting a cross-reactivity of PGI_2 with the thromboxane receptor (351, 288).

In veins, arachidonic acid, acetylcholine, histamine, and serotonin can evoke endothelium-dependent contractions which are mediated by thromboxane A_2 (TxA_2) and prostaglandin H_2 (PGH_2); TxA_2 and PGH_2 activate the thromboxane receptor in vascular smooth muscle and platelets, counteracting the actions of NO and PGI_2 in both cell types (289).

In venous tissues, all types of prostanoid receptors were identified (84, 281, 350)(Table 4.V):

- EP receptors (for PGE_2), linked to different transduction pathways, mediating different vascular responses, depending on the distribution of EP receptor subtypes;
- IP receptors (for PGI_2) linked to the activation of adenylyl cyclase, causing mainly vasodilation and inhibition of vascular smooth muscle proliferation;
- DP (for PGD_2);
- TP receptors (for TxA_2) linked to the inositol phosphate pathway, which mediate vasoconstriction;
- FP and (for PGF_{2a}).

Table 4.V. Prostanoid receptors involved in the modulation of human venous tone

Human preparations	Receptors involved in venoconstriction	Receptors involved in venodilation	References
hand vein	TP	IP	18, 19
saphenous vein	TP		232, 154, 369, 388
placental vein	TP		60, 104
pulmonary vein	TP, EP_1	IP, DP, EP?	404, 408

In human hand veins, beside PGE_1, PGE_2, and PGI_2, $PGF_{2\alpha}$ also elicited concentration-dependent relaxant effects. Removal of the endothelium reduced the relaxation induced by $PGF_{2\alpha}$ and PGE_2, but not that elicited by PGE_1 and PGI_2. The order of potency was $PGE_2 \approx PGE_1 \approx PGI_2 > PGF_{2\alpha}$ regardless of the presence or absence of endothelium (20).

The thromboxane agonist U-46619 (0.1 - 30 nM) contracted human saphenous vein, maximal contractions being larger than those caused by ET-1 (247). In these human preparations, eicosanoid metabolism was also involved in the modulation of the potent vasoconstrictor effect of ET-1. Endothelin-1 induced a sustained contraction of the preparation and concomitantly released from the venous tissue a proportional amount of 6-keto-$PGF_{1\alpha}$. The contractile activity of ET-1 was augmented by inhibition of cyclooxygenase enzyme with indomethacin (42).

In human isolated penile circumflex veins PGE_1 did not affect resting tension, while the compound produced venous relaxation after precontraction with noradrenaline. PGE_2 produced the contraction of the preparations, but in case of previous precontraction with noradrenaline, relaxation was noted. $PGF_{2\alpha}$ also induced contraction, with no relaxant responses after precontraction with NA. PGI_2 produced no mechanical effects in unstimulated venous preparations, but after precontraction with noradrenaline, PGI_2 produced relaxation. All these experimental data indicated that local synthesis of prostanoids might influence resting tension and modulate noradrenaline-induced responses in penile circumflex veins smooth muscle (205).

Pathophysiological aspects

Vasoactive prostanoid production was found impaired in some venous disorders, such as varicose veins. Initially, Sinzinger (1985) found no difference in the prostacyclin-synthesizing capacity between normal and varicose saphenous veins (359). Later, Biagi et al. (45, 46) reported a decreased prostacyclin and an increased thromboxane production in varicose veins of the lower limbs, whereas Haynes et al. (175) found an increased in vitro synthesis of both prostacyclin and thromboxane in varicosities. In 1997, Schuller-Petrovic et al. reported that prostacyclin production was significantly reduced in cells from varicose than healthy saphenous veins (351). More recently, the production of prostacyclin and thromboxane in human varicose and nonvaricose veins was assessed by measuring (RIA) media concentrations of 6-ketoprostaglandin F1α, the stable metabolite of prostacyclin, and thromboxane B_2, the stable metabolite of thromboxane A_2; cyclooxygenase 2 was also measured with Western blot analysis. Prostanoid production was not found significantly altered in the varicose veins, but the ratio between 6-ketoprostaglandin-F1α and thromboxane B_2 was two-fold greater in the varicose veins as compared with the control veins, and cyclooxygenase 2 was not present in either the control or the varicose veins. This chemical pathway was considered a modulatory target to affect contraction with venotropic drugs, because in the presence of the Ruscus aculeatus extract, the ratio of 6-ketoprostaglandin-F1α and thromboxane B_2 was identical in both types of veins (285).

The role of locally produced prostanoids in the patency of venous autografts was also studied. One of the reasons for the higher patency of internal mammary artery grafted into coronary artery in comparison with saphenous vein was the increased capacity to release PGI_2 (75). Another important factor to be considered is the surgical preparation of the graft, common surgical techniques being associated with an extensive loss of endothelial cells and impairment of prostaglandin synthesis.

Cysteinyl-leukotrienes

The cysteinyl-leukotrienes act on two receptor subtypes, $CysLT_1$ and $CysLT_2$, causing contractions and/or relaxations of human isolated vascular preparations.

In human pulmonary veins with an intact endothelium, leukotriene D_4 (LTD_4) induced contraction above basal tone, this effect being partially blocked by $CysLT_1$ antagonists (MK 571 and ICI 198615). In human pulmonary veins previously contracted with noradrenaline LTD_4 caused venodilation, which was potentiated by $CysLT_1$ antagonists, but was abolished by removal of the endothelium. These results suggest that contraction of endothelium-intact HPV by LTD_4 was partially mediated via $CysLT_1$ receptors, and the relaxation induced by LTD_4 in precontracted preparations, dependent on the release of nitric oxide, was also mediated, at least in part, via a non-LT_1 receptor (296). $CysLT_2$ receptor was also identified in the smooth muscle of pulmonary veins; its stimulation produced a contraction, which was not blocked by the antagonists known to be effective in airways. In addition, the endothelium was found to contain two receptors: a $CysLT_1$, which is associated with contraction and is blocked by the antagonists, as well as a second receptor $CysLT_2$ associated with relaxation. This latter receptor is also resistant to the antagonists, which block the airway responses (161, 404).

In human saphenous veins, leukotrienes mediate biphasic responses. LTC_4 and LTD_4 caused weak endothelium-dependent relaxations at lower concentrations (1 pM to 1 nM) and powerful endothelium-independent contractions at higher concentrations (3 nM to 0.1 microM). L-NG-monomethyl L-arginine, an inhibitor of nitric oxide formation, prevented the relaxations to LTD_4, but not LT C4, and unmasked endothelium-dependent contractions to LTD_4, with no effect on the LT-induced contractions (8). In undistended saphenous veins, in which cysteinyl-LTs elicited concentration-dependent contractions, the Emax for LT E_4 was significantly less than that observed with either LTC_4 or LTD_4. Furthermore, there was a preferential contraction to leukotrienes in saphenous veins compared with internal mammary arteries, suggesting that endogenous LT production from circulating or infiltrating leukocytes may be an important factor contributing to graft function, especially in case of venous grafts (9).

4.3.2.4. Bradykinin

Kinins, which can derive from a number of different sources, including endothelium, are considered local hormones acting in a autocrine-paracrine manner. In plasma they circulate at very low concentrations, being

rapidly degraded by kininases, kininase I and kininase II, also known as ACE and enkephalinase. High amounts of ACE were identified at the luminal surface of the endothelium; ACE acts as an ecto-enzyme, which seems to be largely responsible for the local proteolytic breakdown of kinins (44). The angiotensin-converting enzyme inhibitor enalaprilat markedly augmented endothelium-dependent relaxations to bradykinin in human saphenous veins, but not in internal mammary arteries; thus, in veins but not in arteries, ACE inactivates bradykinin and thereby blunts endothelium-dependent relaxations to this peptide and converts Ang I to Ang II (428).

Kinins are vasoactive through the release of different autacoids, mainly generated by the endothelial cells; activation of B_2 kinin receptors in endothelia and in the smooth muscle is followed by relaxation through NO (endothelia) and prostanoids (smooth muscle)(323). B_1 receptors mediate bradykinin-induced contraction, but they are thought not to be present in normal tissues, being induced by certain pathological conditions, such as tissue injury or stress (218). Recent studies in human vessels (umbilical vein) have confirmed the existence of contractile B_1 and B_2 receptors in venous smooth muscles (138, 323, 331).

In humans, bradykinin causes mostly endothelium-dependent relaxations of preconstricted veins, such as hand veins (55), and saphenous veins (185, 219)

In human saphenous vein, the EDHF-mediated hyperpolarization induced by bradykinin was significantly lower compared to internal mammary arteries. Moreover, the duration of bradykinin-induced NO release was longer in the artery than in the vein, indicating a superior long-term patency of arterial grafts (219). Endothelium dependent agonist stimulation with bradykinin induced significant increases in cyclic GMP in saphenous veins and internal mammary artery, but the values obtained were significantly greater in arterial than in venous tissue (380).

In saphenous veins, the endothelium-dependent venodilation caused by bradykinin presented variations due to varicosities and smoking. Maximum relaxation in response to bradykinin of rings obtained in both varicose vein surgery and bypass surgery was higher in non-smokers. These data suggested that smoking impairs NO release in response to bradykinin, leading to an increased vasomotor tone, platelet aggregation and smooth muscle proliferation, with a high risk of graft occlusion (185).

4.3.2.5. Histamine

Histamine presents venoconstrictor and venodilator actions, its actions being dependent upon the presence of endothelium and of histaminergic receptors that induce contractions. Generally, histamine caused venoconstriction, in a dose-dependent manner, via H_1 histaminergic receptors; when preincubated with a H_1 receptor antagonist, histamine relaxed precontracted venous preparations. The H_1 receptors mediate their effects via products of inositol phospholipid hydrolysis and increasing intracellular calcium. H_2 receptors are coupled via a G_S protein to adenylate cyclase and stimulate cAMP formation, their activation inducing a decrease of $[Ca^{2+}]i$. Apart from smooth muscle H_1 receptors, stimulation of endothelial H_1 receptors also causes vasodilation (274).

Histamine actions upon venous smooth muscle were investigated on several human preparations:

- histamine caused dose-dependent contraction of saphenous veins. The relative magnitude of control constrictor response was: NA=5-hydroxytryptamine>or=dopamine>histamine>ACh (76). In denuded human saphenous veins obtained during aortocoronary bypass surgery histamine caused a concentration-dependent contraction, which was antagonized by the H_1 receptor antagonists, mepyramine and cicletanine. In the presence of the H_2 receptor antagonist cimetidine (10 μM), concentration-response curves of histamine-induced contractions were significantly shifted to the left, suggesting the presence of H_2 receptors mediating relaxation (349). Histamine caused dose dependent relaxations of precontracted saphenous veins, but only in the presence of a H_1 receptor antagonist, this relaxation being inhibited by cimetidine (349, 290).

- Similar results were reported for human placental chorionic veins. Histamine induced concentration-dependent contractions, which were inhibited by the H_1 antagonist, pyrilamine, whereas cimetidine had no effect (103). The order of different vasoactive agents with regard to their potencies (EC50 values) was: 5-hydroxytryptamine≥noradrenaline≥ histamine>phenylephrine>clonidine7>K^+ (327).
- In human perfused fetal umbilical vein, histamine was a much less potent vasoconstrictor than thromboxane A_2-mimetic substance U46619, serotonin and bradykinin (233).
- Histamine induced concentration dependent contractions in both human pulmonary arteries and veins, but its maximal response was lower in veins than in arteries. Histamine and 2-methyl-histamine had a dual action, demonstrated in vessels precontracted with potassium: at low concentrations caused relaxation (partly mediated through H_1 receptors and partly via other unspecific mechanisms), but at high concentrations produced contractions (mediated via H_1 receptors); veins were more sensitive to the relaxant effect of histamine than arteries (255).

4.3.2.6. Serotonin

The major source of circulating serotonin is represented by platelets, one of its targets being represented by the vessel wall. Acting on specific 5-HT receptors, serotonin may induce both contraction and relaxation of venous smooth muscle.

A contractile response of serotonin was observed in human saphenous veins (399, 428, 27), human pulmonary veins (275), chorionic veins (327), placental veins (292) and hand veins (85).

- Serotonin-induced contraction of human hand veins was influenced by the extracellular concentration of calcium and temperature; a decrease of extracellular calcium reduced the amplitude of the venoconstriction, whereas cooling to 25°C potentiated the contractile response caused by serotonin (in both intact and denuded preparations). In human hand vein, 5-HT1-like receptors mediated its venoconstrictor response (85).

- In human saphenous vein, the contractile response caused by serotonin was completely prevented by pretreatment with the 5-HT_2-receptor antagonist ketanserine, indicating that this type of receptor meditates its venoconstrictor action (113). However, Glusa and Muller-Schweinitzer (1993) reported that in human saphenous veins both 5-HT_1-like and 5-HT_2 receptors are present (158).
- In human chorionic veins 5-HT-induced contractions were largely dependent on extracellular Ca^{2+} and mainly mediated by 5-HT_2 receptors (327).
- Functional and radioligand binding studies in human isolated intrapulmonary arteries and veins have demonstrated a mixed population of 5-$HT_{1B/1D}$ and 5-HT_{2A} receptors mediating vasoconstriction with no evidence of involvement of 5-HT_{1A}, 5-HT_3 and 5-HT_4 receptors (275).

In several mammalian venous territories, a vasodilator action of serotonin was reported. The relaxing action of serotonin could be explained by three mechanisms: inhibition of NE release from sympathetic nerve endings, direct vascular smooth muscle relaxation, and release of EDRF (274). In human saphenous veins, serotonin inhibited NE release from adrenergic perivascular fibers via 5- HT_{1D} (262).

The importance of serotonin is underlined by its possible role in the pathogenic mechanism of portal hypertension. Acute and continuous administration of 5-HT_2-antagonists (ketanserin and ritanserin) was followed by a significant decrease of portal pressure and collateral blood flow in patients with cirrhosis, without changing the hepatic blood flow (215).

4.3.2.7. Substance P

Substance P (SP) is an endothelium-dependent vasodilator neurokinin,, its effect being mediated by NK1 receptors.

All human precontracted veins (with either endothelin-1, norepinephrine or PG $F_{2\alpha}$) responded to SP by relaxation: omental vein (121, 53), superficial hand vein (244, 375), mesenteric vein (386) and saphenous vein (228).

In vivo, in human hand veins preconstricted with the alpha 1-agonist phenylephrine, substance P proved to be the most potent venodilator known thus far (the dose-rate exerting 50% of mean maximum dilation [ED50], geometric mean: 0.105 pmol/min), but with a rapid development of tolerance. Unlike in other vessels, substance P-induced venodilation in hand veins was not mediated through nitric oxide but to a significant extent through activation of ATP-dependent potassium channels on vascular smooth muscle cells and through the release of endothelium-derived hyperpolarizing factor (its effect was reduced by gliburide and acetylsalicylic acid, but not by L-NMME) (375).

Endothelium dependent agonist stimulation with substance P induced significant increases in cyclic GMP native saphenous vein and in internal mammary artery, whereas distended veins showed non-significant changes in response to agonist stimulation, whereas basal levels of cyclic GMP were significantly higher in the artery than either native or distended saphenous vein. These differences between basal and stimulated cyclic GMP activity in arteries and veins could represent an additional protective mechanism against constrictor influences in arterial bypass grafts, compared to venous ones, which may explain their documented better long term performance (380). Similar results were obtained by O'Neil et al. (1991), who showed that gastroepiploic artery had significantly higher resting and substance P-stimulated levels of cyclic guanosine 3',5'-monophosphate than either the internal mammary artery or the saphenous vein (293).

In other species, substance P caused venoconstriction (for instance rat portal vein)(241).

4.3.3. Role of Ions in Local Control of Venous Tone

Most of the data concerning the influence of ionic environment on venous tone were obtained using animal venous preparations and endothelial cell cultures. Just a few studies explored these aspects in human veins, therefore some of the following data were extrapolated from experimental work dealing with mammalian veins.

4.3.3.1. Sodium

Sodium distribution within venous smooth muscle cells seems to be rather uniform, without major differences between its cytoplasmic, nuclear and mitochondrial concentration (367). Sodium and transport systems regulating Na^+ distribution across cell membrane are involved in the regulation of membrane potential of vascular smooth muscle cells.

- The *sodium pump*, which regulates membrane potential by transmembrane transportation of Na^+ and K^+ ions, seems to be present in vascular smooth muscle cells, but in a lower number of sites per cell compared with cardiac and skeletal muscle (7). Experiments performed on human mesenteric vein and artery (ouabain-induced contraction of human mesenteric veins was higher than that produced in mesenteric arteries) suggested that the electrogenic sodium transport may play a greater role in the maintenance of the resting membrane potential in venous than in arterial smooth muscle cells (254).
- Normally, the *Na^+/Ca^{2+} exchanger* transports Ca^{2+} out of the cell at expense of Na^+ influx, which then will be removed by the N^+-K^+ pump. The role of this exchanger seem to be more important in venous smooth muscle cells than in arterial ones; inhibition of N^+-K^+ pump with ouabain induced a pronounced contraction of human placental veins, that could be explained by an increase of intracellular Na^+ concentration, which in turn decreased Na^+/Ca^{2+} exchanger activity with a subsequent rise of intracellular Ca^{2+} level (49, 236).
- Another exchange system involving sodium is *Na^+/H^+ exchanger*, which in most cell types plays an active role in maintaining intracellular pH homeostasis. This exchanger was found to be a major pathway by which cultured HUVEC regulate H^+ extrusion and Na^+ influx (in a 1:1 ratio)(131).
- A *$Na^+/K^+/2Cl^-$ cotransport* system was characterized in human umbilical and saphenous vein endothelial cells cultures, its activity being stimulated by vasopressin and bradykinin (within the range of circulating levels). The magnitude of K^+ influx through this pathway was high enough to suggest that this ion-transport system plays a role in the regulation of the resting membrane potential and/or cell volume (66). The inhibitory effect of frusemide on angiotensin II-induced contraction of human saphenous vein was mediated, at least in part, by inhibition of $Na^+/K^+/2Cl^-$ symport (370).
- *Fast sodium channels* were also identified in venous smooth muscle cells and might be a potentially important sodium entry pathway for vascular cells (393).

4.3.3.2. Potassium

K^+ presents important roles through direct and indirect mechanisms, being involved in the alteration of cell membrane potential directly or through the electrogenic Na^+-K^+ pump, alterations in cell membrane permeability and intracellular sodium, or modulation of norepinephrine release by sympathetic nerves (368).

In venous smooth muscle cells, similar to arterial ones, increased K^+ level induced a divalent response: a moderate K^+ elevation (5-10 mM) produced relaxation, while a pronounced increase, above 15 mM induced venous contraction (human saphenous veins)(286). In human preparations, such as saphenous and hand veins, K^+-induced contraction was influenced by the extracellular Ca^{2+} concentration, suggesting that KCl-induced contraction was due to depolarization and activation of voltage-dependent calcium channels (17, 410).

Venous smooth muscle cell present different types of potassium channels (Table 4.VI)

Table 4.VI. Main characteristics of potassium channels identified in venous tissue (284, 64)

Main attributes	K_{ATP}	BK_{Ca}	K_{DR}	K_{tran}
Properties	inhibited by intracellular ATP, voltage-independent	activated by Ca^{2+} and voltage	activated by depolarization	rapidly activated and inactivated by a positive potential
Blockers	glibenclamide TEA 4 aminopyridine Ba^{2+} PKC activators	Iberiotoxin TEA paxiline apamin	4 aminopyridine quinine intracellular Ca^{2+} vasoconstrictors	4 aminopyridine quinine

TEA = tetraethylammonium

- Calcium-activated potassium channels (BK_{Ca}), which are activated with increased intracellular calcium level, were described as K_L, K_M and K_s (with large, medium, and small conductance)(rabbit and rat portal vein). K_L and K_s were being both voltage- and calcium-dependent, whereas K_M had a weak dependency on voltage and intracellular Ca^{2+}.

This latter current is thought to be essential for the generation of resting membrane potential (194, 198).

- ATP-sensitive potassium channels (K_{ATP}) are inhibited by micromolar concentration of intracellular ATP. The presence of these channels was proved for the human saphenous vein by De Moura and Jasbik (112), and Beattie et al. (32).
- Voltage-gated potassium channels (K_V), which are typified by the delayed rectifier potassium channel and transient potassium current, are found in a variety of vascular tissues. Delayed rectifier potassium channels [I_{dK}] seems to contribute to the repolarization phase of the action potential in some venous smooth muscle cells, such as those from rabbit portal veins (191). Transient outward potassium channels, were also identified using whole patch clamp technique in isolated smooth muscle cells from rabbit portal vein (34).

Potassium channel openers (PCO), a group of antihypertensive and antianginal drugs (pinacidil, cromakalim, nicorandil, minoxidil, diazoxide and other compounds) induce vasodilation by causing hyperpolarization. There are numerous studies, which proved the relaxing effect of these drugs on mammalian and human venous smooth muscle (80). For example, human saphenous vein rings pre-contracted with phenylephrine showed a concentration-dependent relaxation to all the potassium channel openers tested with a potency ranking of: HOE 234>cromakalim >pinacidil>diazoxide (32).

4.3.3.3. Calcium

In venous smooth cells, similar to arterial ones, calcium plays a major role in the initiation of contraction, which depends on the increase of myoplasmic concentration of Ca^{2+}.

Most of the venoactive agents induce changes in intracellular Ca^{2+} concentration ($[Ca^{2+}]$). Calcium may originate from both extracellular and intracellular sources. Calcium influx from the extracellular pool occurs through receptor-activated, voltage-dependent, or stretch-activated calcium channels. Release of Ca^{2+} from the sarcoplasmic reticulum is linked to binding of the second messenger IP_3 to specific receptors on its membrane; IP_3 is released as a consequence of phospholipase C activation by stimuli acting on sarcolemal receptors coupled with a G protein. The G protein-mediated intracellular calcium release may be accompanied by a potentiation of the contractile response to Ca^{2+} (Ca^{2+} sensitization); this process is secondary to an increased 20-kDa myosin light-chain phosphorylation and is not uncoupled by calcium channel blockers. Calcium efflux is elicited through the Ca^{2+}-ATP-ase and a Na^{+}-Ca^{2+}-exchanger. Sarcoplasmic reticulum refilling with calcium is mediated by a Ca^{2+}-ATP-ase on the membrane of sarcoplasmic reticulum (200).

In a few types of venous smooth muscle cells, with the use of whole cell patch-clamp technique, voltage-dependent calcium channels have been characterized. For instance, in rat portal vein and dog saphenous vein myocytes, two types of calcium channels were identified: one activated by small depolarizations and another which required stronger depolarizations for activation (220, 430). In rabbit portal vein smooth muscle cells, one type of calcium channel was identified, with characteristics similar to an L-type calcium channel (96).

Calcium channel blockers (CaCB) include a diverse group of chemical structures that block calcium-selective ion channels in the plasma membranes of a variety of excitable cells, including vascular smooth muscle cells. They act mainly on voltage dependent calcium channels (L-channels being much more sensitive than T channels) and uncouple electromechanically the muscle. In order to block receptor-operated channels, CaCB concentration should be high and this might not be reached in clinical use (56, 294). Several experimental studies revealed their effects on veins.

Verapamil, diltiazem and nifedipine produced concentration-dependent relaxation of human isolated saphenous vein, verapamil being 7 and 5 times as potent as nifedipine and diltiazem, respectively, in producing relaxation of the human saphenous vein. Verapamil, diltiazem and nifedipine also inhibited the contractions produced by noradrenaline, acetylcholine and 5-hydroxytryptamine and to KCl, suggesting that these CaCB may inhibit calcium influx through both potential and receptor-operated calcium ion channels (409, 410). Nisoldipine also caused a marked relaxation in human saphenous veins (298). Other in vitro experiments on healthy human saphenous veins preparations, showed that verapamil relaxed the potassium contraction by 100% and the thromboxane contraction by 75%; verapamil's effect had a delayed onset, but a long duration. Because glyceryl trinitrate presented rapid onset and a short duration of maximal action, which was similar to that induced by verapamil, the administration of a mixture of these two drugs topically and intraluminally during harvesting of the saphenous vein was thought to provide a relaxed conduit for coronary artery bypass grafting (180, 334).

CaCB also produced concentration-dependent inhibition of the contractile responses induced by K^{+} or 5-HT in different human venous preparations, such as chorionic veins and hand veins (17, 237, 328)

Calcium channel blockers, such as amlodipine, verapamil, and diltiazem, also inhibited human vascular smooth muscle cells proliferation in vitro, regardless of whether the cells were grown from graft stenoses or healthy saphenous vein. Thus, CaCB may improve the long-term patency of vein bypass grafts. However, the concentrations at which these calcium channel blockers elicited antiproliferative effects may not be attainable during therapeutic dosing in humans (276).

The use of CaCB may reveal the major source of calcium necessary for venous smooth muscle contraction. For instance, endothelin-2-induced contractions of human saphenous vein preparations required both intracellular and extracellular calcium, whereas the intracellular Ca^{2+} was most important for the contractile action of endothelin-1 (313, 426).

4.3.3.4. Magnesium

Magnesium represents a natural calcium antagonist; it inhibits voltage-dependent, receptor-dependent, and leak channels alike (10, 12).

There are few studies that have investigated the influence of Mg^{2+} concentration on venous smooth muscle tone and contractility, especially in humans. Most experimental data showed that reduction of extracellular Mg^{2+} level increases Ca^{2+} influx into vascular smooth muscle cells with subsequent elevation in tension and reactivity to vasoconstrictors (10, 12, 378).

- In isolated human umbilical veins, decreased magnesium concentration induced an enhancement of basal tension and augmented the contractile response to several vasoactive agents, such as angiotensin II, serotonin, bradykinin and prostaglandin $F_{2\alpha}$, explaining the effectiveness of magnesium sulfate therapy in preeclamptic syndromes (11).
- In vitro experiments on isolated human saphenous veins showed that high Mg^{2+} concentration caused venodilation (77). Our group investigated the effects of progressive Mg^{2+} withdrawal on isometric tension of isolated spirals of human saphenous veins (360). We noted that reducing magnesium concentration in the organ bath produced both endothelium-dependent relaxations and venous smooth muscle contractions. Lowering magnesium concentration from 1.2 to 0.8 and 0.4 mM caused a decrease of norepinephrine and epinephrine-induced contractions and an enhancement of ET-1 induced contractile response. In all cases, the absence of magnesium produced an increase of the contractile action, similar to the initial response in case of norepinephrine and epinephrine, and significantly greater in case of ET-

1 ($p<0.05$). The fact that L-NA abolished the relaxing effects noted in case 0.8 and 0.4 mM Mg, suggested an involvement of NO. Comparative to norepinephrine and epinephrine, graded reduction of magnesium concentration produced just an augmentation of ET-1 induced contractions; this finding agrees to other experimental studies which showed that in saphenous veins contracted with endothelin-1 but not with norepinephrine, the relaxations induced by nitrovasodilators were blunted, suggesting a specific interaction of the peptide with the cGMP-relaxation (425, 225). Both effects, vasodilation and vasoconstriction, induced by magnesium withdrawal seemed to be a consequence of an increase in calcium entry into the endothelial and venous smooth muscle cells, respectively. Moreover, extracellular magnesium could have a direct effect on nitric oxide synthase (NOS) activity. There are studies which suggested that an elevated magnesium concentration inhibits NO release by inhibiting NOS activity and antagonizing intracellular calcium, the precise mechanism and the location of this antagonism being unclear (188).

4.3.3.5. Chloride Ions

Chloride transport across cell membrane is elicited via several mechanisms:

- cotransporters, such as Na^+-Cl^-, K^+-Cl^-, and Na^+-K^+-$2Cl^-$., the latter was identified in human umbilical and saphenous vein endothelial cells cultures being involved in cell volume regulation (66);
- exchangers, such as Na^+-HCO_3^-/Cl^- and HCO_3^-/Cl^-; the Cl^-/HCO_3^- seems to be involved in regulation of intracellular pH (in guinea-pig vena cava, removal of Cl^- was followed by a marked alteration of intracellular pH by a HCO_3^-/Cl^- mechanism)(242).
- chloride channels; for instance, in isolated cells from rat portal vein calcium-activated chloride channels were described (patch-clamp studies)(412).

In some venous preparations (for instance, rat portal vein), activation of chloride channels in response to norepinephrine (via a pertussis toxin-independent G protein) elicited a depolarizing current that induced the opening of voltage-dependent calcium channels with subsequent contraction (301, 302).

4.3.4. Endothelium-Derived Factors and the Regulation of Venous Tone

During the last two decades, scientists in the field of vascular research have focused their attention on endothelium-derived vasoactive factors. Endothelium is responsible for the short-term regulation of vascular tone. It produces vasodilator substances, such as nitric oxide (NO), prostacyclin (PGI_2) and EDHF, and also vasoconstrictor factors, such as endothelin-1, thromboxane A_2 and prostaglandin H_2. These factors were also identified in veins, but they have been extensively studied in arteries.

4.3.4.1. Endothelium-Derived Relaxing Factors

Nitric oxide (NO)

The endothelium-derived relaxing factor (EDRF) has been identified as free radical NO (303, 192). The properties of EDRF from intact arteries and veins suggested that arterial and venous EDRF are similar. NO is formed from the guanidine-nitrogen terminal of L-arginine by endothelial NO synthase (eNOS), which is activated by receptor-dependent (acetylcholine, ATP, bradykinin, serotonin) and -independent agonists (Ca^{2+} ionophore, polications) in a calcium/calmodulin/dependent manner. The activation of eNOS also requires several cofactors, such as nicotinamide adenine dinucleotide (NADPH), 5,6,7,8-tetrahydrobiopterin (BH_4), and flavin adenine mono- and dinucleotides (FMN/FAD)(270, 69). The eNOS is located in the plasmalemma caveola of endothelial cells, close to caveolin-1, a protein that inhibits the enzyme activity (252).

There are at least two different pathways involved in the synthesis of NO: a pertussis toxin-sensitive G protein (Gi_2) pathway and another one mediated by a toxin-insensitive G protein (Gq). Endothelial receptors for serotonin ($5HT_{1B}$), norepinephrine (α_2), and endothelin (ET_B) are coupled to G_{i2} protein, while those for ADP (P_{2Y}), bradykinin (BK_2), and shear stress are coupled to Gq protein. The endothelial thrombin receptor is coupled to both G proteins (146, 151, 397, 355).

NO produced by the endothelium diffuses into the underlying vascular smooth muscle to mediate vascular relaxation by a cGMP-dependent process (277, 193). The process of guanylate cyclase activation by NO requires heme presence. Thus, the heme component of soluble guanylate cyclase may be considered the "receptor" for NO in vascular smooth muscle cells (99). At the transcriptional level, endothelium-derived

NO modulates the regulation of several genes (such as monocyte chemoattractant protein-1, P-selectin and VCAM-1) most probably by direct and/or indirect interaction with transcriptional factors (147).

The majority of studies concerning NO were performed on arterial preparations. In this section, we tried to focus on experiments carried out on veins as well as on comparing arterial and venous endothelial activity.

The magnitude of endothelium-dependent responses varies substantially within the venous system. It seems that venous smooth muscle with a spikelike mechanism of activation differs in sensitivity to EDRF/NO compared with venous smooth muscle with a tonic mechanism of activation (400).

Animal studies and experiments performed on human conduit veins (superficial hand veins and saphenous vein grafts) suggested that although NO activity can be stimulated by endothelium-dependent agonists, basal NO activity is absent, and therefore NO does not contribute to resting venous tone (400, 307, 392, 224, 426). However, recent studies, performed by Blackman et al. (2000) showed that human forearm capacitance veins exhibit both stimulated and basal NO activity, suggesting that endothelium-derived NO contributes not only to the regulation of venous tone but also to resting venous tone in healthy human subjects. This aspect was considered of practical importance in chronic heart failure, in which venous endothelial dysfunction and reduced NO activity might contribute to an increased venous tone (48).

The first *in vivo* study providing direct evidence for an endothelium-dependent relaxation of vascular smooth muscle in man was performed on superficial hand veins (87). Collier and Vallance showed that both, the removal of venous endothelium by a perfusion with distilled water and locally infused L-NMMA, produced a loss of the dilator action of acetylcholine, while the relaxing action of glyceryl trinitrate was not impaired (87, 88, 392). Moreover, the administration of L-NMMA increased arteriolar, but not venous tone (88, 392).

Several studies showed that relaxation of veins to vasoactive agents via NO is generally smaller than that of the arteries. For instance, the ability of some veins to release nitric oxide in response to acetylcholine is smaller than that of arteries, which can be attributed to several factors: a reduced ability of venous endothelial cells to release NO, a depressed responsiveness of venous smooth muscle to this relaxing factor, and the influences exerted by different arterial and venous flow velocity and oxygen tension (which are lower in veins compared to arteries)(424, 426, 335, 396). Liu et al. (2000) performed a direct measurement of NO release (by NO-sensitive electrode) in human saphenous veins and internal mammary arteries. The duration of acetylcholine- and bradykinin-induced NO release was longer in the IMA than in the SV, probably contributing to the superior long-term patency of arterial grafts (219).

In human arteries the NO release from the endothelium is able to suppress completely endothelin-induced contractions, whereas in human veins the maximum of this effect is much lower. This aspect may be important in pathological conditions associated with increased levels of endothelin-1 and in veins used as coronary bypass grafts (225).

Generally, arteries exhibit a more pronounced endothelium-dependent control and a different response profile to endogenous vasoactive substances than veins. For instance, compared to human mammary artery and gastroepiploic artery, in human saphenous veins, endothelium-dependent relaxing agents, such as acetylcholine, bradykinin, histamine and, serotonin caused weak dose-dependent relaxations or had no effect. Endothelium removal and pretreatment with a NOS inhibitor abolished the relaxations completely in saphenous vein but not in arterial preparations (3, 352, 424).

Pathophysiologic aspects

Venous graft spasm

In the last two decades, studies concerning venous endothelium were performed in order to assess the functions of veins grafts, especially saphenous veins. Vein grafts are capable to contract and relax to various vasoactive mediators and the response is dependent on the receptor profile on the endothelium and smooth muscle. An important aspect regards graft spasm in the perioperative or postoperative period, which increases the risk of morbidity and mortality after coronary revascularization. Into this context, and taking into account that most vasodilators act in an endothelium-dependent manner, the preservation of endothelium integrity and function seems to be extremely important in coronary artery bypass surgery. The functional integrity of the endothelium of the grafted vessel is influenced by numerous factors:

- technique of dissection. Experimental studies performed by Fabricius et al. (2000) showed that saphenous veins harvested by minimally invasive techniques have not shown an impaired reactivity of the endothelium compared with the conventional technique (132).
- use of dyes during coronary artery bypass and other vascular procedures concerning the orientation of the grafted vessel. Externally applied methylene blue reduced both endothelium-dependent and -

independent vasodilation of human saphenous veins. In veins exposed to methylene blue both internally and externally the results were similar but the magnitude of impairment greater (27).

- type of distending solution and distending pressure. Human saphenous vein segments are fully distended at perfusion pressures greater than 50 mm Hg, but can dynamically constrict to vasoactive agonists and regulate graft flow at intraluminal pressures as high as 90 mm Hg (340). Forceful distention, required to restore an adequate diameter for grafting, has been shown to damage the intima and media and may predispose to subsequent occlusion of the vein graft (180).
- composition and temperature of storage solutions. There are several studies that prove that the choice of perioperative storage solution may influence the vascular reactivity of the human saphenous vein (212, 213,13). There are studies which have found that the use of normal saline solution may cause important endothelial damage (213), whereas the experimental studies of Laufs et al (1995), suggested that Krebs Ringer solution and heparinized blood of the patient were not as efficient as NaCl in preserving saphenous vein endothelial function (212). A balanced salt solution, the University of Wisconsin solution produced attenuation of acetylcholine relaxation and temperature dependent increased reactivity of venous smooth muscle (13).
- availability of some factors necessary for endothelial nitric oxide production, such as L-arginine or tetrahydrobiopterin (437, 402).

Primary varicose veins

Several causes have been suggested for the pathogenesis of primary varicose veins of the lower limbs, including an intrinsic abnormality of the venous wall endothelium and smooth muscle, leading to dilation and subsequent venous insufficiency.

- In vitro studies, which explored the influence of the endothelium on smooth muscle contraction in normal and varicose veins, showed that in normal veins removal of endothelium significantly reduced the maximal response to noradrenaline (by 40%), whereas in varicose veins no significant reduction could be seen (382). These data suggested that in the human saphenous vein the endothelium has a contraction facilitating effect in response to stimulation with noradrenaline, while in varicose veins the endothelial-mediated enhancement of noradrenaline-induced vasoconstriction is reduced probably because of endothelial damage. However, these data were not supported by other studies; for instance, Lowell et al. (1992) reported no differences in contraction between saphenous vein rings with and without endothelium (222).

- Lowell et al. (1992) also noted that in varicose veins, both endothelium-dependent relaxations, produced by the calcium ionophore A23187, and endothelium-independent relaxations produced by nitric oxide were diminished (89.7% and 86.8%) compared with relaxations in controls (222). These data were confirmed by Schuller-Petrovic et al. (1997), which determined the intracellular accumulation of cGMP, as a measure of nitric oxide production and cGMP level in plasma from patients with primary varicosis and healthy volunteers (351). Although basal cGMP levels were similar, more cyclic GMP accumulated in response to histamine in cells from varicose saphenous veins than in cells from healthy veins. In plasma from patients with varicose veins, levels of cyclic GMP were higher than in healthy controls. All these results showed that in diseased veins the nitric oxide/cyclic GMP system is up regulated which may shift the balance of vasoactive factors towards vasodilatation and contribute to the development of primary varicosis.

Raynaud's disease

An impairment of endothelium-dependent vasodilation was reported in patients with Raynaud's disease. Bedarida et al (1993) showed that the dilation of superficial hand veins in response to bradykinin was reduced in patients with Raynaud's disease, compared to healthy subjects (33).

Nitrovasodilators

Many diseases of the cardiovascular system (hypertension, hypercholesterolemia, atherosclerosis) are associated with abnormalities of the L-arginine pathway, generating an important interest in the possibility that NO replacement therapy would be beneficial. Nitrovasodilators, including GTN and other organic nitrates, are prodrugs, which exert their pharmacodynamic action via a common pathway, the release of nitric oxide (136). The predominant acute hemodynamic effect of clinically useful nitrovasodilators is venodilation (86), although at higher doses, they also dilate arteries and arterioles. The venoselectivity of these NO-donating drugs presents both advantages (efficacy in heart failure and angina therapy) and disadvantages (postural hypotension, headache). The reasons for the relative venoselectivity of nitrovasodilators is not well understood. It was suggested that this property might be a consequence of preferential metabolism of these drugs by venous smooth muscle (181), but several studies support the idea that NO itself might be venoselective, perhaps as a result of up-regulation of guanylate cyclase in venous smooth muscle (392, 269, 229). More recently, Barba et al. (1999) suggested that soluble guanylate cyclase rather than G kinase (a cGMP-dependent protein kinase activated by cGMP, which mediates relaxation) or phosphodiesterase V (which terminates the action of cGMP), represents the second messenger pathway that induces the arteriovenous profile of NO donors (26). They also indicated that the ambient concentration of NO, with increased local NO might down-regulate the dilator response to NO donors.

Because of the reduced endothelial NO production in conduit vessels for coronary artery bypass grafting has been implicated in post-operative complications (e.g. spasm), the brief effects of existing NO donors limits their applicability to improve patency of graft vessels. Development of novel S-nitrosothiols with sustained effects in areas of endothelial damage might improve graft patency in the early post-operative period. For example, RIG200 and S-nitrosoglutathione (GSNO) had prolonged, NO-mediated effects in human saphenous vein (SV) and internal mammary artery (IMA), compared with glyceryl trinitrate (GTN) and sodium nitroprusside (SNP). Relaxation of phenylephrine-precontracted SV and IMA rings to GTN and SNP generally recovered fully on washout, while responses to RIG200 and GSNO were sustained during washout (30 min). Moreover, pretreatment (30 min) of saphenous veins with both S-nitrosothiols inhibited phenylephrine-induced contraction for >180 min, compared with <90 min for GTN (365).

Endothelium-derived hyperpolarizing factors (EDHFs)

Endothelium-dependent relaxations cannot be fully explained by the release of either NO or/and prostacyclin. Furthermore, endothelium-dependent responses, which are resistant to inhibitors of NO synthase and cyclooxygenase, are observed without an increase in intracellular levels of cyclic nucleotides (cGMP and cAMP) in the smooth muscle cells. Under these conditions, other unidentified substances, which hyperpolarize the underlying vascular smooth muscle cells, may contribute to endothelium-dependent relaxations. Hyperpolarization induces relaxation by reducing the open probability of voltage-dependent calcium channels, thereby decreasing calcium influx and lowering calcium levels in smooth muscle cells. Moreover, smooth muscle cells hyperpolarization may decrease the intracellular phosphatidylinositol turnover stimulated by agonist-induced receptor activation (139).

The contribution of EDHF response increases as the vessel size decreases both in animals and humans (390).

The vasodilator effect of EDHF is mediated by the activation of potassium channels on the vascular smooth muscle, the amplitude of this process being inversely related to the extracellular concentration of potassium ions (hyperpolarization disappcars in K^+ concentrations higher than 25 mM)(92, 93). The exact nature of the potassium channels involved may depend on the investigated species.

This phenomenon has been confirmed in various blood vessels from different species, including human veins.

- Liu et al (2000) measured EDHF-mediated hyperpolarization (by intracellular glass microelectrode) in response to acetylcholine and bradykinin, in both human internal mammary artery (IMA) and saphenous vein (SV). The resting membrane potential of the smooth muscle cells from the IMA was significantly higher than that in those from the SV. The EDHF-mediated hyperpolarization induced by acetylcholine and bradykinin was significantly greater in the artery than in the SV (219). The authors suggested that the differences concerning EDHF-mediated hyperpolarization together with the higher and longer duration of acetylcholine- and bradykinin-induced NO release in the IMA compared to the SV, may contribute to the superior long-term patency of IMA grafts. Similar experiments were performed by Yang and He (1997), who noted that EDHF might play a role in the regulation of human saphenous vein tone, hyperpolarization being abolished in case of surgical preparation (422).
- Hyperpolarization in response to substance P was demonstrated in human omental veins; the activation of high conductance Ca^{2+}-activated K^+-channel could be involved in this phenomenon (411).

It has been suggested that EDHF could be: a short-lived metabolite of arachidonic acid produced through the cytochrome P450 monooxygenase pathway, short-lived molecules such as carbon monoxide, hydroxyl radicals and hydrogen peroxide, NO or prostacyclin (207, 71,268, 92, 93).

The identification of EDHF and /or of the specific inhibitors of its synthesis will allow a better understanding of its physiological and pathophysiological roles.

Prostacyclin (PGI_2)

The effects of prostacyclin (PGI_2) were described in chapter 4, subhead 4.3.2.3.

4.3.4.2. Endothelium-Derived Vasoconstrictors

Endothelin-1

The endothelin family consists of three 21 amino-acid peptide isoforms (ET-1, ET-1, and ET-3), all with very similar structure. Endothelin-1 appears to be the predominant member of the family generated by endothelial cells, including venous ones, and also by vascular smooth muscle cells. ET-1 is cleaved from its precursor, bigET-1, by the action of one or more endothelin converting enzymes (ECE)(336). Two distinct ECEs have been cloned and sequenced. Human ECE-1 exists in two isoforms, which differ in the N-terminal sequence and are generated by alternative splicing of the same gene product (348, 354). A second enzyme, ECE-2, possesses approximately 60% homology with ECE-1, is a membrane-bound, phosphoramidon-sensitive metalloprotease, markedly different in its optimum pH (127).

The most important stimuli for ET-1 release are:

- physical factors, such as hypoxia and low shear stress;
- vasoactive substances (epinephrine, angiotensin II, vasopressin, bradykinin);
- growth factors (transforming growth factor β1);
- cytokines (IL-1)(336).

Atrial natriuretic peptide, nitric oxide and high shear stress potently inhibit ET-1 secretion (336).

Vascular smooth muscle cells explanted from adult vessels, including veins, secrete picomolar quantities of immunoreactive mature ET: saphenous vein 69.4±19.9 pM/10^6 cells, human umbilical vein 38.3±4.3 pM/10^6 cells (432). There are studies that showed that during inflammatory states, the vascular smooth muscle cells as well as, the endothelial cells, might be a site of significant ET-1 production in the blood vessel wall. For example, a 48 hours incubation with a mixture of cytokines (10 ng/ml TNFα, 1,000 U/ml interferon-γ, and 500 U/ml IL-1β) and lipopolysaccharide (10 micrograms/ml) markedly elevated the expression of mRNA for ET-1 and the release of ET-1 into a culture of vascular smooth muscle cells derived from human saphenous vein (421).

The existence of ECE in the different layers of the venous wall was investigated in several human veins.

- Maguire et al. (1999) demonstrated the presence of a phosphoramidon-sensitive ECE on the smooth muscle layer of the human umbilical vein, which can convert all forms of big ET to their mature biologically active forms (230).

- In human saphenous veins, Davenport et al. (1998) showed that immunoreactive ECE localized to the endothelium and infiltrating macrophages in vein grafts, but little or no immunoreactivity was detected within the media or proliferated smooth muscle of the occlusive lesion (110).
- Haynes et al. (1995) found that, in contrast to the situation in forearm resistance vessels, there was little or no local ECE activity in human hand veins (178, 179). In addition, Holm and Franco-Cereda (1996) showed that in all human grafts endothelin-1 content was higher than that of endothelin-3; the highest levels were found in the left anterior descending coronary artery, and the lowest in saphenous vein, and cephalic vein (187).
- The conversion of the precursor of ET-1 can occur also in human placental veins (contractions to big ET-1 were inhibited by phosphoramidon, an inhibitor of ECE). The output of big ET-1 in the vessel wall or from surrounding tissues in the placenta is thought to be involved in the regulation of venous tone in this organ (267).

Two types of ET-receptors are present in the vasculature: type A (ET_A) and type B (ET_B). The ET_A receptor is highly selective for ET-1, while the ET_B receptor is equally sensitive for all three endothelins. These two ET receptors mediate both antagonistic and synergistic effects. ET_A receptor is present on vascular smooth muscle cells and predominantly mediated contraction. The ET_B receptor is present both on endothelium, where mediated relaxation through nitric oxide and prostacyclin release, and also on vascular smooth muscle cells, where it mediates vasoconstriction. However, it is believed that ET_A receptors are the major receptor subtype involved in the vasoconstriction induced by ET-1. Thus, the net effect of ET-1 depends mainly on the relative density of ET_A receptors on SMC and endothelial ET_B receptors (336).

Several studies have characterized the distribution of ET receptor subtypes in human veins. These data are summarized in table 4.VII.

Table 4.VII. ET receptors in human veins

Vein	ET receptor subtype	References
central medullary vein	$ET_A : ET_B = 85:15$	109
saphenous vein	ET_A, ET_B; $ET_A > ET_B$ $ET_A : ET_B = 3:1$ in men $ET_A : ET_B = 1:1$ in women	419, 287, 109 130
hand veins	ET_A, ET_B; $ET_A > ET_B$	187, 373
placental veins	ET_B	267

Endothelin-1 was a potent and sustained constrictor of both resistance and capacitance forearm vessels, acting through both types of receptors (373, 178), but venoconstriction was mainly mediated by ET_A receptors (187). Endothelin-1 also potentiated sympathetically mediated hand venoconstriction, but only in hypertensive subjects (178).

The reactivity of human placental veins to ET was also investigated. Both ET-1 and ET-3 caused concentration-dependent contractions, the responses induced by ET-1 being greater than those evoked by ET-3 and were not significantly affected by BQ-123, a selective inhibitor of ET_A receptors. These findings indicated that ET-induced contractions are probably mediated in part by ET_B receptors (267).

Human saphenous vein contains both endothelin ET_A and ET_B contractile receptors (419, 287), but ET_B receptors represented less than 15% of the ET receptors (109). However, contractions mediated by ET_B-subtypes have smaller maximal responses than those mediated by the ET_A-subtypes (287). Ergul et al. (1998) noted gender differences in the expression of endothelin receptors, which might be an important factor to explain some differences in cardiovascular diseases reported in epidemiological studies. Vascular reactivity studies performed with venous rings reflected these differences: at lower doses of ET-1, when only a small fraction of receptors are occupied, there were no significant differences between ET-1-induced contraction in men and women; at saturating levels of ET-1 (1 μM), the contractile response in men was 2-fold higher than that observed in women. These differences were attributed to the greater number of ET_A receptors in men. After endothelium removal, only ET_A receptors were identified, and contractility studies yielded similar results with those performed using endothelium-intact preparations; these data suggest no involvement of ET_B receptor in ET-1-induced contraction in either men or women (130).

Several studies compared the effects of endothelins on large arteries and veins (Table 4.VIII).

Table 4.VIII. Comparative contractile effects of ET-1 in human arteries and veins

Human preparations	References
human forearm vein and internal mammary vein > internal mammary artery	82
saphenous vein > internal mammary artery	95
internal mammary vein > internal mammary artery	425, 225
uterine veins > uterine arteries	153
saphenous vein > gastroepiploic artery	247
saphenous veins > femoral, internal mammary, and gastroepiploic arteries	97, 98

Generally, these studies found that ET-1 is 3- to 10-fold more potent in veins than in arteries, including human preparations (336).

These in vitro observations were also confirmed in vivo. Infusion of 5 pmol/min. ET-1 into human forearm caused significantly more pronounced constriction of dorsal hand veins than arteries. Calcium channel blockers were effective in preventing ET-1 induced vasoconstriction only in arteries but not in hand veins, suggesting differences in signal transduction pathways (176).

Pathophysiologic aspects

Varicose veins

A possible involvement of endothelin-1 in the pathogenesis of primary varicose vein disease was reported. There are experimental data concerning the production of endothelin-1, the number of specific ET receptors and endothelin-1-induced contraction in healthy and varicose veins.

- Data concerning the production of ET-1 in normal and varicose saphenous veins are also available. Lowell et al (1992) found an increase of endothelin content in diseased venous tissue, although the elevation was not statistically significant; this increase was most evident in overtly varicose tributaries where the proportion of endothelin to total protein was more than seven times higher than that of control tissue (222). Mangiafico et al (1997) reported that plasma ET-1 level was higher in varicose than in normal saphenous veins, and it significantly increased in both groups after 10 minutes of venous stasis when compared with baseline. Absolute increase in plasma ET-1 was significantly greater in varicose than in normal saphenous veins (2.8±0.9 pmol/L vs 1.0±0.2 pmol/L)(235). These results suggested that increased local ET-1 release in varicose saphenous veins could be a marker for venous endothelial activation or damage and/or contribute to promote the morphologic alterations of the varicose vein wall by stimulating smooth muscle cell proliferation. On the other hand, increased ET-1 release may represent a compensatory response to maintain venous tone, counterbalancing the varicose venous relaxation and increasing preload in varicose patients via ET-1-induced venoconstriction. We must add that there are authors that reported no change in plasma endothelin from patients with varicose veins (351).

- By measuring receptor binding, Barber et al. (1997) found that the number, but not the affinity of ET-1 receptors was diminished in the varicose veins. They concluded that, as the veins become varicosed there is a specific loss of receptors for ET-1. Experiments using Sarafotoxin S6c (selective agonist for the endothelin-B receptor), receptor binding studies, and competitive inhibition of ^{125}I-endothelin-1 with endothelin-3 (for both A and B receptors) or sarafotoxin S6c (for B receptors only) suggested that the difference in receptor number might be attributable to differences in the endothelin-B receptor subtype (28).

An important reduction in ET-1 contractile activity in the diseased saphenous veins as compared with the control tissues was noted; concentration-dependent contractions in response to ET-1 in rings with and without endothelium did not differed in control and varicose veins (222, 30, 361, 28, 330).

Vein graft intimal hyperplasia

There are studies investigating the role of ET-1 in isolated human saphenous vein smooth muscle cells and in an organ culture of the human saphenous vein. These studies demonstrated that ET-1 is a mediator of intimal hyperplasia in human saphenous vein in vitro, therefore endothelin receptor antagonists may be of therapeutic value in the modulation of vein graft intimal hyperplasia (240).

Peripheral vasospasm/Raynaud's disease

The plasma level of endothelin-1 is locally increased during cooling but the net vasoconstrictor effect will be dependent on temperature effects on the vascular smooth muscle reactivity in response to the polypeptide. Bodelsson et al. (1997) showed that at 37°C, ET-1 induced a concentration-dependent contraction in the human hand, and cooling to 10°C did not alter precontraction achieved by endothelin-1 at 37°C in the human hand veins. The effect of cold was reversible and removal of the endothelium did not alter the response to cooling. The authors concluded that taking into account the maintained reactivity in response to endothelin-1 during cooling, the reported increase in endothelin-1 levels due to local cooling might contribute in the pathophysiology of peripheral vasospasm in humans (52).

Thromboxane A_2 and Prostaglandin H_2

The actions of TxA_2 and PGH_2 were presented in chapter 4, subhead 4.3.2.3.

4.4. OTHER FACTORS INVOLVED IN THE MODULATION OF VENOUS TONE

4.4.1. Reactive Oxygen Species (ROS)

A byproduct of normal aerobic metabolism is the generation of dangerously reactive intermediates of the reduction of O_2. These include O_2^-, H_2O_2, and HO and arise because of the predisposition of O_2 for univalent reductions (223).

ROS are generated mainly at sites of inflammation and injury; low levels of ROS can function as signaling molecules involved in regulation of fundamental cell activities; at higher concentration, these ROS and others that they can engender, threaten all cellular macromolecules, and defenses are needed (223). Among those known to date are:

- superoxide dismutases (SOD) which convert O_2^- into O_2 and H_2O_2;
- catalases, which dismute H_2O_2 into O_2 and H_2O;
- peroxidases, which reduce H_2O_2 into $2H_2O$ and ROOH into ROH and H_2O.

These defenses are aided by enzymes that repair or recycle oxidatively damaged nucleic acids and proteins (152, 223).

In endothelium and/or vascular smooth muscle, the major ROS-producing systems include (163):

- NADH/NADPH oxidases, which are considered the primary physiological producers of ROS in vascular tissue;
- xanthine oxidase, lipooxygenases;
- cyclooxygenase;
- P-450 monooxygenases;
- the enzymes of mitochondrial oxidative;
- NO synthase.

In addition to generation of intracellular O_2^- by these enzymes, extracellular stimuli including lipophilic substrates, membrane permeant oxidants (e.g., H_2O_2), cytokines, and growth factors may modulate cellular redox state (40, 420, 217). In human umbilical vein endothelial cells, depolarization was proved to be an important stimulus of superoxide production, involving a tyrosine phosphorylation-dependent translocation of the small G-protein Rac (366).

Just a few data concerning the effects of ROS on human venous smooth muscle and venous endothelial reactivity are available.

4.4.1.1. Superoxide Anion

Using selective microelectrodes, the release of superoxide anion by cultured human cord vein endothelial cells was demonstrated. Spontaneous O_2^--release from unstimulated cells was undetectable, whereas stimulation with interleukin-1beta caused a gradual increase in superoxide production, this process being suppressed in the presence of superoxide dismutase (316). Berry et al. (2000) showed that basal superoxide production was lower in human saphenous veins than in internal mammary arteries; the major sources of this radical were NAD(P)H oxidase and xanthine oxidase. Besides

endothelium, vascular smooth muscle cells and adventitial fibroblasts were shown to be additional sources of superoxide generation (41).

Venous walls, similar to arterial walls, contain relative high levels of extracellular superoxide dismutase (EC-SOD)(in both media and intima), and only relatively low levels of the cytosolic copper-and-zinc-containing SOD (CuZn-SOD), and the mitochondrial manganese-containing SOD (Mn-SOD). The EC-SOD concentration in the wall extracellular space seems high enough to efficiently suppress the putative pathological effects of the superoxide radical (374). In another study Berry et al. (2000) showed that the amount of Mn-SOD and CuZn-SOD was similar in arteries and veins (41), whereas Oury et al. (1996) reported that EC-SOD levels were significantly higher in human arteries than veins (299).

The importance of cytoprotective measures to preserve saphenous graft endothelial function was also underlined by Khansarinia et al. (2000). They showed that venous endothelial function (appreciated by prostacyclin production) following ischemia, was preserved in case of vein storage in superoxide dismutase and nitroglycerin; when used in combination, the beneficial effect was additive (204).

The major effects of superoxide anions in vascular tissue include: impairment of NO-vasodilation, promotion of smooth muscle proliferation and vessel restenosis after angioplasty (366). Furthermore, superoxide modulates vessel remodeling by the activation of matrix metalloproteinases and influences vascular smooth muscle migration and apoptosis (319, 376, 186).

Few data concerning superoxide action on venous tone are available.

- The influence of superoxide on the relaxation of human saphenous vein rings was suggested by Hamilton et al. (1997), which noted that treatment with SOD potentiated carbachol stimulated relaxation of these preparations (170).
- Differences in superoxide production between Caucasians and African-Americans might explain the higher incidence of cardiovascular diseases (hypertension, coronary artery disease) in the latter group. The production of superoxide in saphenous veins of African-Americans was nearly twice than in Caucasians, whereas SOD levels were similar in the two groups. Since superoxide can inactivate nitric oxide, an increased production of this anion might explain the reduced relaxing capacity of these veins (379).

4.4.1.2. Hydrogen Peroxide

Hydrogen peroxide is a reactive oxygen species that contracts or relaxes vascular smooth muscle, but the molecular basis of these effects remains obscure. In endothelium-intact and denuded isolated human placental veins, exposure to hydrogen peroxide produced vascular contraction that was eliminated or reversed to a modest relaxation by indomethacin, consistent with mediation by prostaglandins (291).

Pathophysiological aspects

Venous graft intimal hyperplasia

An important aspect refers to the involvement of superoxide in venous bypass graft intimal hyperplasia. West et al. (2000) reported that superoxide production was 3-fold higher in experimental vein grafts compared with ungrafted jugular veins, this increase being mediated by NAD(P)H oxidase. Moreover, undifferentiated intimal smooth muscle cells expressing the p22*phox* subunit of NAD(P)H oxidase appeared to be an important source of increased graft production of superoxide (418).

Varicose veins

The role of oxygen-derived free radicals in pathogenesis of varicose veins and the efficiency of antioxidant systems in the venous wall were reveled by several studies.

Because, oxygen-derived free radicals may increase destructive processes in the vein wall and lead to augmentation of varicose veins, Glowinski and Glowinski (2000) assessed the content of lipid peroxidation products in normal and varicose veins (157). The content of lipid peroxidation products (expressed by concentration of thiobarbituric acid-reactive substances/TBARS) in varicose vein wall presented no significant values compared to the normal vein, whereas in varicose veins with thrombophlebitis was significantly higher). The activity of CuZnSOD was significantly lower in varicose vein than in normal vein, and in the varicose vein with thrombophlebitis the activity remains lower. The content of free – SH groups was significantly lower in varicose veins comparing to normal veins, with no significant differences in varicose vein with superficial thrombophlebitis.

A significant decrease of superoxide dismutase (SOD) blood concentrations and an increase of total leukocyte count after venous stasis in patients with varicose veins and with venous hypertension, were reported by Ciuffetti et al. (78). Similar results were obtained by our group (22, 362); in patients with primary varicosities, after 30 minutes of standing position SOD blood concentration fell significantly. In addition, we were the first to report a significant increase in GSH plasmatic level. We considered that SOD decrease could represent a negative factor for the endothelial cell lining the vessel wall: during the following supine position, oxygen free radicals (especially superoxide) production will rise with damaging effects in the endothelium. Therefore, in varicose veins both plasmatic and intracellular levels of SOD seem to decrease during hypoxic conditions. This observation could be important because hydrogen peroxide also modulates the venous tone: lower concentrations of H_2O_2 (10^{-5} - 10^{-4} M) induced contractions of the human saphenous vein preparations, while higher doses caused irreversible venodilation (10^{-3} - 10^{-2} M); the contractile response induced by 10^{-4} M H_2O_2 was partially inhibited by N^G-nitro-l-arginine, indomethacin and/or nordihidroguaiaretic acid (Siska et al., unpublished data).

Furthermore, generation of superoxide anion, SOD activity, and NO formation were all lower in saphenous veins compared to mammary arteries, with a positive correlation between superoxide anion production and SOD activity ($r=0.70$; $p<0.05$) and NO release ($r=0.75$; $p<0.03$). Similar results were observed in case of pulmonary vessels: superoxide anion formation, SOD activity, and NO generation were found to be greater in pulmonary artery than in pulmonary vein segments. Two possible factors accounting for these differences include the fact that arteries, unlike veins, are exposed to pulsatile stretch and carry blood at higher pressure (347).

4.4.2. Cytokines

Just a few cytokines have been tested for their possible role in modulating vascular function, thus being involved in changing blood supply to inflamed or ischemic tissues.

Stem cell factor (maximal response with 1 mM), granulocyte colony-stimulating factor (0, 1 mM) and erythropoietin (1 mM) relaxed, while tumor necrosis factor alpha (0.1 mM), interleukin (IL) 6 (10 mM) and IL-10 (0.1 mM) induced contraction of arterial but not of venous segments (195).

The cytokines (maximal concentration tested was 1 mM) IL-3, IL-5, IL-13, macrophage colony-stimulating factor and granulocyte-macrophage colony-stimulating factor had no apparent effects on either arterial or venous tone. These vascular effects were endothelium-dependent, as denuded arteries did not respond to any cytokine. Immunochemical studies revealed the existence of specific receptors for the active cytokines on the arterial endothelium (195).

Some interleukins, such as IL-1β may influence venous contractility by inducing NO synthase. In isolated human mammary artery an L-arginine/NO pathway inducible by lipopolysaccharide, whereas in human saphenous veins, IL-1β or LPS treatment inhibited contraction by an unidentified system that was not dependent on NO synthase or guanylate cyclase activities (381). Beasley and McGuiggin (1995) reported that IL-1 markedly increased intracellular levels of the vasodilatory mediator, cAMP, in human saphenous vascular smooth muscle cells. IL-1-induced cAMP was associated with a marked increase in prostacyclin production, and was reversed by indomethacin and tranylcypromine, inhibitors of cyclooxygenase and PGI_2 synthetase respectively and methylene blue inhibited IL-1-induced increases in cAMP, suggesting that prostacyclin-dependent cAMP production is responsible for the vasodilatory effects of IL-1 in humans (31). However, a recent study of Bhagat et al. (1999) revealed that IL-1β increased basal NO-induced venodilation in vivo, this effect being sufficient to reduce the constrictor response to exogenous noradrenaline or sympathetic stimulation. The authors explained IL-1β action by its capacity to induce expression of GTP cyclohydrolase-1, leading to increased generation of BH_4 and activation of eNOS (43).

4.4.3. Fibrinogen

Normal plasmatic concentrations of fibrinogen (4-6 μM) are very important for hemostasis control, and not only.

Hicks et al. (1996) reported that physiological levels of fibrinogen might elicit vasomotor responses. Human saphenous vein rings showed an endothelium-dependent relaxation in response to fibrinogen (0-2 μm), this effect being reversed at higher concentrations of fibrinogen. Moreover, when intact veins were incubated with fibrinogen and the supernatant transferred to a venous denuded preparation, gradual relaxation occurred. These experimental data suggested the existence of specific receptors for fibrinogen on human saphenous vein endothelium, which mediate the above- mentioned vasomotor responses. The inhibition of fibrinogen-mediated relaxation by Ba^{2+}, TEA (non-selective inhibitors of K^+ channels) and gliclazide (selective inhibitor of ATP-sensitive K^+ channels) suggested that fibrinogen binding to specific endothelial receptors initiates the opening of ATP-sensitive K^+ channels. Preincubation with Fab1 fragment of a monoclonal antibody to human ICAM-1 induced a dose-dependent inhibition of the human saphenous vein relaxation in response to fibrinogen. The last experiments proved that fibrinogen binding to ICAM-1 on the human saphenous vein endothelium is followed by venodilation (183).

4.4.4. Thrombin

Hicks et al. (1996) showed that thrombin induces endothelium-dependent relaxation of human saphenous vein rings in a dose-dependent manner (183). The relaxing effect increased significantly after addition of fibrinogen. However, Yang et al. (1997) demonstrated different biological effects of thrombin on endothelium and smooth muscle of human internal mammary artery and saphenous vein (429). Although the endothelium and smooth muscle of both arteries and veins expressed the tethered thrombin receptor, activation of the receptor on the endothelium caused endothelium-dependent relaxations (due to release of NO and prostacyclin) in the arteries but not veins. Furthermore, thrombin induced contractions in intact veins but not arteries and induced a much more pronounced proliferation (in cultured smooth muscle cells) in the former than the latter. This was not due to the absence of the tethered thrombin receptor, because its presence could be demonstrated in venous endothelium by RT-PCR and immunohistology. Thus, the thrombin receptor in the SV endothelium-although expressed-is not linked to NO synthase or cyclooxygenase. In quiescent saphenous veins, thrombin caused marked contractions that were similar in preparations with or without endothelium, confirming that thrombin directly contracted saphenous veins smooth muscle cells (429).

4.4.5. Oxidized Low-Density Lipoprotein (ox-LDL)

It has been demonstrated that Ox-LDL impairs endothelium-dependent relaxation of vascular smooth muscle, and enhances agonist induced- vasoconstriction, which may contribute to an alteration of vascular reactivity in atherosclerosis. These aspects were also demonstrated for human saphenous veins. Zhao et al. (1996) showed that ox-LDL alters acetylcholine-induced endothelium-dependent relaxation and increases serotonin-induced endothelium-dependent contraction of human saphenous vein. In this preparation, endothelium-dependent relaxation may be mediated by both NO/EDRF and EDHF, therefore ox-LDL might also inhibit EDHF-mediated relaxation. Furthermore, hypercholesterolemia and ox-LDL increase superoxide production, which in turn might inactivate NO/EDRF (436).

4.4.6. Vasostatins

Beside catecholamines, chromogranin A (CGA), which belongs to a family of highly acidic proteins, is co-stored and co-released from the mammalian adrenal gland and occurs in nmolar concentrations in the human circulation (1, 2).

The collective term vasostatin(s) refers to N-terminal fragments (CGA1-76 and CGA1-113) of apparent molecular weights 7 to 22 kD, to indicate their vascular inhibitory effects (1, 2).

Preincubation with vasostatin, containing the N-terminal domain of CGA inhibited the contractile responses evoked by K^+, noradrenaline, or endothelin-1 in Ca^{2+}-free solution in human saphenous vein. The vasoinhibitory effects were not dependent on an intact endothelium. These data suggest a vascular role for the N-terminal domain of CGA, presumably by inhibiting Ca^{2+} release from intracellular stores in the human vein (1, 2, 15).

4.5. MYOGENIC CONTROL

Just a few investigators have studied stretch-induced myogenic tone in venous vessels, probably because venous intrinsic tone was considered to play just an insignificant role in overall ability of veins to regulate vascular capacity (394).

In vivo and in vitro studies performed in rats showed that acute changes in pressure load can cause a sustained and reversible depolarization of venous smooth muscle cells, which was coupled to active strain and stress generation in the vein wall. This myogenic response was shown to be capable of a 30% regulation of venous capacity in the rat saphenous vein (271, 272, 273). Moderate, chronic increase in hindlimb venous pressure was followed by a significant hyperpolarization of the venous smooth muscle and an increase in total capacity (271)

In humans, myogenic tone was demonstrated in facial (250) and saphenous veins (38, 245).

Human saphenous veins presented an active myogenic capacity response that was of significant magnitude to potentially aid in the regulation of cardiac output. Myogenic tone of human saphenous veins was investigated after both axial stretching and circumferential deformation:

- Stepwise elevation of intraluminal pressure from 2 to 20 mmHg caused an active myogenic response, which was calcium-dependent and endothelium-independent. This alteration in myogenic tone induced in over 120% change in lumen capacity. Human saphenous veins also showed an eight-times more sensitivity to norepinephrine, compared to canine femoral vein, suggesting that human veins may be adapted to the increased hydrostatic load due to orthostatic position (38).
- After 90 minutes of pulsatile arterial perfusion (mean arterial pressure 100mmHg), the mean maximum tension induced by KCl, phenylephrine and serotonin significantly increased, this response being endothelium-independent. The Rho kinase pathway seemed to mediate the increased sensitivity to vasoconstrictors, because the selective Rho kinase inhibitor Y-27632 abrogated these changes (245).

Data concerning the cellular mechanisms involved in venous myogenic response are scarce, compared to those regarding arterial myogenic tone. It was assumed that intraluminal pressure might activate stretch-sensitive cationic channels in vascular smooth muscle cells; such channels were identified in human umbilical vein endothelial cells, but not in saphenous veins (282, 245).

4.6. PHARMACOLOGICAL ASPECTS

4.6.1. Venodilator Drugs

The effects of some venodilators in different venous territories, such as *calcium antagonists, nitrovasodilators, ACE inhibitors* were presented earlier in this chapter.

Endothelin antagonists are new compounds, which specifically interfere with endothelin receptors. Certain of these substances are orally active (for instance, bosentan, SB209670, and PD142893. In human skin microcirculation and the forearm circulation, ET_A-receptor antagonists increased blood flow and inhibited endothelin-induced constriction, demonstrating the existence of endothelin-induced vascular tone in man (81, 417, 177). However, just phase I of clinical studies using such compounds was assessed. There are no present data regarding the benefice of these classes of vasodilators in venous disorders.

4.6.2. Venotonic Drugs

Standard treatment for varicose veins is mechanical compression, sclerotherapy, or surgery. Additionally, in order to improve microcirculation, capillary flow, and vascular tone, and strengthen connective tissue of the perivascular amorphous substrate, venotonic drugs may be useful. Early intervention with such conservative therapies may prevent time-consuming and expensive complications of varicose veins.

The actions of some of the most well known venotonic agents are summarized in table 4.IX.

Table 4. IX. The major effects of some venotonic drugs

Venotonic drugs	Effects	References
Aesculus hippocastanum (Horse chestnut)	- increases venous tone - inhibits hyaluronidase and elastase, retarding breakdown of the proteoglycans (due to escin); - inhibits the production, release, or activity of some of the various chemotactic factors involved in this inflammatory process - reduces enzymatic and nonenzymatic lipid peroxidation and ensuing subcellular damage	165 133 59 324, 297
Ruscus aculeatus (Butcher's Broom)	- increases venous tone (active component = ruscogenin) - decreases capillary filtration rate	61, 133, 338
Centella Asiatica (Gotu Kola)	- improves vascular tone - enhances connective tissue integrity, elevates antioxidant levels in wound healing, and improves capillary permeability	6, 356, 35, 65
Bioflavonoids: Diosmin, Oligomeric proanthocyanidin complexes, Hesperidin	- exhibit phlebotonic activity, vasculoprotective effects, and antagonism of the biochemical mediators of inflammation	94

GENERAL CONCLUSIONS

Studies dealing with veins almost always have been neglected, probably because the physiological and pathophysiological importance of the venous system was underestimated. However, most of the studies (in vivo and/or in vitro) were performed on animal veins, and just a small part of the available experimental data concerned human veins, especially large ones; the control processes in the venular side need further exploration. Beside this, the major part of the investigations was performed in vitro, in vivo studies being performed mainly in case of human hand veins. At the present state of knowledge, it is possible to conclude that the regulation of human venous tone is very complex. Innervation, hormones, metabolic factors, ionic environment, humoral factors, endothelium-derived vasoactive factors, and even reactive oxygen species and cytokines act directly on venous smooth muscle and endothelial cells. Moreover, almost all factors involved in venous control are interrelated, stimulating and/or inhibiting the synthesis and/or the release of other vasoactive agents. In addition, to their vasoconstrictor or vasodilator actions, some of these factors may be involved in other important physiological mechanisms, such as vascular hypertrophy, intimal hyperplasia, and venular permeability. This chapter summarized the experimental data performed on human large veins, trying to deal mainly with the physiological factors involved in the control of venous tone, but also pointing some pathophysiological aspects (such as venous graft pathology or varicose veins). Nevertheless, the new investigation techniques developed in the last years will probably reveal new aspects of venous regulation, clarifying many of the mechanisms debated in this review.

REFERENCES

1. Aardal S, Helle KB. The vasoinhibitory activity of bovine chromogranin A fragment (vasostatin) and its independence of extracellular calcium in isolated segments of human blood vessels. Regul Pept 1992; 41: 9-18
2. Aardal S, Helle KB, Elsayed S, Reed RK, Serck-Hanssen G. Vasostatins, comprising the N-terminal domain of chromogranin A, suppress tension in isolated human blood vessel segments. J Neuroendocrinol 1993; 5: 405-412
3. Akar F, Uydes BS, Ayrancioiglu K, Yener A, Aslamaci S, Arsan M, Tioriuner A, Kanzik I. Endothelial function of human gastroepiploic artery in comparison with saphenous vein. Cardiovasc Res 1994; 28: 500-504
4. Albino-Taxeira A, Azevedo I, Branco D, Osswald W, Purine agonists prevent trophic changes caused by sympathetic denervation, Eur J Pharmacol 1990; 179: 141-149
5. Aldasoro M, Medina P, Vila JM, Otero E, Martinez-Leon JB, Lluch S. Endothelium-dependent relaxation of human saphenous veins in response to vasopressin and desmopressin. J Vasc Surg 1997; 25: 696-703
6. Allegra C, Pollari G, Criscuolo A. Centella asiatica extract in venous disorders of the lower limbs. Comparative clinico-instrumental studies with a placebo. Clin Ter 1981; 99: 507-513. [Article in Italian]
7. Allen JC, Kahn AM, Navran S. Na^+-K^+-ATP-ase in vascular smooth muscle. Am J Physiol 1986; 250: C536-540
8. Allen SP, Chester AH, Piper PJ, Sampson AP, Akl ES, Yacoub MH, Effects of leukotrienes C4 and D4 on human isolated saphenous veins. Br J Clin Pharmacol 1992; 34: 409-414
9. Allen SP, Chester AH, Dashwood MR, Tadjkarimi S, Piper PJ, Yacoub MH. Preferential vasoconstriction to cysteinyl leukotrienes in the human saphenous vein compared with the internal mammary artery. Implications for graft performance. Circulation 1994; 90: 515-524
10. Altura BM, Altura BT. Magnesium ions and contraction of vascular smooth muscles-relationship to some vascular diseases. Federation Proc 1981: 40: 2672-2679
11. Altura BM, Altura BT, Carella A. Magnesium deficiency-induced spasma of umbilical vessels. Relationship to preeclampsia, hypertension, and growth retardation. Science Wash DC 1983; 221: 376-378
12. Altura BM, Altura BT. Interactions of Mg and K on blood vessels-aspects in view of hypertension. Magnesium 1984; 3: 175-194
13. Anastasiou N, Allen S, Paniagua R, Chester A, Yacoub M. Altered endothelial and smooth muscle cell reactivity caused by University of Wisconsin preservation solution in human saphenous vein. J Vasc Surg 1997; 25: 713-721
14. Ando SI, Imaizumi T, Harada S, Hirooka Y, Takeshita A. Atrial natriuretic peptide increases human capillary filtration and venous distensibility. J Hypertension 1992; 10: 451-457
15. Angeletti RH, Aardal S, Serck-Hanssen G, Gee P, Helle KB. Vasoinhibitory activity of synthetic peptides from the amino terminus of chromogranin A. Acta Physiol Scand 1994; 152: 11-19
16. Arnal JF, Tack I, Besombres JP, Pipy B, Negre-Salvayre A. Nitric oxide and superoxide anion production during endothelial cell proliferation, Am J Physiol 1996; 271: C1521-1526

17. Arner M, Högestatt ED, Actions of some vasodilators on isolated human hand veins. Acta Physiol Scand 1987; 130: 671-677
18. Arner M, Högestatt ED. Endothelium-dependent relaxation and effects of prostacyclin, endothelin, and platelet-activating factor in human hand veins and arteries. Acta Physiol Scand 1991; 142: 165-172
19. Arner M, Hogestatt ED, Uski TK. Characterization of contraction-mediating prostanoid receptors in human hand veins: effects of the thromboxane receptor antagonists BM13, 505 and AH23848, Acta Physiol Scand 1991; 141: 79-86
20. Arner M, Uski T, Hogestatt ED, Arner M, Uski T, Hogestatt ED. Endothelium dependence of prostanoid-induced relaxation in human hand veins. Acta Physiol Scand 1994; 150: 267-72
21. Arnold JMO, Lo IK, Response of superficial dorsal hand veins in normal subjects to locally infused angiotensin II (AII) and noradrenaline (NA), Clin Pharmacol Ther 1993; 53: 139 (abstract)
22. Avram J, Siska I-R, Măties R, Avram R, Crîsnic D. Les taux de superoxide dismutase et de glutathion dans le sang des saphenes variqueuses. Phlebologie, 1999; 52: 155-162
23. Baker VL, Chao VA, Murai JT, Zaloudek CJ, Taylor RN. Human umbilical vessels and cultured umbilical vein endothelial and smooth muscle cells lack detectable protein and mRNA encoding estrogen receptors. J Soc Gynecol Investig 1997; 4: 316-324
24. Banks M, Wei CM, Kim CH, Burnett JC si Miller VM. Mechanism of relaxations to C-type natriuretic peptide in veins. Am J Physiol 1996; 217: H1907-1911
25. Bar RS, Peacock ML, Spanheimer RG, Veenstra R, Hoak JC. Differential binding of insulin to human arterial and venous endothelial cells in primary culture. Diabetes 1980; 29: 991-995
26. Barba G, Mullen MJ, Donald A, MacAllister RJ. Determinants of the response of human blood vessels to nitric oxide donors in vivo. J Pharmacol Exp Ther. 1999; 289: 1662-1668.
27. Barber DA, Rubin JW, Zumbro GL, Tackett RL. The use of methylene blue as an extravascular surgical marker impairs vascular responses of human saphenous vein. J Thorac Cardiovasc Surg. 1995; 109: 21-29
28. Barber DA, Wang X, Gloviczki P, Miller VM. Characterization of endothelin receptors in human varicose veins. J Vasc Surg 1997; 26: 61-69
29. Barker JE, Anderson J, Treasure T, Piper PJ, Influence of endothelium and surgical preparation on responses of human saphenous vein and internal thoracic artery to angiotensin II, Br J Clin Pharmacol 1994; 38:57-62
30. Bax W, Bos E, Saxena PR. Heterogeneity of endothelin/sarafotoxin receptors mediating contraction of the human isolated saphenous vein. Eur J Pharmacol 1993; 239: 267-268
31. Beasley D, McGuiggin ME. Interleukin 1 induces prostacyclin-dependent increases in cyclic AMP production and does not affect cyclic GMP production in human vascular smooth muscle cells. Cytokine 1995; 7: 417-426
32. Beattie DK, Gosling M, Davies AH, Powell JT. The effects of potassium channel openers on saphenous vein exposed to arterial flow. Eur J Vasc Endovasc Surg 1998;15: 244-249
33. Bedarida GV, Kim D, Blaskke TF, Hoffman BB. Venodilation in Raynaud's disease. Lancet 1993; 342: 1451-1454
34. Beech DJ, Bolton TB. A voltage-dependent outward current with fast kinetics in single smooth muscle cells isolated from rabbit portal vein. J Physiol Lond 1989; 412: 397-414

35. Belcaro GV, Grimaldi R, Guidi G. Improvement of capillary permeability in patients with venous hypertension after treatment with TTFCA. Angiology 1990; 41: 533-540.
36. Bell D, McDermott BJ. Calcitonin Gene-related Peptide in the Cardiovascular System: Characterization of Receptor populations and Their (Patho) Physiological Significance. Pharm Rev 1996; 48: 254-282
37. Belz GG, Berrmann J, Schloos J, KleinBloesem CH. The effect of oral clazapril and prazosin on the constrictor effects of locally infused angiotensin I and noradrenaline in human hand veins. Br J Clin Pharmacol 1989; 28: 608-611
38. Berczi V, Greene AS, Dornyei G, Csengodi J, Hodi G, Kadar A, Monos E. Venous myogenic tone: studies in human and canine vessels. Am J Physiol 1992; 263: H315-320.
39. Bergqvist A, Bergqvist D, Fernö M. Estrogen and progesterone receptors in vessel walls. Biochemical and immunochemical assays. Acta Obstet Gynecol Scand 1993; 72:10-16
40. Berk BC. Redox signals that regulate the vascular response to injury. Thromb Haemost 1999; 82: 810-817
41. Berry C, Hamilton CA, Brosnan J, Magill FG, Berg GA, McMurray JJV, Dominczak AF. Investigation into the sources of superoxide in human blood vessels. Angiotensin II increases superoxide production in human internal mammary arteries. Circulation 2000; 101: 2206-2212
42. Berti F, Rossoni G, Biasi G, Buschi A, Mandelli V, Tondo C. Defibrotide, by enhancing prostacyclin generation, prevents endothelin-1 induced contraction in human saphenous veins. Prostaglandins 1990; 40: 337-350
43. Bhagat K, Hingorani AD, Palacios M, Charles IG, Vallance P. Cytokine-induced venodilation in humans in vivo: e NOS masquerading as iNOS. Cardiovasc Res 1999; 41: 754-764
44. Bhoola KD, Figueroa CD, Worthy K. Bioregulation of kinins: kallikreins, kininogens, and kininases. Pharmacol Rev 1992; 44: 1-80
45. Biagi G, Coccheri S, Lapilli A, Granso F, Bizarri M, Zendron R, Piccinni L. Prostacyclin and thromboxane production in human varicose saphenous vein. Thromb Haemostasis 1987; 58: 158 (abstract)
46. Biagi G, Lapilli A, Zendron R, Piccinni L, Coccheri S. Prostanoid production in varicose veins: evidence for decreased prostacyclin with increase thromboxane A_2 and prostaglandin E_2 formation. Angiology 1988; 39: 1036-1042
47. Bishop-Bailey D, Pepper JR, Larkin SW, Mitchell JA. Differential induction of cyclooxigenase-2 in human arterial and venous smooth muscle. Role of endogenous prostanoids. Arterioscler Thromb Vasc Biol 1998; 18: 1655-1661
48. Blackman DJ, Morris-Thurgood JA, Atherton JJ, Ellis GR, Anderson RA, Cockcroft JR, Frenneaux MP. Endothelium-derived nitric oxide contributes to the regulation of venous tone in humans. Circulation 2000; 101: 165-170
49. Blaustein MP, Hamlyn JM. Sodium transport inhibition, cell calcium and hypertension. The natriuretic hormone (Na^+-Ca^{2+} exchange) hypertension hypothesis. Am J Med 1984; 77: 45-49
50. Blochl-Daum B, Vierhapper H, Eichler HG, Waldhausl W. Endothelin-induced venoconstriction is unaffected by type 2-diabetes: in vivo effect of histamine on the endothelin action on veins. Arch Int Pharmacodyn Ther 1992; 316: 90-96
51. Bo X, Sexton A, Xiang Z, Nori SL, Burnstock G. Pharmacological and histochemical evidence for P2X receptors in human umbilical vessels. Eur J Pharmacol 1998;353: 59-65

52. Bodelsson M, Tornebrandt K, Arneklo-Nobin B. Effect of cooling on vascular smooth muscle response to endothelin-1 in human and rat veins. Int Angiol 1997; 16: 262-268
53. Bodelsson G, Sandstrom K, Wallerstedt SM, Hidestal J, Tornebrandt K, Bodelsson M. Effects of propofol on substance P-induced relaxation in isolated human omental arteries and veins. Eur J Anaesthesiol 2000; 17: 720-728
54. Bodmer CW, Patrick AW, How TV, Williams G. Exaggerated sensitivity to NE-induced vasoconstriction in IDDM patients with microalbuminuria. Possible etiology and diagnostic implications. Diabetes 1992; 41: 209-214
55. Bonner G, Preis S, Schunk U, Wagmann M, Chrosch R, Toussaint C. Effect of bradykinin on arteries and veins in systemic and pulmonary circulation. J Cardiovasc Pharmacol 1992; 20(suppl.9): S21-27
56. Borchard U. Calcium Antagonists in Comparison: View of the Pharmacologist. J Cardiovasc Pharmacol 1994; 24: S85-91
57. Borland JA, Chester AH, Crabbe S, Parkerson JB, Catravas JD, Yacoub MH. Differential action of angiotensin II and activity of angiotensin-converting enzyme in human bypass grafts. J Thorac Cardiovasc Surg 1998; 116: 206-212
58. Borland JA, Chester AH, Morrison KA, Yacoub MH. Alternative pathways of angiotensin II production in the human saphenous vein. Br J Pharmacol 1998; 125: 423-428
59. Bougelet C, Roland IH, Ninane N, Amould T, Remachle J, Michiels C. Effect of aescine on hypoxia-induced neutrophil adherence to umbilical vein endothelium. Eur J Pharmacol. 1998; 345: 89-95.
60. Boura AL, Gude NM, King RG, Mak KK, Walters WA. Characterization of thromboxane A2 receptors in the human fetal placental vessels and umbilical vein. Clin Exp Pharmacol Physiol 1986;13: 83-86.
61. Bouskela E, Cyrino FZ, Marcelon G. Possible mechanisms for the inhibitory effect of Ruscus extract on increased microvascular permeability induced by histamine in hamster cheek pouch. J Cardiovasc Pharmacol 1994; 24: 281-285.
62. Branco D, Caramona M, Araujo D, Osswald W. The role of monoamine oxidase in the metabolism of exogenous noradrenaline by the human saphenous vein. Fundam Clin Pharmacol 1992; 6: 145-152
63. Brawley L, MacDonald S, Shaw AM. Role of endothelium in classical and atypical β-adrenoceptor mediated vasorelaxation in rat isolated aorta. Br. J Pharmacol 1998; 122: 395-402
64. Brayden JE. Potassium channels in vascular smooth muscle. Clin Exp Pharmacol Physiol 1996; 23: 1069-1076
65. Brinkhaus B, Lindner M, Schuppan D, Hahn EG. Chemical, pharmacological and clinical profile of the East Asian medical plant Centella asiatica. Phytomedicine 2000; 7: 427-448.
66. Brock TA, Brugnara C, Canessa M, Gimbrone MA. Bradykinin and vasopressin stimulate Na+-K+-Cl- cotransport in cultured endothelial cells. Am J Physiol 1986; 250: C888-895
67. Bryan LJ, Cole JJ, O'Donell SR, Wanstall JC. A study designed to explore the hypothesis that beta-1 adrenoceptors are "innervated" receptors and beta-2 adrenoceptors are "hormobal" receptors. J Pharmacol Exp Ther 1981; 216: 395-400
68. Burroughs AK, McCormick PA. Randomized trial for variceal bleeding. Z Gastroenterol 1988; 26: 24-35
69. Busse R, Mulsch A, Fleming I, Hecker M. Mechanisms of nitric oxide release from the vascular endothelium. Circulation 1993; 87: V18-25

70. Calcagno D, Bei M, Ross SA, Klein A, Foegh ML. Effects of estrogen on vein grafts. J Cardiovasc Surg 1992; 33: 579-584
71. Campbell WB, Gebremedhin D, Pratt PF, Harder DR. Idendification of epoxyeicosatrienoic acids as endothelium-derived hyperpolarizing factor. Circ Res 1996; 78: 415-423
72. Cario-Toumaniantz C, Loirand G, Ladoux A, Pacaud P. P2X7 receptor activation-induced contraction and lysis in human saphenous vein smooth muscle. Circ Res 1998; 27; 83: 196-203
73. Carter AJ, Bevan JA, Hanley SP, Morgan WE, Turner DR. A comparison of human pulmonary arterial and venous prostacyclin and thromboxane synthesis. Effect of a thromboxane synthase inhibitor. Thromb Haemostasis 1984; 51: 257-260
74. Caulfield MP, Birdsall NJ. International Union of Pharmacology. XVII. Classification of Muscarinic Acetylcholine Receptors. Pharm Rev 1998; 50: 279-288
75. Chaikouni A, Crawford FA, Kochel PJ, Olanoff LS, Haluschka PV. Human internal mammary artery produces more prostacyclin than saphenous vein. J Thorac Cardiovasc Surg 1986; 92: 88-91
76. Chester AH, O'Neil GS, Tadjakarimi S, Borland JA, Yacoub MH. Effect of peri-operative storage solution on the vascular reactivity of the human saphenous vein. Eur J Cardiothorac Surg 1993; 7: 399-404
77. Chiavarelli M, Fabi F, Stati T, Chiavarelli R, Del Basso P. Effects of cardioplegic solution and their components on human saphenous vein contractility. Ann Thorac Surg 1992; 53: 455-459
78. Ciuffetti G, Mannarino E, Paltriccia R, Malagigi V, Sergi F, Paulisch P, Pasqualini L, Lupattelli G. Leucocyte activity in chronic venous insufficiency. Int Angiol 1994; 13: 312-316
79. Civantos Calzada B, Aleixandre de Artinano A. Alpha-adrenoceptor subtypes, Pharmacol Res 2001; 44: 195-208
80. Clapp LH, Tinker A. Potassium channels in the vasculature. Curr Opin Nephrol Hypertension 1988; 7: 91-98
81. Clozel M, Breu V, Burri K. Pathophysiologic role of endothelin reversed by the first orally active endothelin receptor antagonist. Nature 1993; 365: 759-761
82. Cocks TM, Faulkner LN, Sudhir K, Angus J. Reactivity of endothelin 1 on human and canine large veins compared with large arteries in vitro. Eur J Pharmacol 1989; 171: 17-24
83. Cohen J. Insufficience veineuse et contraception orale. Rev Fr Gynecol Obstet 1991; 86: 187-189
84. Coleman RA, Smith WL, Narumyia S. VIIIth International Union of Pharmacology Classification of Prostanoid Receptors: Properties, Distribution, and Structure of the Receptors and their Subtypes. Pharmacol Rev 1994; 46: 206-224
85. Collier JG, Nachev C, Robinson BF. Effect of catecholamines and other vasoactive substances on superficial hand veins, Clin Sci 1972; 43: 455-467
86. Collier J, Lorge RE, Robinson BF. Comparison of effects of tolmexoside (RX71107), diazoxide, hydralazine, prazosin, glyceriltrinitrate and sodium nitroprusside on forearm arteries and dorsal hand veins in man. Br J Pharmacol 1978; 5: 35-44
87. Collier J, Vallance P. Endothelium-derived relaxing factor is an endogenous vasodilator in man. Br J Pharmacol 1989, 97: 639-641
88. Collier J, Vallance P. L-NMMA increase arteriolar but not venous tone in humans: The mechansim appears to be independent of sympathetic tone, J Cardiovasc Pharmacol 1991; 17(Suppl.3): S182-185

89. Collins P, Meale CM, Rosano MC. Oestrogen as a calcium channel blocker. Eur Heart J 1996; 17(suppl D): 27-31
90. Communi D, Parmentier M, Boeynaems JM. Les recepteurs P2: une famille en pleine expansion. MedSci 1996; 12: 614-619
91. Cordi AA, Lacoste JM, Descombes JJ, Courchay C, Vanhoutte PM, Laubie M, Verbeuren TJ. Design, synthesis, and structure-activity relationships of a new series of alpha-adrenergic agonists: spiro [(1,3 – diazacyclopent – 1 - ene) - 5,2 '- (1', 2', 3', 4 '- tetrahydronaphthalene)]. J Med Chem 1995; 38: 4056-4069
92. Corriu C, Feletou M, Canet E, Vanhoutte PM. Endothelium-derived factors and hypepolarizations of isolated carotid artery of the guinea pig. Br J Pharmacol 1996; 119: 959-964
93. Corriu C, Feletou M, Canet E, Vanhoutte PM. Inhibitors of the cytochrome P-450monooxygenase and endothelium-dependent hyperpolarizations in the guinea pig isolated carotid artery. Br J Pharmacol 1996;107: 607-610
94. Cospite M. Double blind, placebo-controlled evaluation of clinical activity and safety of Daflon 500 mg in the treatment of acute hemorrhoids. Angiology 1994; 45: 566-573.
95. Costello KB, Stewart DJ, Baffour R. Endothelin is a potent constrictor of human vessels used in coronary revascularization surgery. Eur J Pharmacol 1990; 186: 311-314
96. Cox RH, Katzka D, Morad M. Characteristics of calcium currents in rabbit portal vein myocytes. Am J Physiol 1992; 263: H453-463
97. Cracowski JL, Stanke-Labesque F, Sessa C, Hunt M, Chavanon O, Devillier P, Bessard G. Functional comparison of the human isolated femoral artery, internal mammary artery, gastroepiploic artery, and saphenous vein. Can J Physiol Pharmacol 1999; 77: 770-776
98. Cracowski JL, Stanke-Labesque F, Chavanon O, Corompt E, Veitl S, Blin D, Bessard G, Devillier P. Thromboxane A(2) modulates cyclic AMP relaxation and production in human internal mammary artery. Eur J Pharmacol 2000; 387: 295-302
99. Craven PA, DeRubertis FR. Restoration of the responsiveness of purified guanylate cyclase to nitrosoguanidine, nitric oxide, and related activators by heme and hemeproteins. Evidence for involvement of the paramagnetic nitrosyl-heme complex in enzyme activation. J Biol Chem. 1978; 253: 8433-8443.
100. Creager MA, Liang C, Coffman JD. Beta-adrenergic mediated vasodilator response to insulin in the human forearm. J Pharmacol Exp Ther 1985; 235: 709-714
101. Crossman D, McEwan J, MacDermot J, MacIntyre I, Dollery CT. Human calcitonin gene-related peptide activates adenylate cyclase and releases prostacyclin from human umbilical vein endothelial cells. Br J Pharmacol. 1987; 92: 695-701.
102. Crowe R, Burnstock G, Dickinson IK, Pryor JP. The human penis: an unusual penetration of NPY-immunoreactive nerves within the medial muscle coat of the deep dorsal vein. J Urol 1991; 145: 1292-1296
103. Cruz MA, Gonzalez C, Sepulveda WH, Rudolph MI. Effect of histamine on human placental chorionic veins: interaction with serotonin. Pharmacology 1991; 42: 86-90.
104. Cruz MA, Gallardo V, Miguel P, Carrasco G, Gonzalez C. Serotonin-induced vasoconstriction is mediated by thromboxane release and action in the human fetal-placental circulation. Placenta 1997; 18: 197-204.
105. Curtis SB, Hewitt J, Yakubovitz S, Anzarut A, Hsiang YN, Buchan AM. Somatostatin receptor subtype expression and function in human vascular tissue. Am J Physiol Heart Circ Physiol 2000; 278: H1815-1822

106. Daly RN, Hieble JP. Neuropeptide Y modulates adrenergic neurotransmission by an endothelium dependent mechanism. Eur J Pharmacol. 1987; 138: 445-446.
107. Danesi R, Del Tacca M. The effects of the somatostatin analog octreotide on angiogenesis in vitro. Metabolism 1996; 45(8 Suppl 1): 49-50
108. Danser JAH. Local Renin-angiotensin systems. Moll Cell Biochem 1996; 157: 211-216
109. Davenport AP, Kuc RE, Maguire JJ, Harland SP. ETA receptors predominate in the human vasculature and mediate constriction. J Cardiovasc Pharmacol 1995; 26 (Suppl 3): S265-267
110. Davenport AP, Kuc RE, Mockridge JW. Endothelin-converting enzyme in the human vasculature: evidence for differential conversion of big endothelin-3 by endothelial and smooth-muscle cells. J Cardiovasc Pharmacol 1998; 83: S1-3
111. Dawes M, Chowienczyk PJ, Ritter JM. Effects of inhibition of the L-arginine/nitric oxide pathway on vasodilation caused by β-adrenergic agonists in human forearm. Circulation 1997; 95: 2293-2297
112. De Moura RS, Jasbik W. Actions of cromakalim in isolated human saphenous vein. Hypertension 1992; 19(2 Suppl):II121-124
113. Dhein S, Reiss N, Gerwin R, Borowski A, Korb H, Klaus W, de Vivie ER. Endothelial function and contractility of human vena saphena magna prepared for aortocoronary bypass grafting. Thorac Cardiovasc Surg 1991; 39: 66-69
114. Diehl NL, Shreeve SM. Identification of the alpha 1c-adrenoceptor in rabbit arteries and the human saphenous vein using the polymerase chain reaction. Eur J Pharmacol 1994; 268: 393-398
115. Dimech J, Feniuk W, Latimer RD, Humphrey PP. Somatostatin-induced contraction of human isolated saphenous vein involves sst2 receptor-mediated activation of L-type calcium channels. J Cardiovasc Pharmacol 1995; 26: 721-728
116. Docherty JR. Aging and vasoconstrictor responses mediated by alpha 2-adrenoceptors and 5-HT1 and 5-HT2 receptors. Ann N Y Acad Sci 1994; 717: 282-292
117. Docherty JR. Subtypes of functional alpha1- and alpha2-adrenoceptors. Eur J Pharmacol. 1998; 361: 1-15.
118. Drouet L, Baudin B, Baumann FC, Caen JP. Serum angiotensin-converting enzyme. An endothelial cell marker. J Lab Clin Med 1988; 112: 450-457
119. Dubiak GR, El-Moatassim C. Signal transduction via P2-purinergic receptors for extracellular ATP and other nucleotides. Am J Physiol 1993; 265: C577-606
120. Dzau VJ, Re R., Tissue Angiotensin System in Cardiovascular Medicine. A Paradigm Shift? Circulation 1994; 89: 493-498
121. Edvinsson L, Hakanson R, Steen S, Sundler F, Uddman R, Wahlestedt C, Edvinsson L, Hakanson R, Steen S, Sundler F, Uddman R, Wahlestedt C., Innervation of human omental arteries and veins and vasomotor response to noradrenaline, neuropeptide Y, substance P and vasoactive intestinal peptide. Regul Pept 1985; 12: 67-79
122. Edwards RM, Stack EJ, Trizna W. CGRP stimulates adenylate cyclase and relaxes intracerebral arterioles. J Pharmacol Exp Ther 1991; 257: 1020-1024
123. Eglen RM, Hedge SS, Watson N. Muscarinic receptor subtypes and smooth muscle function. Pharm Rev 1996; 48: 532-556
124. Eichler HG, Blochl-Daum B, Kyrle PA, Gasic S. Cilazapril and enalapril inhibit local angiotensin I conversion in human veins but lack direct venodilating properties. J Cardiovasc Pharmacol 1989; 14: 248-252
125. Eichler HG, Blaschke TF, Hoffman BB. Decreased responsiveness of superficial hand veins to phenylephrine in black normotensive males. J Cardiovasc Pharmacol 1990; 16: 177-181

126. Eichler HG, Blaschke TF, Kraemer FB, Ford GA, Blochl-Daum B, Hoffman BB. Responsiveness of superficial hand veins to α-adrenoceptor agonists in insulin-dependent diabetic patients. Clin Sci 1992; 82: 163-168
127. Emoto N, Yanagisawa M. Endothelin-converting enzyme-2 is a membrane bound, phosphoramidon-sensitive metalloprotease with acidic pH optimum. J Biol Chem 1995; 270: 15262-15268
128. Enero MA, Saidman BQ. Possible feedback inhibition of noradrenaline release by purine compounds. Naunyn Schmiedebergs Arch Pharmacol 1977;297: 39-46
129. Enero MA. Further evidence for the purinergic inhibition of adrenergic neurotransmission in the rat portal vein. Acta Physiol Lat Am 1981; 31: 93-103
130. Ergul A, Shoemaker K, Puett D, Tackett RL. Gender differences in the expression of endothelin receptors in human saphenous veins in vitro. J Pharmacol Exp Ther 1998; 285: 511- 517
131. Escobales N, Longo E, Cragoe EJ, Danthuluri NR, Brock T. Osmotic activation of Na-H exchange in human endothelial cells. Am J Physiol 1990; 259: C640-646
132. Fabricius AM, Oser A, Diegeler A, Rauch T, Mohr FW. Endothelial function of human vena saphena magna prepared with different minimally invasive harvesting techniques. Eur J Cardiothorac Surg 2000;18: 400-403
133. Facino RM, Carini M, Stefani R. Anti-elastase and anti-hyaluronidase activities of saponins and sapogenins from Hedera helix, Aesculus hippocastanum, and Ruscus aculeatus: factors contributing to their efficacy in the treatment of venous insufficiency. Arch Pharm (Weinheim) 1995;328: 720-724.
134. Falkenhahn M, Gohlke P, Paul M. The Renin-Angiotensin System in the Heart and Vascular Wall: New Therapeutic Aspects. J Cardiovasc Pharm 1994; 24(suppl 2): S6-13
135. Farhat MY, Abi-Younes S, Dingaan B, Vargas R, Ramwell PW. Estradiol increases cyclic adenosine monophosphate in rat pulmonary vascular smooth muscle cells by a nongenomic mechanism. J Pharmacol Exp Ther 1996; 276: 652-657
136. Feelisch M. Biotransformation to nitric oxide of organic nitrates - comparison to other nitrovasodilators. Eur Heart J 1993; 14: I123-132
137. Feldman RD, Bierbrier GS. Insulin-mediated vasodilation: impairment with increased blood pressure and body mass, Lancet 1993; 342: 707-709
138. Feletou M, Martin CA, Molimard M, Naline E, Germain M, Thurieau C, Fauchere JL, Canet E, Advenier C. In vitro effects of HOE 140 in human bronchial and vascular tissue. Eur J Pharmacol 1995; 274: 57-64
139. Feletou M, Vanhoutte PM. The alternative: EDHF. J Moll Cell Cardiol 1999; 31: 15-22
140. Ferro A, Kaumann AJ, Brown MJ. Beta 1- and beta 2-adrenoceptor-mediated relaxation in human internal mammary artery and saphenous vein: unchanged beta- and alpha-adrenoceptor responsiveness after chronic beta 1-adrenoceptor blockade. Br J Pharmacol 1993; 109 : 1053-1058
141. Ferro A, Queen LR, Priest RM, Xu B, Ritter JM, Poston L, Ward JPT. Activation of the nitric oxide synthase by β2-adrenoceptors in human umbilical vein endothelium in vitro. Br J Pharmacol 1999; 126: 1872-1880
142. Figueroa R, Omar HA, Tejani N, Wolin MS. Gestational diabetes alters human placental vascular responses to changes in oxygen tension. Am J Obstet Gynecol 1993; 168: 1616-1622
143. Figueroa R, Martinez E, Fayngersh RP, Jiang H, Omar HA, Tejani N, Wolin MS. Absence of relaxation to lactate in human placental vessels of pregnancies with severe preeclampsia. Am J Obstet Gynecol 1995; 173: 1800-1806

144. Flavahan NA, Vanhoutte PM. Sympathetic purinergic vasoconstriction and thermosensitivity in acanine cutaneous vein. J Pharm Exp Ther 1986; 239: 784-789
145. Flavahan NA, Miller VM, Aarhus LL, Vanhoutte PM. Dennervation augments alpha-2 but not alpha-1 adrenergic responses in canine saphenous vein. J Pharmacol Exp Ther 1987; 240: 589-593
146. Flavahan NA, Shimokawa H, Vanhoutte PM. Pertussis toxin inhibits endothelium-dependent relaxations to certain antagonists in porcine coronary arteries J Physiol 1989; 408: 549-560
147. Fleming I, Bauersachs J, Busse R. Pracrine functions of the coronary vascular endothelium. Moll Cell Biochem 1996; 157: 137-145
148. Foegh ML, Ramwell PW. Cardiovascular effects of estrogen: implications of the discovery of the estrogen receptor subtype beta. Curr Opin Nephr Hypertens 1998; 7: 83-89
149. Ford GA, Hoffman BB, Vestal RE, Blaschke TF. Age-related changes in adenosine and beta-adrenoceptor responsiveness of vascular smooth muscle in man. Br J Clin Pharmacol 1992 ; 33: 83-87
150. Franco-Cereceda A, Liska J. Neuropeptide Y Y1 receptors in vascular pharmacology. Eur J Pharmacol 1998; 349: 1-14
151. Freeman JE, Kuo WY, Milligan G, Lowenstein CJ, Levine MA, Flavahan NA. Analysis of the pertussis toxin-sensitive receptor: G protein interactions in native porcine endothelial cells. Endothelium 1995; 3:321-330
152. Fridovich I. Fundamental aspects of reactive oxygen species, or what's the matter with oxygen? Ann N Y Acad Sci 1999; 893:13-18
153. Fried G, Samuelson U. Endothelin and neuropeptide Y are vasoconstrictors in human uterine blood vessels. Am J Obstet Gynecol 1991; 164: 1330-1336
154. Furci L, Fitzgerald DJ, Fitzgerald GA. Heterogeneity of prostaglandin H_2/thromboxane A_2 receptors: distinct subtypes mediate vascular smooth muscle contraction and platelet aggregation. J Pharmacol Exp Ther 1991; 258: 74-81
155. Gardner DG. Molecular Biology of Natriuretic Peptides. TCM 1994; 4: 159-164
156. Gavin KT, Colgan MP, Moore D, Shanik G, Docherty JR. Alpha 2C-adrenoceptors mediate contractile responses to noradrenaline in the human saphenous vein. Naunyn Schmiedebergs Arch Pharmacol 1997; 355: 406-411
157. Glowinski J, Glowinski S. Role of oxygen-derived free radicals in pathogenesis of varicose veins. Przeglad Flebologiczny 2000; 8: 5-9 (abstract)
158. Glusa E, Muller-Schweinitzer E. Heterogeneity of 5-HT receptor subtypes in isolated human femoral and saphenous veins, Naunyn Schmiedebergs Arch Pharmacol 1993; 347: 133-136
159. Goodfraind TL, Elliott ME, Catt KJ. Angiotensin receptors and their antagonists New Engl J Med 1995; 334: 1649-1654
160. Goodrich SM, Wood JE. Peropheral venous distensibility and velocity of venous blood flow during pregnancy or during oral contraceptive therapy. Am J Obstet Gynecol 1964; 90: 740-744
161. Gorenne I, Labat C, Gascard JP, Brink C. Antigen stimulation of human pulmonary smooth muscle: an in vitro model of inflammation. Cell Biol Toxicol 1996; 12: 239-44
162. Gothert M, Molderings GJ, Fink K, Schlicker E. Heterogeneity of presynaptic serotonin receptors on sympathetic neurones in blood vessels. Blood Vessels. 1991; 28: 11-18.
163. Griendling KK, Sorescu D, Lassegue B, Ushio-Fukai M. Modulation of Protein-kinase activity and gene expression by reactive oxygen species and their role in vascular physiology and pathophysiology. Arteriscler Thromb Vasc Biol 2000; 20: 2175-2183

164. Grunenberger F. Calcitonin gene-related peptide (CGRP): a vasodilator neuropeptide with many potential applications. Pathol Biol (Paris). 1993; 41: 936-942
165. Guillaume M, Padioleau F. Veinotonic effect, vascular protection, antiinflammatory and free radical scavenging properties of horse chestnut extract. Arzneimittelforschung 1994; 44: 25-35.
166. Guimaraes S, Moura D. Vascular Adrenoceptors: An Update. Phamacol Rev 2001; 53: 319-356
167. Haefeli WE, Srivastava N, Kongpatanakul S, Blaschke TF, Hoffman BB. Lack of role of endothelium-derived relaxing factor in effects of alpha-adrenergic agonists in cutaneous veins in humans. Am J Physiol 1993; 264: H364-369
168. Haegerstrand A, Dalsgaard CJ, Jonzon B, Larsson O, Nilsson J., Calcitonin gene-related peptide stimulates proliferation of human endothelial cells, Proc Natl Acad Sci U S A. 1990; 87: 3299-3303.
169. Hamilton CA, Reid JL. The effect of 6-hydroxydopamine on rabbit peropheral alpha adrenoceptors in vivo and in vitro. Br J Pharmacol 1981; 72: 119P
170. Hamilton CA, Berg G, Mcintyre M, Mcphaden AR, Reid JL, Dominiczak AF. Effects of nitric oxide and superoxide on relaxation in human artery and vein. Atherosclerosis 1997; 133: 77-86
171. Hanley SP, Bevan J. Inhibition by aspirin of human arterial and venous prostacyclin synthesis. Prostaglandin Leukotriene Med 1985; 20: 141-149
172. Harada K, Ohashi K, Kumagai Y, Ohmori M, Fujimura A. Influence of age on venodilator effect of isoproterenol and amrinone. Eur J Clin Pharmacol 1996; 50 : 37-40
173. Harker CT, Ousley PJ, Harris EJ, Edwards JM, Taylor LM, Porter JM. The effects of cooling on human saphenous vein reactivity to adrenergic agonists. J Vasc Surg 1990; 12: 45-49
174. Harker CT, Bowman CJ, Taylor LM Jr, Porter JM. Cooling augments human saphenous vein reactivity to electrical stimulation. J Cardiovasc Pharmacol 1994; 23: 453-457
175. Haynes DF, Kersten MD, Rish DS, Kadowitz PJ, McNamara DB. Increased prostacyclin (PGI_2) on thromboxane A_2 (TxA_2) formation by segments of varicose vein. Br J Surg 1988; 75: 1236-1240
176. Haynes WG, Clarke JG, Cockcroft JR, Webb DJ. Pharmacology of endothelin-1 in vivo in humans. J Cardiovasc Pharmacol. 1991; 17 Suppl 7: S284-286
177. Haynes WG, Webb DJ. Contribution of endogenous generation of endothelin-1 to basal vascular tone. Lancet 1994; 344: 852-854
178. Haynes WG. Endothelins as regulators of vascular tone in man, Clin Sci 1995; 88: 509-517
179. Haynes WG, Moffat S, Webb DJ. An investigation into the direct and indirect venoconstrictor effects of endothelin-1 and big endothelin-1 in man. Br J Clin Pharmacol 1995; 40: 307-311
180. He GW, Rosenfeldt FL, Angus JA. Pharmacological relaxation of the saphenous vein during harvesting for coronary artery bypass grafting. Ann Thorac Surg 1993; 5: 1210-1217
181. Henderson AH. Endothelium in control. Br Heart J 1991; 65: 116-125
182. Herbst WM, Eberle KP, Ozen Y, Hornstein OP. The innervation of the great saphenous vein: an immunohistochemical study with special regard to regulatory peptides. Vasa 1992; 21: 253-257

183. Hicks RCJ, Golledge J, Mir-Hasseine R, Poewll JT. Vasoactive effects of fibrinogen on saphenous vein. Nature 1996; 379: 818-820
184. Hicks RC, Moss J, Higman DJ, Greenhalgh RM, Powell JT. The influence of diabetes on the vasomotor responses of saphenous vein and the development of infra-inguinal vein graft stenosis. Diabetes 1997; 46: 113-118
185. Higman DJ, Greenhalgh RM, Powell JT. Smoking impairs endothelium-dependent relaxation of saphenous vein. Br J Surg 1993; 80: 1242-1245
186. Hiraoka W, Vazquez N, Nieves-Neira W, Chanock SJ, Pommier Y. Role of oxygen radicals generated by NADPH oxidase in apoptosis induced in human leukemia cells. J Clin Invest 1998; 102: 1961-1968
187. Holm P, Franco-Cereceda A. Tissue concentrations of endothelins and functional effects of endothelin-receptor activation in human arteries and veins. J Thorac Cardiovasc Surg 1996; 112: 264-272
188. Howard AB, Alexander RWl, Taylor WR. Effects of magnesium on nitric oxide synthase activity in endothelial cells. Am J Physiol 1995; 269: C612-618
189. Hu RM, Levin ER, Pedram A, Frank HJ. Insulin stimulates production and secretion of endothelin from bovine endothelial cells. Diabetes 1993; 42: 351-358.
190. Hull RW, Hasbargen JA, Fall S, O'Barr TP. Conjugated estrogens reduce endothelial prostacyclin production and fail to reduce postbypass blood loss. Chest 1991; 99: 1116-1119
191. Hume JR, Leblanc N. Macroscopic K^+ currents in single smooth muscle cells of the rabbit portal vein. J Physiol Lond 1989; 413: 49-73
192. Ignarro LJ, Byrns RE, Buga GM, Wood KS. Endothelium-derived relaxing factor from pulmonary artery and vein possesses pharmacologic and chemical properties identical to those of nitric oxide radical. Circ Res 1987; 61: 866-879
193. Ignarro LJ. Heme-dependent activation of guanilate-cyclase by nitric oxide: a nivel signal transduction mechanism. Blood Vessels 1991; 28: 67-73
194. Inoue R, Okabe K, Kitamura K, Kuriyama H. Two Ca^{2+}-dependent K^+-channels classified by the application of tetraethylammonium distribute to smooth muscle membrane of single cells dispersed from the rabbit portal vein. Pfluegers Arch 1986; 406: 138-143
195. Iversen PO, Nicolaysen A, Kvernebo K, Benestad HB, Nicolaysen G. Human cytokines modulate arterial vascular tone via endothelial receptors. Pflugers Arch 1999; 439: 93-100
196. Izhar U, Hasdai D, Richardson DM, Cohen P, Lerman A. Insulin and insulin-like growth factor-I cause vasorelaxation in human vessels in vitro. Coron Artery Dis 2000; 11: 69-76
197. Jilma B, Wolzt H, Wagner OF, Zweytek B, Monitzer B, Schuller-Petrovic S, Eichler HG. In vivo study of the effect of exogenous estradiol on α-adrenoceptor responsiveness of human veins. J Cardiovasc Pharmacol 1994; 23: 859-863
198. Kajioka S, Oike M, Kitamura K. Nicorandil opens a calcium-dependent potassium channel in smooth muscle cells from rat portal vein. J Pharmacol Exp Ther 1990; 254; 905-913
199. Kalsner S. Cholinergic constriction in the general circulation and its role in coronary artery spasm. Circ Res. 1989; 65: 237-257.
200. Karaki H, Ozaki H, Hori M, Mitsui-Sato M, Amano K-I, Hrada K-I, Miyamoto S, Nakazawa H, Won K-J, Sato K. Calcium movements, distribution, and functions in smooth muscle. Pharmacol Rev 1997; 49: 158-220

201. Karas RH, Patterson BL, Mendelsohn ME. Human vascular smooth muscle cells contain functional estrogen receptor. Circulation 1994; 89: 1943-1950
202. Karas RH, Baur WE, van Eickles M, Mendelsohn ME. Human vascular smooth muscle cells express an estrogen receptor isoform. FEBS Lett 1995; 377: 103-108
203. Karasu C, Soncul H, Altan VM. Effects of non-insulin dependent diabetes mellitus on the reactivity of human internal mammary artery and human saphenous vein. Life Sci 1995; 57: 103-112
204. Khansarinia S, Dennis J, Sekharan J, Veldenz H, Ceithaml E, Edwards F. Cytoprotective effects of nitric oxide and superoxide dismutase on ischemic saphenous vein endothelium. Jacksonville Medicine 2000; 295 (abstract)
205. Kirkeby HJ, Andersson KE, Forman A. Comparison of the effects of prostanoids on human penile circumflex veins and corpus cavernosum tissue. Br J Urol 1993; 72: 220-225
206. Kohno M, Yasunari K, Yokokawa K, Murkawa K, Horio T, Takeda T. Inhibition by atrial and brain natriuretic peptides of endothelin-1 secretion after stimulation with angiotensin II and thrombin of cultured human endothelial cells. J Clin Invest 1991; 87: 1999-2004
207. Komori K, Vanhoutte PM. Endothelium-derived hyperpolarizing factor. Blood Vessels 1990; 27: 238-245
208. Krasner LJ, Wendling WW, Cooper SC, Chen D, Hellmann SK, Eldridge CJ, McClurken JB, Jeevanandam V, Carlsson C. Direct effects of triiodothyronine on human internal mammary artery and saphenous veins. J Cardiothorac Vasc Anesth 1997; 11: 463-466
209. Kummer W, Haberberger R. Extrinsic and intrinsic cholinergic systems of the vascular wall. Eur J Morphol. 1999; 37: 223-226.
210. Kuriyama H, Kitamura K, Nabata H. Pharmacological and Physiopathological significance of ion channels and factors that modulate them in vascular tissues. Pharm Rev 1995; 47: 387-573
211. Langer SZ. Presynaptic regulation of the releaser of catecholamines. Pharmacol Rev 1981; 32: 337-362
212. Laufs U, La Fata V, Plutzky J, Liao JK. Effect of solutions of preservation on the vascular reactivity of human saphenous veins. Ann Chir 1995; 97: 728-734
213. Lawrie GM. Endothelial preservation in human saphenous veins (letter). J Thorac Cardiovasc Surg 1990; 100: 149-150
214. Le SQ, Wasserstrum N, Mombouli JV, Vanhoutte PM. Contractile effect of endothelin in human placental veins: role of endothelium prostaglandins and thromboxane. Am J Obstet Gynecol 1993; 169: 919-924
215. Lebrec D. Portal hypertension. Serotonin and pathogenesis. Cariovasc Drugs Ther 1990; 4: 33-35
216. Li Q, Feenstra M, Pfaffendorf M, Eijsman L, van Zwieten PA, Comparative vasoconstrictor effects of angiotensin II, III, and IV in human isolated saphenous vein, J Cardiovasc Pharmacol 1997; 29: 451-456
217. Li WG, Miller FJ Jr, Zhang HJ, Spitz DR, Oberley LW, Weintraub NL H2O2-induced O_2 production by a non-phagocytic NAD(P)H oxidase causes oxidant injury. J Biol Chem 2001; 276: 29251-29256
218. Linz W, Wiemer G, Gohlke P, Unger T, Scholkens BA. Contribution of kinins to the cardiovascular actions of angiotensin-Converting Enzyme Inhibitors. Pharm Rev 1995; 47: 25-49

219. Liu ZG, Ge ZD, He GW. Difference in endothelium-derived hyperpolarizing factor-mediated hyperpolarization and nitric oxide release between human internal mammary artery and saphenous vein. Circulation 2000; 102(Suppl 3): III296-301
220. Loirand G, Mironneau C, Mironneau J, Pacaud P. Two types of calcium currents in single smooth muscle cells from rat portal vein. J Physiol Lond 1989; 412: 333-349
221. Loirand G, Pacaud P. Mechanism of the ATP-induced rise in cytosolic Ca2+ in freshly isolated smooth muscle cells from human saphenous vein. Pflugers Arch 1995; 430: 429-436
222. Lowell RC, Gloviczki P, Miller VM. In vitro evaluation of endothelial and smooth muscle function of primary varicose veins. J Vasc Surg 1992;16: 679-686
223. Lum H, Roebuck KA. Oxidant stress and endothelial cell dysfunction. Am J Physiol Cell Physiol 2001; 280: C719-741
224. Lüscher TF, Diedrich D, Siebenmann R, Lehmann K, Stulz P, von Segesser L, Yang Z, Turina M, Gradel E, Weber E, Bühler FR. Difference between endothelium-dependent relaxation in arterial and in venous coronary bypass grafts. New Engl J Med 1988; 319: 462-467
225. Lüscher TF, Yang Z, Tschudi M, von Segesser L, Stulz P, Boulanger C, Siebenmann R, Turina M, Bühler FR, Interaction between endothelin-1 and endothelium-derived relaxing factor in human arteries and veins. Circ Res 1990; 66: 1088-1094
226. Luthra A, Borkowski KR, Carruthers SG. Genetic aspects of variability in superficial vein responsiveness to norepinephrine, Clin Pharmacol Ther 1991; 49: 355-361
227. Luthra A, Borkowski KR, Carruthers SG. Variability of superficial vein responsiveness to noradrenaline. Clin Paharmacol Ther 1990; 47: 178-180
228. Luu TN, Chester AH, O'Neil GS, Tadjkarimi S, Yacoub MH. Effects of vasoactive neuropeptides on human saphenous veins. Br Heart J 1992; 67: 474-477
229. MacAllister RJ, Calver AL, Riezebos J, Collier J, Vallance P. Relative potency and arteriovenous selectivity of nitrovasodilators on human blood vessels: an insight into the targeting of nitric oxide delivery. J Pharmacol Exp Ther 1995; 273: 154-60
230. Maguire JJ, Johnson CM, Mockridge JW, Davenport AP. Endothelin converting enzyme (ECE) activity in human vascular smooth muscle. Br J Pharmacol 1997; 122: 1647-1654
231. Maigaard S, Forman A, Andersson KE. Differential effects of angiotensin, vasopressin, and oxytocin on various smooth muscle tissues within the human uteroplacental unit. Acta Physiol Scand 1986; 128: 23-31
232. Mais DE, Dunlap C, Hamanaka N, Halushka PV. Further studies on the effects of epimers of thromboxane A2 antagonists on platelets and veins. Eur J Pharmacol. 1985; 111: 125-128.
233. Mak KK, Gude NM, Walters WA, Boura AL. Effects of vasoactive autacoids on the human umbilical-fetal placental vasculature. Br J Obstet Gynaecol 1984; 91: 99-106
234. Malmqvist U, Arner A, Uvelius B. Lactate dehydrogenase activity and isoform distribution in normal and hypertrophic smooth muscle tissue from the rat. Pfluegers Arch, 1991; 419: 230-234
235. Mangiafico RA, Malatino LS, Santonocito M, Spada RS, Benedetto FA. Plasma endothelin-1 release in normal and varicose saphenous veins. Angiology 1997; 48: 769-774
236. Marin J, Reviriego J. Effect pf nicardipine on human placental vasculature. Arch Int Pharmacodyn Ther 1989; 302; 209-219

237. Marin J, Fernandez-Alfonso MS, Sanchez-Ferrer CF. Sodium pump activity and contractile effect of ouabain in human placental veins. Eur J Pharmacol 1991; 201: 75-82
238. Martinez MC, Aldasoro M, Vila JM, Medina P, Lluch S. Responses to vasopressin and desmopressin of human cerebral arteries. J Pharmacol Exp Ther 1994; 270: 622-627
239. Mashiah A, Berman V, Thole HH, Rose SS, Pasik S, Schwarz H, Ben-Hur H. Estrogen and progesterone receptors in normal and varicose saphenous veins. Cardiovasc Surg 1999; 7: 327-331
240. Masood I, Porter KE, London NJ. Endothelin-1 is a mediator of intimal hyperplasia in organ culture of human saphenous vein. Br J Surg 1997; 84: 499-503
241. Mastrangelo D, Mathison R, Huggel H. Postjunctional localization of substance P receptors on the rat portal vein. Pharmacology 1983; 27: 305-318
242. Matsumoto T, Tomita T. Intracellular alkalinization caused by chloride removal in the smooth muscle of guinea-pig vena cava. Jpn J Physiol 1993; 43: 67-73
243. McCormack DG, Mak JC, Coupe MO, Barnes PJ. Calcitonin gene-related peptide vasodilation of human pulmonary vessels, J Appl Physiol 1989; 67: 1265-1270
244. McEwan JR, Benjamin N, Larkin S, Fuller RW, Dollery CT, MacIntyre I. Vasodilatation by calcitonin gene-related peptide and by substance P: a comparison of their effects on resistance and capacitance vessels of human forearms. Circulation 1988; 77:1072-1080
245. McGregor E, Gosling M, Beattie DK, Ribbons DM, Davies AH, Powell JT. Circumferential stretching of saphenous vein smooth muscle enhances vasoconstrictor responses by Rho kinase-dependent pathways. Cardiovasc Res 2002; 53: 219-226
246. McKay MK, Hester RL. Role of nitric oxide, adenosine and ATP-sensitive potassium channels in insulin-induced vasodilation. Hypertension 1996; 28: 202-208
247. McNamara, DB, Light JT, Minkes RK, Saroyan RM, Kvamme P, Rowe N, Webb WR, Fox L, Kersten MD, Mills NL, Kadowitz PJ. Comparative effects of endothelin (ET-1) and U 46619 on human saphenous vein and gastroepiploic artery, sources of human autologous graftS, Mol Cell Biochem. 1992; 117: 81-85
248. Mehta P, Mehta J, Crews F, Roy L, Ostrowski N, Horalek C. Comparison of umbilical vein models from measurement of relative prostacyclin and thromboxane production. Prostaglandins 1982; 24: 743-749
249. Mehta J, Roberts A. Human vascular tissue produce thromboxane as well as prostacyclin. Am J Physiol 1983; 244: R839-844
250. Mellander S, Andersson PO, Afzelius LE, Hellstrand P. Neural beta-adrenergic dilatation of the facial vein in man. Possible mechanism in emotional blushing. Acta Physiol Scand. 1982; 114: 393-399
251. Metsarinne K, Saijonmaa O, Yki-Jarvinen H, Fyhrquist F. Insulin increases the release of endothelin in endothelial cell cultures in vitro but not in vivo. Metabolism 1994; 43: 878-882
252. Michel JB, Feron O, Sase K, Prabhakar P, Michel T. Caveolin versus calmodulin. Counterbalancing allosteric modulators of endothelial nitric oxide synthase. J Biol Chem 1997; 272: 25907-25912
253. Michiels C, Arnould T, Knott I, Dieu M, Remacle J. Stimulation of prostaglandin synthesis by human endothelial cells exposed to hypoxia. Am J Physiol 1993; 264: C866-874
254. Mikkelsen E, Andersson KE, Pedersen OL. Effects of digoxin on isolated human mesenteric vessels. Acta Pharmacol Toxicol 1979; 45: 25-31

255. Mikkelsen E, Sakr AM, Jespersen LT, Studies on the effect of histamine in isolated human pulmonary arteries and veins, Acta Pharmacol Toxicol (Copenh) 1984; 54: 86-93
256. Miller VM, Vanhoutte PM. Endothelial α_2-adrenoceptors in canine pulmonary and systemic blood vessels. Eur J Pharmacol 1985; 118: 123-129
257. Miller VM, Rud KS, Gloviczki P. Pharmacological assessment of adrenergic receptors in human varicose veins. Int Angiol 2000; 19: 176-183
258. Milesi V, Rebolledo A, Ayala Paredes F, Sanz N, Tommasi J, Rinaldi GJ, Grassi AO. Mechanical properties of human saphenous veins from normotensive and hypertensive patients. Ann Thorac Surg 1998; 66: 455-461
259. Milton SG, Knutson VP. Insulin receptor characterization and function in bovine aorta endothelial cells: insulin degradation by a plasma membrane, protease-resistant insulin receptor. J Cell Physiol. 1993; 157: 333-343.
260. Mizuno K, Niimura S, Tani SM, Haga H, Inagami T, Fukuchii S. Direct proof for local generation and release of angiotensin II in peripheral human vascular tissue. Am J Hypertens 1991; 4 (suppl): S67-72
261. Molderings GJ, Likungu J, Hentrich F, Gothert M. Facilitatory presynaptic angiotensin receptors on the sympathetic nerves of the human saphenous vein and pulmonary artery. Potential involvement in beta-adrenoceptor-mediated facilitation of noradrenaline release. Naunyn Schmiedebergs Arch Pharmacol 1988; 338: 228-233
262. Molderings GJ, Werner K, Likungu J, Gothert M. Inhibition of noradrenaline release from the sympathetic nerves of the human saphenous vein via presynaptic 5-HT receptors similar to the 5-HT 1D subtype. Naunyn Schmiedebergs Arch Pharmacol 1990; 342: 371-377
263. Molderings GJ, Weissenborn G, Schlicker E, Likungu J, Göthert M. Inhibition of noradrenaline release from the sympathetic nerves of the human saphenous vein by presynaptic histamine H_3 receptors. Naunyn Schmiedebergs Arch Pharmacol 1992; 346: 46-50
264. Molderings GJ, Colling E, Likungu J, Jakschik J, Gothert M. Modulation of noradrenaline release from the sympathetic nerves of the human saphenous vein and pulmonary artery by presynaptic EP_3- and DP-receptors. Br J Pharmacol 1994; 111: 733-738
265. Molderings GJ, Gothert M. Subtype determination of presynaptic alpha 2-autoreceptors in the rabbit pulmonary artery and human saphenous vein. Naunyn Schmiedebergs Arch Pharmacol 1995; 352: 483-490.
266. Molenaar P, Malta E, Jones CR, Buxton BF, Summers RJ. Autoradiographic localization and function of beta-adrenoceptors on the human internal mammary artery and saphenous vein. Br J Pharmacol 1988; 95: 225-233
267. Mombouli JV; Le SQ; Wasserstrum N; Vanhoutte PM. Endothelins 1 and 3 and big endothelin-1 contract isolated human placental veins. J Cardiovasc Pharmacol 1993; 22 (Suppl 8): S278-281
268. Mombouli J-V, Vanhoutte PM. Endothelium-dependent hyperpolarizing factor(s): updating the unknown. Trends Pharmacol Sci 1997; 18: 252-256
269. Moncada S, Rees DD, Schultz R, Palmer RMJ. Development and mechanism of a specific supersensitivity to nitrovasodilators after inhibition of vascular nitric oxide synthesis in vivo. Proc Natl Acad Sci USA 1991; 88: 2166-2170
270. Moncada S, Higgs A. The L-arginine-nitric oxide pathway. N Engl J Med 1993; 329: 2002-2012

271. Monos E, Contney S, Cowley AW, Stekiel WJ. Effect of long-term tilt on mechanical and electrical properties of rat saphenous vein, Am J Physiol 1989; 256: H1185-1191
272. Monos E, Contney S, Cowley AW, Stekiel WJ. Axial extension of vein induces endothelium-dependent cell membrane hyperpolarization in the smooth muscle in vivo. Pfluegers Arch 1992; 384: 177-182
273. Monos E. How does the vein respond to pressure. NIPS 1993; 8: 124-128
274. Monos E, Berczi V, Nadasy G. Local Control of veins: Biomechanical, Metabolic and Humoral Aspects, Physiological Reviews 1995; 75: 616-619
275. Morcillo EJ, Cortijo J. Species differences in the responses of pulmonary vascular preparations to 5-hydroxytryptamine. Therapie 1999; 54: 93-97
276. Munro E, Patel M, Chan P, Betteridge L, Gallagher K, Schachter M, Wolfe J, Sever P. Effect of calcium channel blockers on the growth of human vascular smooth muscle cells derived from saphenous vein and vascular graft stenoses. J Cardiovasc Pharmacol 1994; 23: 779-784
277. Murad E, Waldman S, Molina C, Bennett B, Leitman D. Regulation and role of guanylate cyclase-cyclic GMP in vascular relaxation. Prog Clin Biol Res 1987; 249: 65-76
278. Nadasy GL, Szekacs B, Juhasz I, Feher J, Kowach AGB, Monos E. Role of endothelium, oxygen and ionic milieu in the prostacyclin and thromboxane production of rat aortic tissue slices. Acta Physiol Hung 1991; 78: 77-87
279. Nakakita K. Peptidergic innervation in the cerebral blood vessels of the guinea pig: an immunohistochemical study. J Cereb Blood Flow Metab. 1990; 10: 819-826.
280. Nakazato Y, Ohga A, Shigei T, Uematsu T. Extrinsic innervation of the canine abdominal vena cava and the origin of cholinergic vasoconstrictor nerves. J Physiol 1982; 328: 191-203
281. Narumiya S, Sugimoto Y, Ushikubi F. Prostanoid recepotrs: structures, properties, and functions. Physiol Rev 1999; 79: 1193-1226
282. Naruse K, Sokabe M. Involvement of stretch-activated ion channels in Ca^{2+} mobilization to mechanical stretch in endothelial cells. Am J Physiol 1993;264: C1037-1044
283. Nath RG, Lokhandwala MF, McCalden TA. Evidence for presynaptic dopaminergic inhibition of noradrenergic transmission in the rat portal vein. Proc West Pharmacol Soc. 1983; 26: 377-379
284. Nelson MT, Quayle JM. Physiological roles and properties of potassium channels in arterial smooth muscle. Am J Physiol 1995; 268: C799-822
285. Nemcova S, Gloviczki P, Rud KS, Miller VM. Cyclic nucleotides and production of prostanoids in human varicose veins. J Vasc Surg 1999; 30: 876-883
286. Nguyen DH, Voss U, Brecht K, The effect of potassium on isolated bovine facial and human saphenous veins. Experientia Basel 1980; 36: 975-976
287. Nishiyama M, Takahara Y, Masaki T, Nakajima N, Kimura S. Pharmacological heterogeneity of both endothelin ET_A- and ET_B-receptors in the human saphenous vein. Jpn J Pharmacol 1995; 69; 391-398 (abstract)
288. Noll G, Buhler FR, Yang Z, Lüscher TF. Different potency of endothelium-derived relaxing factors against thromboxane, endothelin, and potassium chloride in intramyocardial porcine coronary arteries. J Cardiovasc Pharmacol. 1991; 18: 120-126
289. Noll G, Lüscher TF. The endothelium in acute coronary syndromes. Eur Heart J 1998; 19(suppl C): C30-38
290. Ochiai M, Ohno M, Taguchi J, Hara K, Suma H, Isshiki T, Yamaguchi T, Kurokawa K. Responses of human gastroepiploic arteries to vasoactive substances: comparison with

responses of internal mammary arteries and saphenous veins. J Thorac Cardiovasc Surg 1992; 104: 453-458
291. Omar HA, Figueroa R, Omar RA, Tejani N, Wolin MS. Hydrogen peroxide and reoxygenation cause prostaglandin-mediated contraction of human placental arteries and veins. Am J Obstet Gynecol 1992; 167: 201-207
292. Omar HA, Ramirez R, Gibson M. Properties of a progesterone-induced relaxation in human placental arteries and veins. J Clin Endocrinol Metab 1995; 80: 370-373
293. O'Neil GS, Chester AH, Allen SP, Luu TN, Tadjkarimi S, Ridley P, Khagani A, Musumeci F, Yacoub MH. Endothelial function of human gastroepiploic artery. Implications for its use as a bypass graft. J Thorac Cardiovasc Surg 1991; 102: 561-565
294. Opie LH. Pharmacological differences between calcium antagonists. Eur Heart J 1997; 18(supl. A): A71-79
295. Orimo A, Inoue S, Ouchi Y, Orima H. Vascular smooth muscle cells possess estrogen receptor and respond to estrogen. Ann NY Acad Sci 1995; 748: 592-594
296. Ortiz JL, Gorenne I, Cortijo J, Seller A, Labat C, Sarria B, Abram TS, Gardiner PJ, Morcillo E, Brink C. Leukotriene receptors on human pulmonary vascular endothelium. Br J Pharmacol 1995; 115: 1382-1386
297. Ottillinger B, Greeske K. Rational therapy of chronic venous insufficiency – chances and limits of the therapeutic use of horse-chestnut seeds extract. BMC Cardiovascular Disorders 2001; 1: 5-10
298. Ottosson AM, Josefsson M, Ahlner J. Inhibition of nisoldipine on bovine mesenteric arteries and veins and on human peripheral veins. Arzneimittelforschung. 1995;45: 777-780.
299. Oury T, Day BJ, Crapo JD. Extracellular superoxide dismutase in vessels of airways of humans and baboons. Free Radic Biol Chem 1996; 20: 957-965
300. Öztürk Y, Melih Altan V, Yildizoglu-Ari N. Effects of Experimental Diabetes and Insulin on Smooth Muscle Functions. Pharm Rev 1996; 48: 70-100
301. Pacaud P, Loirand G, Mironneau C, Mironneau J. Noradrenaline activates a calcium-activated chloride conductance and increases the voltage-dependent calcium current in cultured single cells of rat portal vein. Br J Pharmacol 1989; 97: 139-146
302. Pacaud P, Loirand G, Gregoire G, Mironneau C, Mironneau J. Calcium-dependence of the calcium-activated chloride current in smooth muscle cells of rat portal vein. Pfluegers Arch 1992; 421: 125-130
303. Palmer RM, Ferrige AG, Moncada S. Nitric oxide release accounts for the biological activity of endothelium-derived relaxing factor. Nature. 1987;327: 524-526.
304. Panconesi A, Del Bianco PL, Franchi G, Anselmi B, Andreini R. Somatostatin. Peripheral venoconstrictive activity and interaction with monoamine in man. Regul Pept 1987; 18: 267-276
305. Park TC, Harker CT, Edwards JM, Moneta GL, Taylor LM, Porter JM. Human saphenous vein grafts explanted from the arterial circulation demonstrate altered smooth-muscle and endothelial responses. J Vasc Surg 1993; 18: 61-69
306. Paul M, Wagner J, Dzau VJ. Gene expression of the renin-angiotensin system in human tissues. Quantitative analysis by the polymerase chain reaction. J Clin Invest 1993; 91: 2058-2064
307. Pawloski JT, Chapnick BM. Leukotrienes C_4 and D_4 are potent endothelium-dependent relaxing agents in canine splachnic venous capacitance vessels. Circ Res 1993; 73: 395-404

308. Pernow J, Lundberg JM. Modulation of noradrenaline and neuropeptide Y (NPY) release in the pig kidney in vivo: involvement of alpha 2, NPY and angiotensin II receptors, Naunyn Schmiedebergs Arch Pharmacol 1989; 340: 379-385.
309. Perrot-Applanat M, Dacquet C, Finet M, Pichon MF, Milgrom E. Estradiol and progesterone action in human and rabbit saphenous veins. Proceedings of the Ninth International Congress of Endocrinology. Nice, France; 1992: 525.
310. Perrot-Applanat M, Deng M, Fernandez H, Lelaidier C, Meduri G, Bouchard P. Immunohistochemical localization of estradiol and progesterone receptors in human uterus throughout pregnancy: expression in endometrial blood vessels. J Clin Endocrinol Metab 1994; 78: 216-224
311. Perrot-Applanat M, Cohen-Solal K, Milgrom E, Finet M. Progesterone receptor expression in human saphenous veins. Circulation 1995; 92: 2975-2983
312. Perrot-Applanat M. Estrogen receptors in the cardiovascular system. Steroids 1996; 61: 212-215
313. Poli E, Casoli C, Spaggiari I, Starcich R, Bertaccini G. Contractile effect of endothelin-2 on the isolated human saphenous vein. Arch Int Pharmacodyn Ther 1991; 313: 108-119
314. Preibisz JJ. Calcitonin Gene-Related Peptide and regulation of human cardiovascular homeostasis. Am J Hypertens 1993; 6: 434-450
315. Prieto D, Benedito S, Simonsen U, Nyborg NC. Regional heterogeneity in the contractile and potentiating effects of neuropeptide Y in rat isolated coronary arteries: modulatory action of the endothelium. Br J Pharmacol 1991;102: 754-758.
316. Privat C, Stepien O, David-Dufilho M, Brunet A, Bedioui F, Marche P, Devynck J, Devynck MA. Superoxide release from interleukin-1B-stimulated human vascular cells: in situ electrochemical measurement. Free Radic Biol Med 1999; 27: 554-559
317. Protter AA, Wallace AM, Ferraris VA, Weishaar RE. Relaxant effect of human brain natriuretic peptide on human artery and vein tissue. Am J Hypertens 1996; 9: 432-436
318. Racchi H, Irarrazabal MJ, Howard M, Moran S, Zalaquett R, Huidobro-Toro JP. Adenosine 5'-triphosphate and neuropeptide Y are co-transmitters in conjunction with noradrenaline in the human saphenous vein. Br J Pharmacol 1999;126: 1175-1185
319. Rajagopalan S, Meng XP, Ramasamy S, Harisson DG, Galis ZS. Reactive oxygen species produced by macrophage-derived foam cells regulate the activity of vascular matrix metalloproteinases in vitro: implications for atherosclerotic plaque stability. J Clin Invest 1996; 98: 2572-2579
320. Ralevic V, Burnstock G. Roles of P_2-Purinoceptors in the Cardiovascular System. Circulation 1991; 84: 1-10
321. Regoli D, Boudon A, Fauchere JL. Receptors and antagonists for substance P and related peptides, Pharm Rev 1994; 46: 551-589
322. Regoli D, Jukic D, Gobeil F. Kinin B1 and B2 receptor antagonists and therapeutic perspectives. Therapie 1995; 50: 9-18
323. Regoli D, Pheng LH, Allogho SN, Nguyen-Le XK, Gobeil F. Receptors for kinins: from classical pharmacology to molecular biology. Immunopharmacology 1996; 33: 116-122
324. Rehn D, Unkauf M, Klein, P, Jost, V, L'ucker PW. Comparative clinical efficacy and tolerability of oxerutins and horse chestnut extract in patients with chronic venous insufficiency. Arzneimittelforschung. 1996; 46: 483-487
325. Remie R, Coppes RP, Meurs H, Roffel AF, Zaagsma J. Characterization of presynaptic vascular muscarinic receptors inhibiting endogenous noradrenaline overflow in the portal vein of the freely moving rat, Br J Pharmacol. 1990; 99: 223-226.

326. Reubi JC, Horisberger U, Laissue J. High density of somatostatin receptors in veins surrounding human cancer tissue: role in tumor-host interaction? Int J Cancer 1994; 56: 681-688
327. Reviriego J, Fernandez-Alfonso MS, Marin J. Actions of vasoactive drugs on human placental vascular smooth muscle. Gen Pharmacol 1990; 21:719-727
328. Reviriego J, JM, Fernandez-Alfonso MS, Guerra P, Marin J. Effects of Ca^{2+} antagonists' nifedipine and diltiazem on isolated human chorionic arteries and veins. J Cardiovasc Pharmacol 1990; 16: 128-138
329. Rice TL. Treatment of esophageal varices. Clin Pharm 1989; 8: 122-131
330. Rizzi A, Quaglio D, Vasquez G, Mascoli F, Amadesi S, Calo G, Regoli D, Zamboni P. Effects of vasoactive agents in healthy and diseased human saphenous veins. J Vasc Surg 1998; 28: 855-861
331. Rizzi A, Rizzi C, Amadesi S, Calo' G, Varani K, Inamura N, Regoli D. Pharmacological characterisation of the first non-peptide bradykinin B2 receptor agonist FR 190997: an in vitro study on human, rabbit and pig vascular B2 receptors. Naunyn Schmiedebergs Arch Pharmacol 1999; 360: 361-367
332. Rogerson FM, Chai SY, Schlawe I, Murray WK, Marley PD, Mendelsohn FA. Presence of angiotensin converting enzyme in the adventitia of large blood vessels. J Hypertens 1992; 10: 615-620
333. Rorie DK, Rusch NJ, Shepherd JT, Vanhoutte PM, Tyce GM. Prejunctional inhibition of norepinephrine release caused by acetylcholine in the human saphenous vein. Circ Res 1981; 49:337-41
334. Roubos N, Rosenfeldt FL, Richards SM, Conyers RA, Davis BB. Improved preservation of saphenous vein grafts by the use of glyceryl trinitrate-verapamil solution during harvesting. Circulation 1995; 92: II31-36
335. Rubanyi GM, Vanhoutte PM. Heterogeneity of endothelium-dependent responses to acetylcholine in canine femoral arteries and veins. Blood vessels 1988; 25: 407-415
336. Rubanyi GM, Polokoff MA. Endothelins: Molecular Biology, Biochemistry, Pharmacology, Physiology, and Pathophysiology. Pharm Rev, 1994; 46: 328-394
337. Rudner XL, Berkowitz DE, Booth JV, Funk BL, Cozart KL, D'Amico EB, El-Moalem H, Page SO, Richardson CD, Winters B, Marucci L, Schwinn DA. Subtype specific regulation of human vascular alpha(1)-adrenergic receptors by vessel bed and age. Circulation. 1999; 100: 2336-2343.
338. Rudofsky G. Return Circulation and Norepinepherine: An Update. Paris: John Libbey Eurotext; 1991: 219-224.
339. Rump LC, von Kugelgen I. A study of ATP as a sympathetic cotransmitter in human saphenous vein. Br J Pharmacol 1994; 111: 65-72
340. Rusch NJ, Wooldridge TA, Kulig CC, Almassi GH, Nicolosi AC, Olinger GN, Boerboom LE. Reactivity of human saphenous veins at arterial perfusion pressures. J Thorac Cardiovasc Surg 1995; 97: 1005-1012
341. Russell KS, Haynes MP, Caulin-Glaser T, Rosneck J, Sessa WC, Bender JR. Estrogen stimulates heat shock protein 90 binding to endothelial nitric oxide synthase in human vascular endothelial cells. Effects on calcium sensitivity and NO release. J Biol Chem 2000; 275: E571-583
342. Sabouni MH, Brown GL, Kotake AN, Douglas FL, Mustafa SJ. Effects of CGS-159434 on the relaxations produced by adenosine analogs in human blood vessels. Eur J Pharmacol 1990; 187: 525-530

343. Saetrum Opgaard O, Gulbenkian S, Bergdahl A, Barroso CP, Andrade NC, Polak JM, Queiroz e Melo JQ, Edvinsson L. Innervation of human epicardial coronary veins: immunohistochemistry and vasomotility. Cardiovasc Res 1995; 29: 463-468
344. Saris JJ, van Dijk MA, Kroon I, Schalekamp MA, Danser AH. Functional importance of angiotensin-converting enzyme-dependent in situ angiotensin II generation in the human forearm. Hypertension 2000; 35: 764-768
345. Scherrer U, Randin D, Vollenweider P, Vollenweider L, Nicod P. Nitric oxide release accounts for insulin effects in humans. J Clin Invest 1995; 94: 2511-2515
346. Schimke I, Griesmacher G, Weigel G, Holzhutter HG, Muller MM. Effects of reactive oxygen species on eicosanoid metabolism in human endothelial cells. Prostaglandins 1992; 43: 281-292
347. Schmalfuss CM, Chen LY, Bott JN, Staples ED, Mehta JL. Superoxide anion generation, superoxide dismutase activity, and nitric oxide release in human internal mammary artery and saphenous vein segments. J Cardiovasc Pharmacol Ther 1999; 4: 249-257
348. Schmidt M, Kroger B, Jacob E., Seulberger H, Subkowski T, Otter R, Meyer T, Schmalzing G, Hillen H. Molecular characterization of human and bovine endothelin-converting enzyme (ECE-1). FEBS Lett, 1994; 356: 238-243
349. Schoeffter P, Godfraind T. Histamine receptors in the smooth muscle of human internal mammary artery and saphenous vein. Pharmacol Toxicol 1989; 64: 64-71
350. Schror K, Schröder H. "Eicosanoids and Smooth Muscle Function". In *Pharmacology of Smooth Muscle.* Szekeres L, Papp JGY, ed. Springer-Verlag, 1994; 127-154
351. Schuller-Petrovic S, Siedler S, Kern T, Meinhart J, Schmidt K, Brunner F. Imbalance between the endothelial cell-derived contracting factors prostacyclin and angiotensin II and nitric oxide/cyclic GMP in human primary varicosis. Br J Pharmacol 1997;122: 772-778
352. Schwartz LB, Radic ZS, O'Donohoe MK, Mikat EM, McCann RL, Hagen PO. Saphenous vein endothelium-dependent relaxation in patients with peripheral vascular disease. Ann Vasc Surg 1992; 6:425-432
353. Sheehan DW, Fahri LE, Russell JA. Prolonged lobar hypoxia in vivo enhances the responsivity of isolated pulmonary veins to hypoxia. Am Rev Respir Dis 1992; 145: 640-645
354. Shimada K, Matsushita Y, Wakabayashi K, Takahashi M, Matsubara A, Iijima A, Tanzawa K. Cloning and functional expression of endothelin-converting enzyme cDNA. Biochem Biophys Res Commun 1995; 207: 807-812
355. Shimokawa H, Flavahan NA, Vanhoutte PM. Natural course of the impairment of endothelium-dependent relaxations after baloon endothelium removal in porcine coronary arteries. Possible dysfunction of an apertussis toxin-sensitive G protein. Circ Res 1989; 65: 740-753
356. Shukla A, Rasik AM, Dhawan BN. Asiaticoside-induced elevation of antioxidant levels in healing wounds. Phytother Res 1999; 13: 50-54
357. Sidawy AN, Hakim FS, Neville RF, Korman LY. Autoradiographic mapping and characterization of insulin-like growth factor-I receptor binding in human greater saphenous vein. J Vasc Surg 1993; 18: 947-952
358. Sinzinger H, Fitscha P. Prostacyclin contracts normal and varicose human saphenous veins. Vasa 1984; 13: 228-230
359. Sinzinger H. The effect of dihydroergotamine on various platelet function tests and venous prostacyclin-formation in men. Thromb Haemost 1985; 53: 285-286.

360. Siska I-R, Avram J., Crisnic D, Tanasie G, Tatu C, Bunu C, Schneider Fr. Magnesium modulates human saphenous vein smooth muscle contractility. Proceedings of the 3rd International Symposium on Metal Elements in Environment, Medicine and Biology; Timisoara-Romania, October 26-28, 1998. Z.Gârban, P.Dragan, ed. Eurobit Publishing House Timisoara-Romania, 1998; 353-358
361. Siska I. -R., Avram J, Tatu C, Tanasie G, Bunu C. In vitro evaluation of smooth muscle contractility and endothelium function in primary varicose veins. Physiol Res 1999; 48(suppl.1): S118
362. Siska I-R, Avram J, Tatu C, Bunu C, Schneider Fr, Maties R. "Some aspects concerning the antioxidant capacity of venous blood in lower limbs varicose veins". In *Oxygen Transport to Tissue XXI*. D.Delpy, A.Eke, ed. Kluwer Academic/Plenum Publishers NY, 1999: 445-452
363. Smith K, Connaughton S, Docherty JR. Investigations of the subtype of alpha 2-adrenoceptor mediating contractions of the human saphenous vein. Br J Pharmacol 1992; 106: 447-451
364. Sneddon P, Westfall TD, Todorov LD, Mihaylova-Todorova S, Westfall DP, Kennedy C. Modulation of purinergic neurotransmission. Prog Brain Res 1999; 120: 11-20
365. Sogo N, Campanella C, Webb DJ, Megson IL. S-Nitrosothiols cause prolonged, nitric oxide-mediated relaxation in human saphenous vein and internal mammary artery: therapeutic potential in bypass surgery. Br J Pharmacol 2000;131: 1236-1244
366. Sohn H-Y, Keller M, Gloe T, Morawitz H, Rueckschloss U, Pohl U. The small G-protein Rac mediates depolarization-induced formation in human endothelial cells. J Biol Chem 2000; 275: 18745-18750
367. Somlyo Apm Somlyo AV, Shuman H. Electron probe analysis of vascular smooth muscle. Composition of mitochondria, nuclei, and cytoplasm. J Cell Biol 1979; 81: 316-335
368. Sparks HV. "Effect of local metabolic factors on vascular smooth muscle". In *Handbook of Physiology. The Cardiovascular System. Vascular Smooth Muscle.* Volume II. Bethesda, MD: Am Physiol Soc 1980; 475-513
369. Stanke F, Cracowski JL, Chavanon O, Magne JL, Blin D, Bessard G, Devillier P. Glibenclamide inhibits thromboxane A2-induced contraction in human internal mammary artery and saphenous vein. Eur J Pharmacol 1998; 341: 65-71
370. Stanke F, Devillier P, Breant D, Chavanon O, Sessa C, Bricca G, Bessard G. Frusemide inhibits angiotensin II-induced contraction on human vascular smooth muscle. Br J Clin Pharmacol 1998; 46: 571-575
371. Steinberg HM, Brechtel G, Johnson A, Fineberg N, Baron AD. Insulin-mediated skeletal muscle vasodilation is nitric oxide dependent. J Clin Invest 1994; 94: 1172-1179
372. Stones RW; Beard RW; Burnstock G. Pharmacology of the human ovarian vein: responses to putative neurotransmitters and endothelin-1. Br J Obstet Gynaecol 1994; 101: 701-706
373. Strachan FE; Haynes WG; Webb DJ. Endothelium-dependent modulation of venoconstriction to sarafotoxin S6c in human veins in vivo. J Cardiovasc Pharmacol 1995; 26 (Suppl 3): S180-182
374. Stralin P, Karlsson K, Johansson BO, Marklund SL. The interstitium of the human arterial wall contains very large amounts of extracellular superoxide dismutase. Arterioscler Thromb Vasc Biol 1995; 15: 2032-2036

375. Strobel WM, Lüscher TF, Simper D, Linder L, Haefeli WE. Substance P in human hand veins in vivo: tolerance, efficacy, potency, and mechanism of venodilator action. Clin Pharmacol Ther 1996; 60: 435-443
376. Sundaresan M, Zu-Xi Y, Ferrans VJ, Irani K, Finkel T. Requirement for generation of H_2O_2 for platelet-derived growth factor signal transduction. Science 1995; 270: 296-299
377. Suzuki S., Takeshita A, Imaizumi T, Hirooka Y, Yoshida M, Ando S. Biphasic forearm vascular responses to intraarterial arginine vasopressin. J Clin Invest 1989; 84: 427-434
378. Szabo C, Berczi V, Schneider F, Kovacs AGB, Monos E. Role of endothelium in the response of the vein wall to magnesium withdrawal. Pflugers Arch 1992; 420: 140-145
379. Tadjkarimi S, O'Neil GS, Luu TN, Allen SP, Schyns CJ, Chester AH, Yacoub MH. Comparison of cyclic GMP in human internal mammary artery and saphenous vein: implications for coronary artery bypass graft patency, Cardiovasc Res 1992; 26: 297-300
380. Tackett RL, Zumbro G, Rubin J. Increased superoxide production in vasculature of African Americans impairs endothelial-mediated relaxation. Circulation 1997; 97: I-375 (abstract)
381. Thorin-Trescases N, Hamilton CA, Reid JL, McPherson KL, Jardine E, Berg G, Bohr D, Dominiczak AF. Inducible L-arginine/nitric oxide pathway in human internam mammary artery and saphenous vein. Am J Physiol 1995; 268: H1122-1132
382. Thulesius O, Said S, Shuhaiber H, Neglen P, Gjores JE. Endothelial mediated enhancement of noradrenaline-induced vasoconstriction in normal and varicose veins. Clin Physiol 1991; 11: 153-159
383. Tirupattur PR, Ram JL, Standley PR, Sowers JR. Regulation of Na^{+}·K^{+}-ATPase gene expression by insulin in vascular smooth muscle cells. Am J Hypertens. 1993;6: 626-629.
384. Toda N, Kimura T, Okamura T. Nitroxidergic nerve stimulation relaxes human uterine vein. J Auton Nerv Syst 1995; 55: 189-192
385. Toda N; Yoshida K; Okamura T. Involvement of nitroxidergic and noradrenergic nerves in the relaxation of dog and monkey temporal veins, J Cardiovasc Pharmacol 1995; 25 ; 741-747
386. Tornebrandt K, Nobin A, Owman C. Contractile and dilatory action of neuropeptides on isolated human mesenteric blood vessels. Peptides 1987; 8: 251-256
387. Touyz RM, Schiffrin EL. Signal transduction mechanisms mediating the physiological and pathophysiological actions of angiotensin II in vascular smooth muscle cells. Pharmacol Rev 2000; 52: 639-672
388. Tripodi F, Stanke-Labesque F, Devillier P, Chavanon O, Sessa C, Bessard G. Antagonistic effects of losartan on thromboxane A2-receptors in human isolated gastroepiploic artery and saphenous vein. J Cardiovasc Pharmacol 1999; 34: 734-740
389. Tsuru H, Matsukado Y, Shigei T. Evidence for the excitatory cholinergic innervation in the rabbit portal vein. Jpn J Pharmacol 1994; 66: 393-396
390. Urakami-Harasawa L, Shimokawa H, Nakashima H, Egashira K, Takeshira A. Importance of endothelium-derived hyperpolarizing factor in human arteries. J Clin Invest 1996; 100: 2793-2799
391. Vajo Z, Szekacs B, Dachman W. Evidence for genetic variability in venous responsiveness. Acta Physiol Hung 1996; 84: 353-360
392. Vallance P, Collier J, Moncada S. Nitric oxide synthesized from L-arginine mediates endothelium dependent dilation in human veins in vivo. Cardiovasc Res 1989; 23: 1053-1057

393. Van Renterghem C, Lazdunski M. A new non-voltage-dependent, epithelial-like Na^+ channel in vascular smooth muscle cells. Pfluegers Arch 1991; 419: 401-408
394. Vanhoutte PM, Janssens WJ. Local control of venous function,. Microvasc Res 1978; 16: 144-146
395. Vanhoutte PM, Shepherd JT. Muscarinic and beta-adrenergic prejunctional modulation of adrenergic neurotransmission in the blood vessel wall. Gen Pharmacol 1983; 14: 35-37
396. Vanhoutte PM. The role of the systemic veins: an update. Phlebology 1988; 3(suppl.1): 13-25
397. Vanhoutte PM, Shimokawa H. Endothelium-derived relaxing factor and coronary vasospasm. Circulation 1989; 80: 1-9
398. Vanhoutte PM, Lüscher TF, Graser T. Endothelium dependent contractions. Blood vessels 1991; 28: 74-83
399. Vashisht R, Sian M, Sharp EJ, Leathard HL, O'Malley MK. Serotonin-induced contractility in human saphenous vein is inhibited by naftidrofuryl. Br J Surg 1992; 79: 1154-1156
400. Vedernikov YP, Graser T, Tiedt N, Vikhert M. Heterogeneity of the response of venous smooth muscle to arterial endothelium-derived relaxing factor (EDRF) in respect of the role of nitric oxide. Basic Res Cardiol 1988; 83: 122-127
401. Verbeuren TJ, Lopez RR, Aarhus LL, Shepherd TJ, Vanhoutte PM. Prejunctional beta-adrenoceptors in human and canine saphenous veins. J Anatomic Nervous System 1983; 8: 261-271
402. Verma S, Lovren F, Dumont AS, Mather KJ, Maitland A, Kieser TM, Triggle CR, Anderson TJ. Tetrahydrobiopterin improves endothelial function in human saphenous veins. J Thorac Cardiovasc Surg 2000; 120: 668-671
403. Vesely DL. Atrial Natriuretic Peptides. Kidney: A Current Survey of World Literature, 1994; 3: 4-8
404. Walch L, Taisne C, Gascard JP, Nashashibi N, Brink C, Norel X. Cholinesterase activity in human pulmonary arteries and veins. Br J Pharmacol 1997; 121: 986-990
405. Walch L, Norel X, Gascard JP, Brink C. Cysteinyl-leukotriene receptors in pulmonary vessels. J Physiol Pharmacol 1999; 50: 567-573
406. Walch L, Norel X, Leconte B, Gascard JP, Brink C. Cholinergic control of human and animal pulmonary vascular tone. Therapie 1999; 54: 99-102
407. Walch L, Gascard JP, Dulmet E, Brink C, Norel X. Evidence for a M_1 muscarinic receptor on the endothelium of human pulmonary veins. Br J Pharmacol 2000;130: 73-78
408. Walch L, de Montpreville V, Brink C, Norel X.Prostanoid EP(1)- and TP-receptors involved in the contraction of human pulmonary veins. Br J Pharmacol. 2001; 134: 1671-1678.
409. Wali FA, Suer AH, Greenidge E. Verapamil, diltiazem and nifedipine inhibit vascular responses to noradrenaline, acetylcholine and 5-hydroxytryptamine in human saphenous vein. Pharmacol Res Commun 1986; 18:1123-1138
410. Wali FA, Greenridge E, Tugwell AC. Effect of verapamil on the contraction produced by high potassium and by noradrenaline in human isolated saphenous vein. Acta Physiol Hung 1988; 72: 115-121
411. Wallerstedt SM, Bodelsson M. Endothelium-dependent relaxation by substance P in human isolated omental arteries and veins: relative contribution of prostanoids, nitric oxide and hyperpolarization. Br J Pharmacol 1997; 120: 25-30
412. Wang Q, Hogg RC, Large WA. Properties of spontaneous inward currents recorded in

smooth muscle cells isolated from the rabbit portal vein. J Physiol Lond 1992; 451: 525-537
413. Webb DJ, Benjamin N, Allen MJ, Brown J, O'Flynn M, Cockcroft JR. Vascular responses to local atrial natriuretic peptide infusion in man. Br J Clin Pharmac 1988; 26: 245-251
414. Webb DJ, Benjamin N, Cockcroft JR, Collier JG. Augmentation of sympathetic venoconstriction by angiotensin II in human dorsal hand veins. Am J Hypertens 1989; 2: 721-723
415. Weiner N, Molinoff PB, "Catecholamines" In *Basic Neurochemistry: Molecular, Cellular and Medical Aspects*, 4th edition. Siegel GJ et al., ed. Raven Press NY, 1989; 233-251
416. Weinstein JS, Grossman W, Weintraub RM, Thurer RL, Johnson RG, Morgan KG. Differences in alpha-adrenergic responsiveness between human internal mammary arteries and saphenous veins. Circulation 1989; 79: 1264-1267
417. Wenzel RR, Noll G, Lüscher TF. Endothelin receptor antagonists inhibit endothelin in human skin microcirculation. Hypertension 1994; 23: 581-586
418. West NEJ, Guzik TJ, Black E, Channon KM. Enhanced superoxide production in experimental venous bypass graft intimal hyperplasia. Role of NAD(P)H oxidase. Arterioscler Thromb Vasc Biol 2001; 21: 189-194
419. White DG, Garratt H, Mundin JW, Sumner MJ, Vallance PJ, Watts IS. Human saphenous vein contains both endothelin ETA and ETB contractile receptors. Eur J Pharmacol 1994; 257: 307-310
420. Wolin MS. Interactions of oxidants with vascular signaling systems. Arterioscler Thromb Vasc Biol 2000; 20: 1430-1442
421. Woods M, Bishop-Bailey D, Pepper JR, Evans TW, Mitchell JA, Warner TD. Cytokine and lipopolysaccharide stimulation of endothelin-1 release from human internal mammary artery and saphenous vein smooth-muscle cells, J Cardiovasc Pharmacol 1998; 83: S348-350
422. Yang JA, He GW. Surgical preparation abolishes endothelium-derived hyperpolarizing factor-mediated hyperpolarization in the human saphenous vein. Ann Thorac Surg 1997; 63: 429-433
423. Yang Z, Luscher TF. Endothelium-dependent regulatory mechanisms in human coronary bypass grafts: possible clinical implications. Z Kardiol. 1989;78 Suppl 6: 80-84
424. Yang ZH, Diederich D, Schneider K, Siebenmann R, Stulz P, von Segesser L, Turina M, Bühler FR, Lüscher TF. Endothelium-derived relaxing factor and protection against contractions induced by histamine and serotonin in the human internal mammary artery and in the saphenous vein. Circulation 1989; 80:1041-1048
425. Yang ZH, Bühler FR, Diederich D, Lüscher TF. Different effects of endothelin-1 on cAMP- and cGMP-mediated vascular relaxation in human arteries and veins: comparison with norepinephrine. J Cardiovasc Pharmacol 1989; 13 (Suppl 5): S129-123
426. Yang ZH, von Segesser L, Bauer E, Stulz P, Turina M, Lüscher TF. Different activation of the endothelial L-arginine and cyclooxygenase pathway in the human internal mammary artery and saphenous vein. Circ Res 1991; 68: 52-60
427. Yang Z, Arnet U, von Segesser L, Siebenmann R, Turina M, Lüscher TF. Different effects of angiotensin-converting enzyme inhibition in human arteries and veins. J Cardiovasc Pharmacol 1993; 22 (suppl 5): S17-22
428. Yang Z, Lüscher TF. Basic cellular mechanisms of coronary bypass graft disease, Eur

Heart J 1993; 14 (suppl I): 193-197
429. Yang Z, Ruschitzka F, Rabelink TJ, Noll G, Julmy F, Joch H, Gafner V, Aleksic I, Althaus U, Lüscher TF. Different effects of thrombin receptor activation on endothelium and smooth muscle cells of human coronary bypass vessels implications for venous bypass graft failure. Circulation. 1997; 95: 1870-1876
430. Yatani A, Seidel CL, Allen J, Brown AM. Whole-cell and single-cell calcium currents of isolated smooth muscle cells from saphenous vein. Curc Res 1987; 60: 523-533
431. Yoshioka K, Furuta T, Hayakawa A, Ishikawa N, Shigei T. Excitatory cholinergic innervation in canine portal and mesenteric veins. Am J Physiol 1988;255: H288-294.
432. Yu JC, Davenport AP. Secretion of endothelin-1 and endothelin-3 by human cultured vascular smooth muscle cells. Br J Pharmacol 1995; 114 : 551-557
433. Zhang LM, Castresana MR, McDonald MH, Johnson JH, Newman WH. Response of human artery, vein, and cultured smooth muscle cells to atrial and C-type natriuretic peptides. Crit Care Med 1996; 24: 306-310
434. Zhao Y, Packer CS, Rhoades RA. Pulmonary vein contracts in response to hypoxia. Am J Physiol 1993; 265: L87-92
435. Zhao Y, Packer CS, Rhoades RA. Chronic hypoxia impairs pulmonary venous smooth muscle contraction. Respir Physiol 1995; 100: 75-82
436. Zhao M, Bo X, Burnstock G. Distribution of [3H] alpha, beta-methylene ATP binding sites in pulmonary blood vessels of different species. Pulm Pharmacol 1996; 9: 167-174
437. Zhao L, Tackett RL. Oxidized low-density lipoprotein inhibits acetylcholine-induced vasorelaxation and increases 5-HT-induced vasoconstriction in isolated human saphenous vein. J Pharmacol Exp Ther 1998; 284: 637-643.
438. Zurowska-Grojec Z, Pruszcyk P, Colton C, Yao J, Shen GH, Myers AK, Wahlestedt C. Mitogenic effect of neuropeptide Y in rat vascular smooth muscle cells. Peptides 1993; 14: 263-268

CHAPTER 5

VARICOSE DISEASE

TAKE HOME MESSAGES

- The varicose disease is a frequent illness with great economical and social impact; it may be congenital, primary or secondary.
- The development of primary varicose veins is determined by venous wall changes "wall disease" or by valves incompetence "ostial disease" influenced by local and general factors. The genetic implications have been demonstrated, the apoptosis may occur and the inflammation has an important role according to the latest researches.
- Clinical examination is insufficient to identify the extension of the varicose vein and determine the proper treatment.
- Echo-Doppler is the main noninvasive screening test and it is sufficient in not complicated cases. Pletismography and ambulatory venous pressure or invasive tests such as phlebography, phleboscopy are useful for research purpose and for surgery of the varicose disease.
- Benefits of the medical treatment are controversial although some trials demonstrated that phlebotonic and phlebotrophic drugs are useful. The external compression is a compulsory measure together with physical exercises, changes of life style and the loss of weight. In selected cases the sclerotherapy and different surgical methods are indicated with good late results.

5.1. GENERALITIES

5.1.1. Definition

The varicose are the permanent twisted, ropelike saccular vein dilatation of the epifascial veins of the lower limbs, including alterations of the vein walls and hemodynamic vein disturbances. The same disease affects other veins of the body, as the veins of the upper limbs, the esophageal, pelvic or spermatic veins. R.L.Kistner stated in 2001 " that the venous field is alive and dynamic and that progress is rampant at all levels from molecular science through pharmaceutical manipulation of clotting and fibrinolytic system of coagulation to the aggressive clinical treatment of specifically diagnosed disease states".

Nowadays the importance of varicose disease is increased by the worldwide conception that the female legs are "a secondary sexual characteristic".

5.1.2. Frequency

Varicose is a very frequent disease. It affects 30-50% or even 60% of the adult population. In Western countries 1 from 2 women and 1 from 4 men present varicose disease but some recent studies have suggested that in fact men and women are equally affected. In the well-known Framingham study, the incidence of varicose disease per year was 2.6% in women and 1.9% in men per year; in two years time varicose affects 5.2% women and 3.9% men. (7, 76) The men/women ratio is 1 to 2-3, except the Widmer study where the ratio was 1 to 1. Probably the difference between sexes is present till the age of 50 and than equalization appears. Burkitt found a decreased frequency of varicose at African (3.2%), at Indian (9.7%) and Arabian (1.5%) people. The prevalence of the varicose disease increases with age although the primary evolution of the disease is not well known. (Fowkes-27) Except congenital varicose, the presence of the primitive varicosities is rare in children and adolescents. Children develope varicosities at the age of 10 when important familial history of disease is present. The hereditary factor is important, the incidence is 27-53% in the absence of heredity, and 44-65% in the presence of this factor. The studies demonstrated the "vertical inheritance", with a familiar predisposition of 85%. Only 22% present the absence of inheritance (Wienert V, Scott T).

Cornu-Thenard communicates that the risk of varicose veins at child is 90% if both parents suffers from venous insufficiency, 25% for boys and 62% for girls if one parent is affected and 20% in the absence of family history. (Ramelet-93) The "horizontal inheritance" is not yet demonstrated. The prevalence of varicosities increases linearly with age: 7-35% in men and 20-60% in women between ages of 35-40, respectively 15-55% in men and 40-78% in women over 60. Due to the increasing of old population in Europe the importance and the incidence of this disease will increase in the future. Open venous ulcers occur in about 0.3% of the adult population and a history of open or healed ulceration occurs in 1%. The risk of ulceration is related to the severity of varicosities and venous insufficiency and it is increased after the deep venous thrombosis. (Fowkes-27)

5.1.3. Genesis

The genesis of vascular system is complex and depends on a lot of factors. In the last few years more classes of molecules that react with specific receptors from the vascular endothelium were discovered. This interaction determines the appearance and proliferation of vessels. There are differences among arteries, veins and lymphatics. The receptors VEGF-1 and VEGF-2 are present in the endothelium of the small arteries and veins and they stimulate VEGFA ligand and so they induce the development of arteries at the end of the veins and the dilation of postcapillary small veins. VEGF-C ligand activating VEGFR-2 and VEGFR-3 induces marked limphangiogenesis and much lesser arterial and venous angiogenesis. Recently was demonstated that VEGF level increase when the hart rate is lower. (Tomanek R.J., Zheng W. in Bauer- 4)

Transmembranar Ephrin-B-2 is present in the arterial endothelium and Ephrin-B-4 in venous endothelium. When a vein is put in the place of an artery it will determine the appearance of Ephrin-B-2 in venous endothelium. The specific marker for lymphatics is the transcription factor Prox-1. The lymphatic system would not develop when the gene Prox-1 is experimentally destroyed. (Wigle, Oliver 1999) In embryo, the superficial and deep lymphatic network is tied to venous system in the presence of Prox-1. Prox-1 is present in melanomas that produce growth factor VEGF-C in an increased amount. Prox-1 is absent in hemangioma. Prox-1 is present and CD-34 is absent in lymphangioma.

Some genetic mutations have been identified in varicose disease such as: mutations in the distal promoter region of the thrombomodulin gene (nucleotides 300 to 2052). Paris Thrombosis Study (PATHROS) showed two frequent mutations: 1748G/C and 1208/1209 del TT.
Embriologically the reticular "X" veins on the lateral surface of the leg and thigh represent the primary venous network that develops in embryo. Later in development these veins normally regress and they are replaced by the saphenous and deep venous networks.

Aging of the venous wall is characterized by: thickening of the wall, decrease of elastic fibres, atrophy of intimal and medial structure and hypertrophy of the adventiceal layer. The decrease in number of venous valves in the aging process is not confirmed. Calcification of venous intima occurs rarely in long lasting CVI and venous ossification is exceptionally. The veins of the soleus muscle have efficient valve cusps till the age of 30. Then they suffer parietal and valves degeneration and the veins became varicose and sinusoidal. In case of increased venous pressure the most vulnerable vein region is the place where the valves are inserted (because of a thinner venous wall). Therefore this region suffers a greater distension than the rest of the vein. (Ramelet- 93)

5.2. ETIOPATHOGENY

The etiology and pathogeny of venous disease is still poorly understood. According to many researches varicose veins have a multi-factorial origin, linked to heredity, environment and age. Some studies showed clearly that telangiectasiae are an important indicator for the progressive venous degeneration. So, these patients require a meticulous phlebological examination (duplex scanner) and a long lasting supervision. An appropriate treatment can slow down the progression of the dilative illness of the deep veins.
The varicose veins can be classified into three groups:

- congenital: agenesia or hypoplasia, agenesia or defect of valves of the deep veins or persistence of abnormal veins at newborns;
- primary: venous dilatation without a previous cause but with the presence of some favorable factors;

- secondary varicose veins are represented by:
  - postthrombotic varicose veins are the result of deep thrombosis on the main veins, with the compensatory secondary dilatation of the perforating and superficial veins and with its sequelae as a result of the valve destruction; these are the most frequent secondary varicosities;
  - the compression of the main vein trunks (tumors, adenopathies, tissue sclerosis after radiotherapy, vicious scars); the frequency is low and easy to be recognized;
  - external trauma of the veins (a blow kick in the thigh at football) and internal trauma (vein catheter with the destruction of the valves); the incidence is very low;
  - artery and vein shunts and fistulas: posttraumatic or as results of surgical operation.

5.3. PRIMARY VARICOSE VEINS (HYDROSTATICS)

The following local and general factors determine the development of varicose disease:

- local factors: the gravitation, the topography of the epiphascial veins above the fascia and inside the subcutaneous lax tissue, which have insufficient valves, and no muscular support;
- general factors:
  - internal (hereditary): obesity, tall people, endocrine factors and pregnancies;
  - external (of the environment): profession (prolonged, orthostatic position; important effort), heat, humidity, avitaminosis, infections and diet factors combined with bowel habit (according to a few well-conducted studies), smoking (Framingham study finds a link but only in men, Basel study doesn't take this into account).

The arterial hypertension had not been demonstrated to determine the varicose disease and the CVI. The long lasting upright or standing posture, the high temperature at workplace has correlation with CVI. (Hobson) The economic and social standard of patients is important for the evolution of the disease and the healing of the complication, especially of the venous ulcer (50). The tight closes (especially jeans) and high heels favor the appearance of varicose disease.

There are several conflicting theories concerned with the etiopathogeny and the development of the varicose disease:

- classic theory: varicose disease usually starts at junction's points, where superficial veins connect to the deep veins. These points are the saphenofemural, the saphenopopliteal junction and the main perforating veins. The first step of the disease is represented by the valvular incompetence. Than the increased hydrostatic pressure determines the dilatation and the elongation of the veins. The simple dilatation of the vein determines the appearance of a distance between the normal leaflets of the valve. Harvey considered the descending valve incompetence as the trigger of varicose; Trendelenburg, Hesse and Schaack sustained the role of aplasia of the valves in saphena vein; Hach and Kistner discussed about the initial role of valvular lesions in saphena or femoral veins. The result is the blood retrograde reflux and the venous hypertension. This fact determines first the dilatation of the main veins and than the dilatation of the collateral veins, from top to the bottom, step by step, proportionally with the development of the valvular incompetence;
- hydrostatic theory: human bipedal position causes the opening of the venous valves and the increase of the vein pressure at long standing position with veins dilation and secondary valvular incompetence in the lower limbs;
- theory of the intrinsic constitutional biochemical deficiency of the vein walls: biochemical deficiency, alters the physical properties of the collagen and elastic fibers of the veins determining abnormal distensibility of the connective tissue. Probably the patient's veins with varicosities are more distendable than those of healthy people. This fact explains the frequent association between varicose, hemorrhoid disease, hernias and flat foot. Recent theories incriminated the anomalies of muscular layers and endothelium. More than that, the colagenous infiltrates separate the smooth muscles cells. These segmentations block the reaction of the muscle to different stimuli as a whole, and the venous tonus decrease. So the veins dilate, the valves are not competent any more and they don't close. The microscopic parietal abnormalities are: vacuoleted endothelium with picnotic nuclei, thinning and disorganising of the media, swelling and helical splitting of the collagen fibers. Experimental studies on human veins demonstrate that contraction of the varicose veins is lesser than that of

the normal veins answering to stimulation with norepinephrine, serotonine, histamin or passive stretch. Another argument is that degeneration of the venous wall is not uniform but disseminated at patients with varices. The vein wall can be thickened and fibrous or very thin, with aneurismal dilatations, in alternation with normal calibrated veins. But even the "normal" calibrated veins have structural abnormalities. The normal veins introduced as graft in arterial circulation become "arterialized " with hypertrophy and thickening of the wall. The varicose veins answer at hyperpressure with dilatation. Certain segments of the varicose veins dilate under local parietal and hemodynamic conditions determining fusiform varicosities between competent valves, collateral dilatations, real telangiectasies and dilated collateral veins;

- theory of the arterio-venous communications (AVC), which by-pass the capillaries and transfer the increased arterial pressure in the distal veins. The peripheral venous hyperpressure determines the vein dilatation and starts the varicosis development (Haimovici- 40). The AVCs were discovered by Sucquet in 1862 and confirmed in 1877 by Hoyer. In 1929 Blalock records a high oxygen saturation of the blood in the varicose veins and discussed the presence of the AVCs. In 1949 Pratt found many throbbing AVCs with arterial blood. Pratt described "the arterial varices", which are an important cause of the early relapse of varicose after correct operation. Schalin (1981) dissected and described the AVCs as pulsating arteries in the aria of "hot spot" with varicose veins. The diameter of AVCs was between 0.1-2.0 mm with a media of 0.6 mm. The connection between AVC and the vein is extrafascial (Pulaches and Vidal-Barraquer-1953; Gius-1960; Haeger-1963) or subfascial (Schalin-1981). The arterial sources of AVCs are the tibial arteries and muscular gastrocnemian arteries. The venous ends were in the extrafascial varicosities or in the subfascial parts of the perforans veins (Haimovici- 40). Haimovici considered that the AVCs in varicose disease are the result of the dysfunction of the arterio-venous (AV) shunts, which have the diameter of 30-60 μm. The arteriographies with early venous return and Doppler exam with venous pulse image demonstrate the presence of AVCs (Haimovici- 40). The congenital or acquired AV fistulae are large morphologic abnormalities. According to this theory the interruption or the excision of the AVCs for preventing early relapsing of the varicose disease are considered the most effective treatment;

- theory of the enzymatic anomalies: enzyme abnormalities reflect metabolic changes in the venous wall; patiens with varicose veins may have high blood levels of β-glucuronidase, β-N-acetylglucaseaminidase and arylsulfatase; this levels decrease after surgical treatment of varicose veins; (Ramelet- 93)
- theory of the disturbance of the endothelial prostanoids and endothelin production;
- theory of smooth vein muscle disfunction: the evaluation of smooth muscle contractility and endothelium function in primary varicose veins show that histamine caused only weak or absent endothelium-dependent relaxation of the normal veins compared to varicose veins where histamine induces dose-dependent relaxations (J.Avram, I.Siska- 3);
- theory of hypoxia in varicose disease genesis: Michiels et al. explained the alterations of the pathological veins as consequence of hypoxia that determines the activation of endothelial cells, which release inflammatory activators and also growth factors for smooth muscle cells. These processes lead to structural and functional modifications of the venous wall. The continuous exposure to blood components, including pro-oxidant agents, makes the venous wall susceptible to oxidative stress and free radical mediated reactions. Under pathological conditions, excessive amount of macromolecules is broken down by free radicals and proteases, the varicose saphenous vein loosing as much as 60% of the collagen in its wall. (Robert 1992) Some of the systems, which can protect the cells against oxidative injury are: reduced glutathion (GSH) and superoxide-dismutase. The glutathion redox cycle is sufficient to detoxify normal amounts of intracellular oxidants in catalase-deficient cells, but hydrogen peroxide in non-toxic concentration may overcome this single system and thus contribute to "in vitro" cellular damage. According to our data the plasmatic level of GSH increases significantly after 30 minutes of venous stasis in patients with lower limbs varicosities that could be due to a decrease of intracellular GSH stores. (I.Siska, J.Avram- 3) Hydrogen peroxid modulates the venous tone: lower concentration of H_2O_2 induces contractions of the saphenous vein, while higher doses are followed by venous dilation. The cells cultured at the low oxygen tension have significantly lower antioxidant activities than the cells cultured at the high oxygen tension suggesting that postcapillary venous endothelial cells should have lower antioxidant enzyme activities than the precapillary arterial ones. (Li et al. 1992)

- genetic implication: defects in the valves or in the venous wall;
- theory of apoptosis: in other studies it was observed the significance of apoptosis in varicose veins, compared to the healthy ones, indicating that deregulated apoptosis has a role in the pathogenesis of varicosities. In addition, significant differences are noted in the expression and subcellular localization of the cell cycle regulatory protein, cyclinD1, in varicose tissue, as compared with controls. (Jacob- 51) The entry of smooth muscle cells into the apoptotic pathway may be regulated by the induction of bax (a molecular mediator of apoptosis), because there is a significant presence of this pro-apoptotic protein in healthy veins. Both bax and PARP (poly ADP-ribose polymerase) are down regulated in varicose veins, as compared with healthy veins and so this may play a significant role in the pathogenesis of varicose veins. (Jacob- 51)
- theory of inflammation: experimentally Ono T. and Bergan J. (79) demonstrated that the venous hypertension may trigger the infiltration of the valves by leukocytes. Than the result is a proteolitic breakdown of the valvular structures combined with apoptosis of the cells in this area. The valves become atrophied and inefficient. There are also valves of the deep veins that are initially and congenitally affected by elongation and insufficient closing. Rothfuss (2001) demonstrated on endothelial cells cultures from umbilical vein that the increasing pressure determines a higher granulocytes adherence at the endothelial cells.

The orthostatic venous hyperpressure actions on GSV and on the collateral veins but greater dilatations occur in the saphenous tributaries in primary varicose. The explanation is the presence of the double fascial sheeting of the GSV. A.Caggiati (9) described the saphenous fascia formed by the interlacing of the hypodermal connective sheets, which fuses with the muscular fascia. A second fascia originates from the outer adventitia of the long saphenous vein and anchors it to the opposite face of the compartment. These two fascias oppose to the pressure acting on GSV.

The presence of reflux from pelvic veins through vulvar varices can favor the development of the lower limb varices even in the absence of incompetence of sapheno-femoral junction or perforans reflux. This happens to women with several pregnancies and hemorrhoids and vulvar varicosities at the same time. The symptoms of pelvic congestion, uterine retroversion and dispareunia are present.

Recent studies showed that monocytes / macrophages migrate into the venous wall and valves where they play a role in the pathogenesis of primary venous insufficiency. For the appearance of the varicose disease and chronic venous insufficiency the following processes are important: rolling, adherences and migration of leucocytes through the venous wall. Moyses (72) reported sequestration of leukocytes in the circulation of lower limbs after venous hypertension. Coleridge-Smith (14) considered that leukocytes trapping cause a reduction in capillary blood flow because of an increase in venous pressure. The sequestrated activated population of neutrophiles and monocytes in the microcirculation, remained bind to the endothelium when venous hypertension is reversed. An important element in these studies has been the interaction between the monocytes and the endothelium as a precursor of damage to venous valves and the venous walls. The study indicates that not only luminal venous endothelium but also endothelium in the vasa vasorum of refluxing saphenous veins is activated, as indicated by the upregulation of ICAM-1. (Takase- 111) Patients with chronic venous disease show increased leukocytes priming. The primed leukocytes show increased surface CD62L (involved in the initial "rolling"), CD11B (ligand for firm leukocytes adhesion and then diapedesis). Ono T., Bergan J., Schmid Schonbein and Takase S. put in evidence the inflammatory mechanism in the damage of the venous valve for varicose disease. (79)

It is observed that the balance between proteases and their inhibitors is temporally destroyed through the induction of matrix metalloproteinase gene expression or the secretion of enzymes of inflammatory cells. Smooth muscle cells, the most numerous cells in vascular walls have the capacity to respond to injury through their ability to synthetis extracellular matrix molecules and protease inhibitors. In conclusion, the protease/inhibitor balance must be perfectly controlled, because an accumulation of abnormal extra cellular matrix may have unforeseen side effects. (Jacob- 51)

The Edinburg Vein Study contains 1566 men and women aged 18-64 years who were selected at random from the age-sex registers of 12 general practices. Fiber intake, intestinal transit time, defecation frequency and the prevalence of straining at stool were all found to be significantly different between the two sexes. Men who reported that they strained to start passing motion showed a higher prevalence of mild and severe trunk varices compared to men who did not strain. In contrast, no consistent relationships were seen among women. An association between dietary fiber, constipation and the presence or severity of varicose veins was not supported. (Lee- 63)

The altered expression of glypican (a proteoglycan) and syndecan-1and-4 (another proteoglycan) in chronic ulcers reflect their possible roles during inflammation and cell proliferation. Hence, analysis of proteoglycans expression should be of interest in future study on normal as well as defective wound healing. (Lundqvist- 66)

Since haemostatic factors are involved in the processes of fibrinolysis and platelet aggregation, it is conceivable that such processes may be implicated in the pathology of varicose veins and chronic venous insufficiency. (Lee- 63)

In case of varicose disease without complication, changes of micro-vessels are considered to be compensatory adaptation. Patients suffering from a complicated type of varicose disease and postthrombotic syndrome have "failure" of compensatory adaptation reaction.

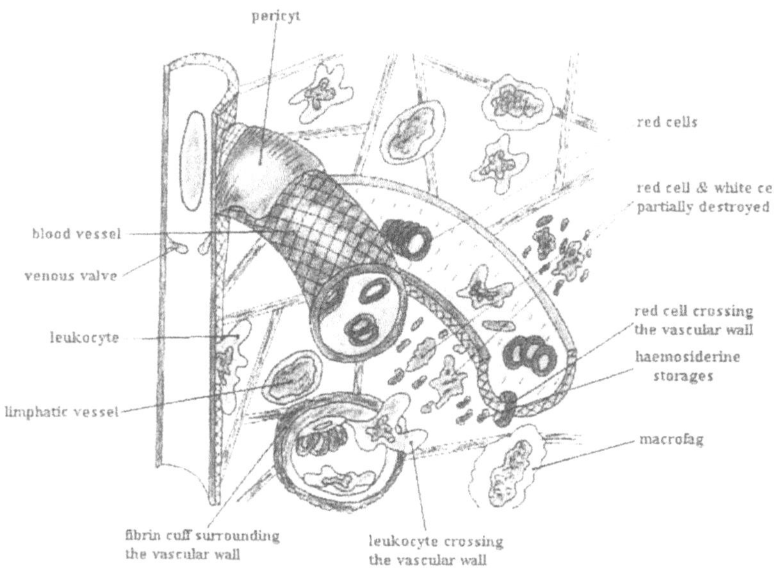

Fig.5.1. Pathophysiology of venous disease: the role of inflammation.

5.3.1. Morphopathology

The dilated and elongated veins become sinuous forming varicose packets; the dilatation is not homogenous (there are very dilated zones and normal zones). The valves are atrophied and the wall has adenoid endophlebitis plaques. The microscopic aspect is the phlebosclerosis of the walls. The connective tissue dysplasia of the vein wall is characterized by the irregular display of the fibers and by the change of the contractile myocites into metabolic myocites. This process debases the secretion of some enzymes. Around the veins there are sclerosis lesions of the surrounding subcutaneous tissue and of the skin lymphatic vessels. In the varicose veins the three tunics are still distinguishable but with great difficulty. The normal layers are disrupted by the fibrosis in varicose veins and the muscle layers are disorganized. The mesh-like bundles of smooth muscle cells are irregular, sometimes dispersed pell-mell, interrupted by bands of fibrosis in varying amounts. The elastic network is diminished and atrophied. In addition to the classical alterations of the varicose walls, mast cells were noted; they were oval, large, with numerous metachromatic granules stained with toluidine blue; the number of mast cells noted in the varicose segments was significantly higher that in the normal-looking portions. The cells were gathered in groups and were present especially in the adventitia, around in vasa vasorum. In some histological preparations a few mast cells were noted in the media.(J.Avram and I.Siska - 3)

5.3.2. Physiopathology

5.3.2.1. Soleus-Gastrocnemius Muscular Pump

The soleus muscles compress the soleus veins and push the blood into the tibio-fibular system and from the gastrocnemius veins into the popliteal vein. The thigh muscular pump compresses and evacuates the deep femoral vein and it is less important. The pumps work sometimes non simultaneous and so hyperpressure areas are formed and they are amortized through the perforans veins system, through the capacity systems. This system takes the hyperpressure through the special soleus vessels system. The tonus of the intrinsic vascular muscles adapts itself regulating the distensibility of the system. So it is embedded the venous stasis in the inferior limb in orthostatic position and the decrease of the arterial pressure that can cause faint.

The muscular pump looses its efficiency with aging, lack of exercises, ankle ankylosis and fibrosis of Achiles tendon.

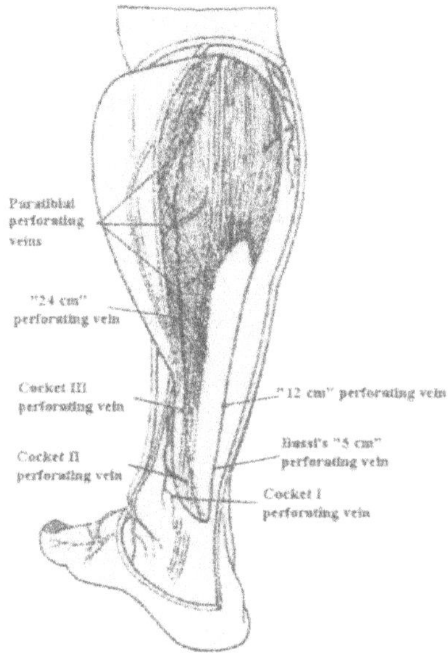

Fig.5.2. Perforating veins of the calf.

5.3.2.2. Cycle of the Walking Process is divided into (Partsch, Cappelli - 82):

- 2/3 for the anterior tibial muscle which maintains the foot in balance and does not determine the evacuation of the perforans veins;
- 1/3 for the contraction of the calf muscles, which initially empties the distal dilated veins, than the proximal ones and finally the muscular veins to the popliteal vein.

5.3.2.3. Superficial, Deep and Mixed Vein Insufficiency

Venous hemodynamic is altered by the varicose disease. The pressure in the lower limbs veins, in orthostatism and in movement, at healthy people has a low value, because the competent valves divide the blood column from heart to lower limb veins. The blood stasis in orthostatic position is followed by the opening and after that by the insufficiency of the vein valves. In this situation the veins are no more segmented by the insufficient valves. The blood flows backwards from top to bottom at the level of the crossing junctions, namely from the deep venous system to the superficial one. The ostial valvular insufficiency at the sapheno-femoral or saphenopopliteal confluent allows the blood to return from the deep venous system to the superficial one. That blood overloads the superficial venous system and induces the dilatation and the development of the varicose veins. The result is a vicious circle that overloads by the route of perforating veins the deep venous system with more blood. Thus the ostial vein insufficiency has an effect on the superficial venous system whose valves become incompetent and the superficial vein insufficiency overloads the deep venous system. Overloading of some perforating veins induces their dilatation and the perforating veins valves become insufficient. The finally result of this process is a vein insufficiency (superficial, deep or mixed) with a permanent increase of the vein pressure (phlebohypertonia).

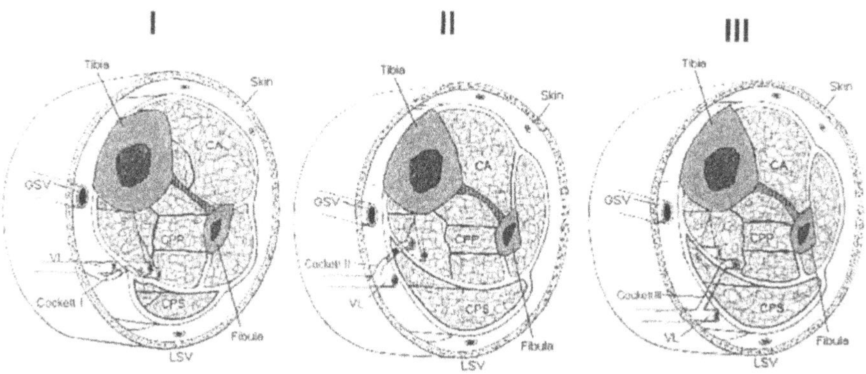

Fig.5.3. The tophography of perforans veins Cocket
(after P. Glovitscky-modified)

There is also a primary valvular insufficiency caused by congenital, thin and elongated valves. Its functionality is affected and the vein valves are inefficient.

5.3.2.4. Siphon Effect

When a venous segment is dilated the blood flow increase upstream by suction as in a siphon system and it appears a proximal functional valve deficiency. The destroy of the dilated vein restore the normal venous function and determine the disappearance of the siphon effect. (Ramelet-93)

5.3.2.5. Territorial Steal

It is represented by incompetence at the junction of a LSV, which drains in the territory of the GSV.

5.3.3. Physical Examination

5.3.3.1. Evolution Stages of the Varicose Disease

- The subjective signs of the pre-varicose period: heaviness in the calf while walking or in a prolonged orthostatic position, complaining of paresthesias and pains, sometimes juxtamalleolar or calf edema more intense in the evening. Calf edema is diminished while resting, especially in cases when one elevates the lower limbs above the horizontal level ("the American position of rest").
- The period of constituted varicose veins has the same subjective signs like those already mentioned: dull aching, heaviness, cramping, swelling in the lower part of the leg, but this time more emphasized and it has also the classical objective signs. The clinical examinations in orthostatic position done comparatively for both lower limbs proves irregular dilated venous girdles that can be seen under the skin. Sometimes there are folded veins displayed in packets. In the case of incompetence of a perforating vein it appears a subcutaneous ampullary dilatation named "blow-out". Another manifestations are the "varicose pearls": small, raised, ampullary dilatations covered with thin skin, which appears along of varicose veins.
- The period of complications: chronic vein insufficiency with dermatosclerosis, discoloration, inflammation, thrombosis, ulcers and bleeding. In lipodermatosclerosis the varicose veins are deeply embedded in fibrosis like a river passing through a canyon, therefore they are named "canyon" varicose veins.

The predictable increase of symptoms of varicose veins is correlated with aging in both sexes. In women there was a better correlation between the trunk varices and heaviness, tension, aching and itching as in men (Bradbury- 6).

5.3.3.2. Types of Varicose Veins

1. Telangiectasiae (dilated intradermal venules up to 1 mm in diameter) can be noticed as a "spider web" venectasias, especially on women's thighs. The German word for it is "Besenreisenvarizen" that means a broomstick - like varices. Perimalleolar and paraplantar teleangiectatic varicosities are also named "corona phlebectatica paraplantaris". There are four types of telangiectasies:
   - essential telangiectasiae: a fine bright-red capillary hairy pattern,
   - solitary teleangiectatic varicosities,
   - sheet telangiectasiae dependent upon a feeder vein,
   - secondary telangiectasiae (neotelangiectasiae, matting): small, congestive, localized angiomatose telangiectasiae developed after contusion, sclerosis of varicose vein or surgery; probably a hormonal factor is needed but determinant seems to be some unknown factors which trigger the angiogenesis. (Ramelet- 93)
2. Reticular varices are dilated veins under the derma that are 1-4 mm in diameter. These are not touchable. In the last classification - CEAP, 1994 - at clinical stage, the reticular veins and the telangiectasiae are separated from the varicose veins because they do not produce ulceration.
3. Varices of the collaterals of the saphena vein are subcutaneous, dilated and palpable and they are over 4 mm in diameter.
4. The varices of the great superficial veins are varicose of the two main venous collectors, the GSV and LSV. Only the varicose veins can produce varicose ulcer.
5. Superficial varices located in the area of insufficient perforating veins (Cockett, Dodd, Boyd, May, Kuster and Hach) as a "blow up" varicose. In the European classical view there are two types of anastomosis between veins:
   - communicating veins that connect either two deep or two superficial veins and thus never cross the deep fascias,
   - perforating veins cross the compartmental fascia and connect a superficial and a deep vein directly (direct perforating vein) or create a connection with a muscular vein (indirect perforating vein).

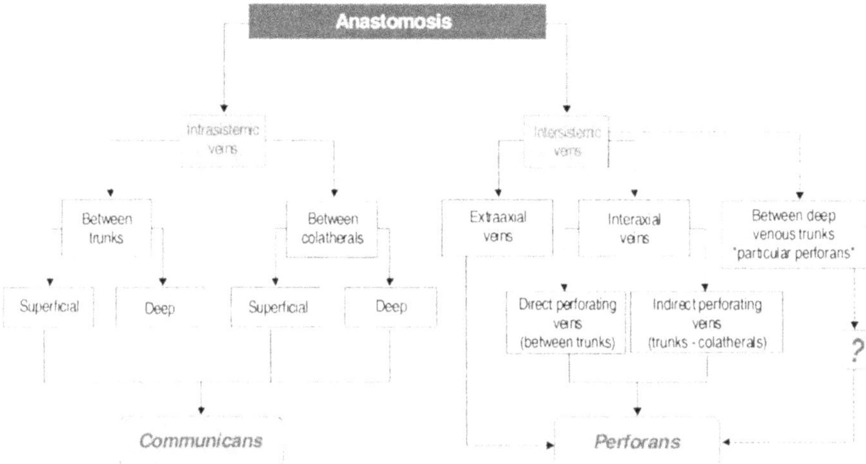

Fig.5.4. Inferior limb venous network – European classification.

Generally the British and American phlebologists don't respect the European schedule and they make not difference between anastomosing, perforating and communicating veins. There are variants of drainage from the superficial venous territory. The Leonardo's vein (posterior leg vein) drains the three Cockett veins and the "24 cm perforating vein"; they all are find in a vertical straight line from the posterior border of the medial maleolus upwards (Linton's line). The intersaphenous anastomosis creates communication between GSV and LSV territory and explains the diversity of clinical aspects observed in CVI. The duplication of the main vein such as popliteal, superficial femoral or GSV are frequent. Along the border of the Achilles tendon we can find Bassi's perforating vein and the "12 cm perforating vein". Bassi's perforating vein is located 5 cm above the tuberosity of the calcaneum and drains the blood from the LSV to peronial veins. The "12 cm perforating vein" is located 12 cm above the level of the tuberosity of the calcaneum and connects the LSV territory or the adjacent collaterals with the peroneal veins. (Ramelet- 93)

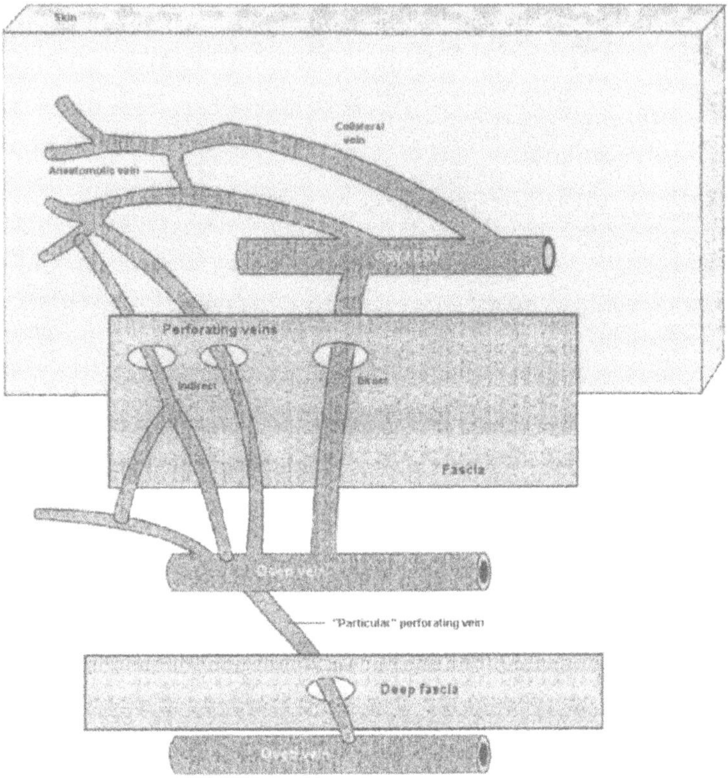

Fig.5.5. The venous network of the inferior limb – schedule representation

The varicose dilatations may appear either along the main saphenous axes or outside them. In both cases the venous dilatations may appear between competent valves (there are no valves disorders but the venous wall is affected primarily). Dilatation of sciatic vein (a remnant of an embryonic axis) determines a pseudosciatica syndrome by distending the nerve fibres. (Ramelet- 93)

5.3.3.3. Hach Classification of the GSV Insufficiency

- grade I: the opening of the ostial valve of GSV with the dilation of its initial segment at thigh (the Giacomini vein connects the GSV with the external saphena in obliquely "scarf" on thigh);

- grade II: the backward dilation of the saphena at the thigh level with valvular insufficiency and aneurysm dilation from the sapheno-femoral junction to the knee;
- grade III: the varicosis extends on the calf below the knee;
- grade IV: reflux and dilation of the superficial veins distal of malleola and varicosis that measure one finger in thickness.

The clinical examination records: cutaneous trophic changes (pigmentation, dermoepidermitis areas, white atrophy areas), calf ulcer and edemas. The compression by palpation determines the vein emptying. The arterial pulse is felt and the differential diagnosis of arteritis can be rejected. By percussion one can detect the vein trajectories hidden in the fat at obese patients. The palpation and auscultation of the lower limb veins records a frolement and a bruit when standing in orthostatic position at patients with venous reflux, important valvular insufficiency and giant varices.

5.3.3.4. CEAP Classification System of the Inferior Limbs Varicose

In 1994 in Maui (Hawaii) an international group of agreement has elaborated a new scoring system and gradation of the lower limb varicose disease. The CEAP system is based on 4 types of classification criteria, a score of the vein dysfunction and a methodology for diagnosis procedures. The classification criteria are:

- C - clinical
- E - etiologic
- A - anatomical
- P - physiopathological dysfunction

Clinical Classification(C)

- Class 0 - without any visible or palpable signs of varicose disease;
- Class 1 - telangiectasias or reticular veins;
- Class 2 - varicose veins;
- Class 3 - edema;
- Class 4 - cutaneous modifications due to the vein disease (pigmentation, venous eczema, lipodermatoslerosis);
- Class 5 - cutaneous modifications like those mentioned above with healed ulcer;
- Class 6 - cutaneous modifications like those mentioned above with active ulcer.

Etiologic Classification(E)

- Congenital (EC);
- Primary (EP) caused by undetermined factors;
- Secondary (ES) caused by determined factors.

Anatomical Classification(A)

Superficial veins (AS): 1.Telangiectasias/reticular veins;
2.Vena saphena magna above the knee;
3.Vena saphena magna below the knee;
4.Vena saphena parva;
5.Non-saphena;

Deep veins (AD)-Profound: 6.Vena cava inferior;
7.Vena iliaca communis;
8.Vena iliaca interna;
9.Vena iliaca externa;
10.Pelvo-gonadals venae, veins of the broad ligament, others;
11.Vena femoralis communis;
12.The deep femoralis vein;
13.Vena femoralis superficial;
14.Vena poplitea;
15.Vena tibiales anterior, tibiales posterior, peroneae;
16.Muscular veins - gastrocnemius, soleus, others;

Perforans veins (AP): 17.Thigh;
18.Calf.

Pathophysiologic Classification (P)

- Reflux (PR);
- Obstruction (PO);
- Obstruction and reflux (PRO).

The treatment can modify the clinical signs and symptoms. In that case the disease must be reevaluated. The physiopathologic classification may show the precise type of lesion in every vein from the anatomical table.

Score of the chronic vein dysfunction

It offers a numerical basis for an exact comparison of the patients with inferior limb vein diseases. This score is based on three individual criteria:

1. anatomical score: the sum of the anatomical segments, each being scored by 1 point;
2. clinical score:
   - pain: 0=absent; 1=moderate (there is no need for analgesics), 2=severe (analgesics are required);
   - edema: 0=absent, 1=moderate, 2=severe;
   - vein claudication: 0=absent, 1=moderate, 2=severe;
   - pigmentation: 0=absent, 1=circumscribed, 2=extended;
   - lipodermatosis: 0=absent, 1=circumscribed, 2=extended;
   - ulcer size: 0=absent, 1=↓2cm in diameter; 2=↑2cm in diameter;
   - duration in time of the ulcer: 0=absent, 1=↓3 months, 2=↑3 months;
   - ulcer recurrence: 0=absent, 1=once, 2=more than once;
   - number of ulcers: 0=absent, 1=unic, 2=multiple.
3. incapacity score:
   - 0= without any symptoms;
   - 1= symptomatic, the patient can work without any devices;
   - 2= the patient can work 8 hours a day only by using devices;
   - 3= the patient is unable to work, even if he has the supporting devices.

At the World Congress of Angiology Rome (2001) the CEAP classification was discussed, and it was proposed for some modifications. This improvement may be used especially in scientific studies on treatment efficiency.

5.3.4. Functional Vein Tests

- **Trendelenburg-Brodie Test**

  The patient is placed in dorsal decubitus and he is examined with the inferior limb approximately in vertical position waiting and softly massaging and "milking" upward the limb until the superficial veins get empty. Then we should manually compress the sapheno-femoral junction or we put a tourniquet at the bottom of the thigh. During this process the patient should stand up in orthostatic position. We can quickly evaluate the vein filling. The inferior limb veins get visible below the tourniquets in orthostatic position after 45-60 seconds due to the normal vein filling with blood from the peripheral to the proximal part. The quick filling from the proximal part while taking off the tourniquet proves the ostial insufficiency (the Trendelenburg I sign). The quick visualization of the calf veins with the maintained tourniquet proves the insufficiency of some perforating veins (the Trendelenburg II sign).

- **Mahorner-Ochsner Test ("3 Tourniquets")**
  It resembles to the Trendelenburg test but there are 3 tourniquets put on: at the bottom of the thigh, just above the knee and below the knee. It allows us to detect more precisely the reflux and the insufficient perforating veins. We successively take off the tourniquets in orthostatic position and thus the insufficient perforating veins can easily be observed.
- **Perthes Test**
  The patient is in orthostatic position and we put on a tourniquet in the distal third part of the thigh above the knee. Then the patient must walk. The varicose veins of the calf get empty while the patients walking. This fact indicates the permeability of the deep vein system; the increase in volume of the calf, and the dilated veins indicate an obstructed deep vein system.
- **Pratt Test**
  The test for the communicating veins: the patient is in the dorsal decubitus with the inferior limb raised for emptying the veins. The inferior limb must be wrapped up with a bandage. Then the patient stands up in an orthostatic position and we progressively unroll the bandage from the distal to the proximal part. At the same time we roll a second bandage from the distal part. We notice the vein refilling, located in the free area between the two bandages and thus we track down the insufficient communicating veins.
- **Linton Test**
  The tourniquet is applied below the knee. When the patient is in dorsal decubitus with the inferior limb elevated, the varicose veins can get empty very quickly if the deep vein system is permeable.
- **Schwartz Test (Tap sign/Wave test)**
  The percussion of a visible vein transmits proximally the venous wave and so we can locate the subcutaneous vein trajectories, which are

invisible at inspection. In the case of valve insufficiency of the superficial veins, the wave is transmitted towards the distal part.

- **Cough Test**
  In case of patients suffering from ostial insufficiency of the GSV we can palpate the vein reflux at the junction level when they cough.
- **Marmasse Test**
  Performing the percussion in the popliteal region at a patient in orthostatism with a partially bent knee (the resting position of the athlets) allows us to locate a dilated crossa of the varicose vena saphena parva.

5.3.5. Investigations (see 7.6)

- **Ambulatory venous pressure:** the importance of venous hypertension was recognized since the late 19th century (Perthes 1895). In 1949 Pollack and Wood recorded the venous pressure in saphenous vein at the ankle level in men during exercise and changes in position. The recordings were performed especially in the superficial venous system (Höjensgard and Starup-1952; P.Brinzeu –1954; Arnoldi-1966).
  Nicolaides and Zukowski (1986) considered that "pressure changes occurring in the deep system were almost identical to those in the superficial system". This statement is true only when the incompetent perforating veins transmit the pressure and the concept is erroneous in other situations. In 1994 Alimi measured the venous popliteal pressure and GSV pressure at healthy people with special devices.
  The technique of measuring the ambulatory venous pressure: a scalp needle is inserted into a dorsal vein and the pressure is measured at rest and after exercise or at standardized compression of the calf. The pressure curve is continuously recorded.
  The ambulatory venous pressure is the "gold standard " of hemodynamic measurement of venous circulation of lower limbs. The ambulatory venous measurements do not always reflect the regional hemodynamic changes that can occur in the deep or superficial venous system. Raju and Neglen (92) found different pressure values in the deep venous system compared with the pressure found in the dorsal vein. The pressure curves show clearly the differences between the deep and superficial venous systems recorded data.

The ambulatory venous pressure is the result of many parameters: arterial inflow, compliance of veins and valves competence, muscle pump ejection fraction, mobility of ankle joint, overall venous volume, degree of venous outflow obstruction.
The technique has a degree of aggression. Ambulatory venous pressure is helpful for the preoperative evaluation of patients proposed for venous reconstructive procedures and for postoperative controls.

- **Continuous Doppler ultrasonography, echo-Doppler and Doppler duplex** are non-invasive methods that are used for diagnosis. These methods help us to decide whether the intervention is needed or not. The vascular test has somehow limitations of indications and an important cost. Therefore the physician must select the real needed investigations at the patients. Clinical examination is very important and sufficient for not complicated cases associated with ultrasound explorations. We must detect the permeability of the deep veins, the sites of reflux or obstruction. For the indication of operation the evaluation must be carefully led.
- **Phlebography** is indicated in selected cases, it is a minimum invasive method and allows the exact visualization of the superficial and deep vein system in order to minimize the risk of errors.
- **Phleboscopy**: the phleboscope is a 2.3-2.8 mm in diameter angioscope with optic fiber and a fine coaxial irrigation channel. A pump controls the irrigation flow with normal saline serum and maintains the visibility in the vein. The phleboscope is introduced through a little incision in the inguinal region in the GSV and in the popliteal region in the LSV. The advance of the phleboscope is controlled by the transdermal illumination that is visible on the surface of the skin. Phleboscopy controls the presence and the function of the valves and the junctions of collaterals. Phleboscopy helps to perform external valvuloplasty, the obliteration of the incompetent collateral or perforans junctions and to preserve GSV or LSV for reconstructive surgery. The limitations of the method are the difficulty to pass the venous tortuosities and the stop of the phleboscope when it meets the first competent valve.

5.3.6. Diagnosis

5.3.6.1. Positive Diagnosis

On the basis of the clinical examination that locates the dilated superficial veins we can easily establish the positive diagnosis. Besides this we must know if:

- the symptoms are determined by the varicose;
- exists an ostial insufficiency or a perforans veins insufficiency and its location;
- the deep vein system is permeable or not.

5.3.6.2. Differential Diagnosis

a) First we establish the differential diagnosis taking into account the types of varicose that can be primary or secondary (of multiple causes). In addition to that we shall establish the differential diagnosis with other diseases that could be the cause of the symptoms (pain, local swelling, ulceration or edema):
   - crural hernia, inguinal adenopathy, hypodermic tumors (lipoma), epidermoid cyst, synovial cyst, onchocercosis;
   - lumbosciatic pains, arterial acute and chronic obstruction, osseous pain in ostheomielitis, joint pains in arthritis;
   - other affections which can cause calf ulcer are: peripheral arterial diseases, neuropaties, ulcerated malignant tumors, arterial hypertension etc.

b) The differential diagnosis of the edema:
   - edemas of general causes: cardiac, renal, hepatic, endocrine, hypoproteic (denutrition) are bilateral and easy to be differentiated from the edema of varicose disease cause;
   - the chronic vein edemas can appear at patients with important varicosis, with insufficient communicating veins and progresive varicose edemas progressive withdrawing at rest in bed; the edema caused by acute thrombophlebitis is accompanied by a specific pain;
   - the edema caused by an arterial insufficiency can be recognized by a lack of pulse and it is accompanied by pains at walking or even at rest;

- lipodistrophies increases the volume of the inferior limbs, but that does not depend on the position, the skin is normal;
- the acute or chronic lymphedema; in elephantiasis the edema is more stabile, it does not diminish at bed rest, the skin is characteristic, the Stemmer sign is present.

5.3.7. Evolution and Complications of Varicose Disease

Varicose disease that is not treated develops continuously and slowly. Different acute complications can appear in case of chronic insufficiency:

- chronic vein insufficiency is the late result of the aggravation of the disease in more than 15 years of evolution in cases with primary varicose disease but more faster (in only 2-3 years) in the PTS. The superficial insufficiency overloads the deep system and increases the diameter of the popliteal and superficial femoral veins with secondary valve insufficiency. The trophic lesions are: dermite ocre, lipodermatosclerosis, atrophie blanche and ulcer.
- varicose thrombophlebitis: predisposed by stasis.
- spontaneous or posttraumatic rupture of the varicose veins with bleeding:
    - subtegumental hematomas;
    - intramuscular = deep subfascial hematoma;
    - external = abundant hemorrhage, increased in the orthostatic position that often determines the patient's panic.
- calcification of the venous wall(venous sclerosis)

The varicose thrombophlebitis brings about located pains at the level of some thrombosed varicose packets, which formally were permeable. The tegument placed above the thrombosed vein has eritema and edema at inspection. By palpating the thrombosed vein you can feel something like an acute girdle incompressible with acute pain sensibility. The substratum is the thrombosis of the blood in a varicose packet, determined by the prolonged stasis and endothelial alteration. The thrombosis is usually located at the level of some important varicose packets and the thrombus adheres to the altered wall of the vein. Sometimes the process of thrombosis largely extends to the vena saphena magna or parva and it can affect the crossa as well. Through the insufficient thrombosed perforans' veins or through the thrombosed junction, the process of thrombophlebitis can extend itself to the deep vein system. As a result of this process the pain is being increased, the edemas are extended to calf and thigh. This is accompanied by functional impotence that is characteristic to the deep thrombophlebitis. In this situation a pulmonary embolism may occur at any time.

5.3.8. Treatment

The varicose disease is an evolutionary illness which progresses naturally with age, therefore the therapy must stop, slow or prevent the varices development.

I. Prophylactic: you have to avoid obesity, sedentary, orthostatic position, constipation, sports which require static physical effort (volleyball, weight lifting) and the increasing of the abdominal pressure; you have to protect the foot by elastic stocking or bandage which keep the superficial veins empty and reduce the effect of the venous hypertension; walking and swimming are indicated as sports.

II. Curative: etiologic treatment of primary varicose is not known. The treatment takes into consideration morphological alterations and clinical symptoms and it does not affect the history and the natural evolution of the varicose disease (50). The aim of the treatment is functional (the suppressing of the reflux), morphological (the suppressing of all varicose veins) and esthetic. There are many methods of treatment and they must be applied for the rest of the life because varicose disease is evolving and has recurrent characteristics. Due to this fact the patient must come to periodical check over examination and each time we shall establish the appropriate treatment.

Balneophysiotherapic, life hygiene, weight loss;

Medical:

- phlebotonic and phlebotrophic (vitamin C and vitamin E, flavonoids preferable micronized, extracts of Gingo Biloba) which induce the increase of vein tonus and quality of the vein wall by re-establishing the capillary permeability, by improving the lymphatic drainage, by decreasing the edemas;
- non - steroids anti-inflammatory drugs: phenylbutasone; the usage of non-steroids anti-inflammatory drugs

improves the symptomatology but it has a lot of secondary effects and risks;

- steroid anti-inflamatory drugs: too risky for a real benefit.

Compressive: elastic stockings, elastic / non-elastic or special bandages;
Sclerotherapeutical: Polidocanol (Aethoxisclerol), sodium tetradecyl sulfate only for un-systematized varicose or associated with surgical treatment for important varicose; sclerotherapy brings about the edema or irritates and damages the vein endothelium with a local thrombosis of the injected vein; this is followed by a fibrosis and the vein lumen disappears. Endo-venous inclusions with catgut are introduced intraoperatory for the remaining varicose. This determines the sclerosis of the remained varicose packets after the surgery. The last technique is the sclerotherapy with foam;

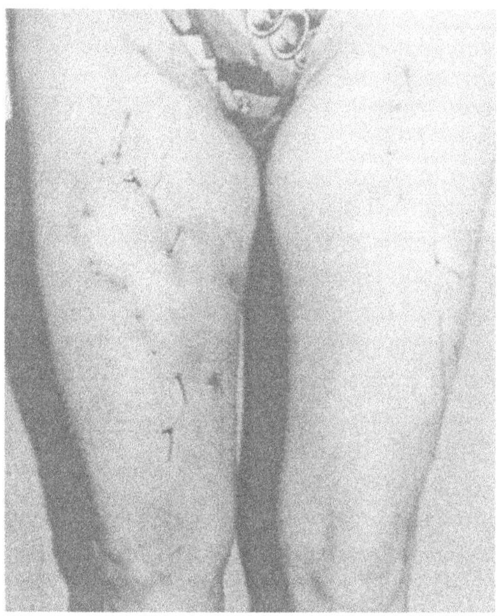

Fig.5.6. Sclerotherapy with catgut

Surgical treatment of venous disease consists in:

Classical methods:

- suppressing the reflux:
  - crossectomies at the level of GSV's and LSV's junctions;
  - ligature of insufficient perforating veins through direct procedures, underfascial or laparoscopic procedures-SEPS.

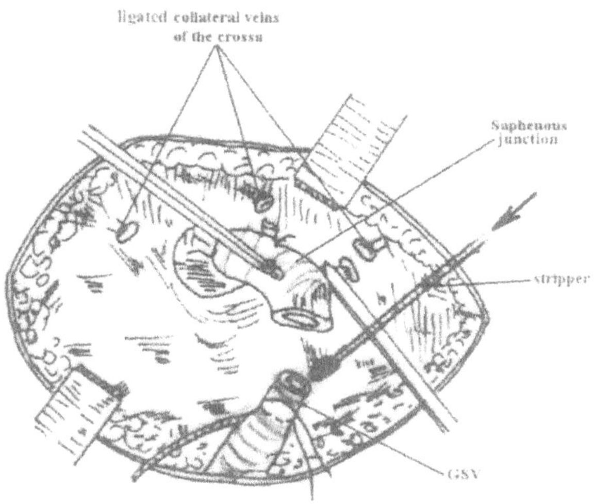

Fig.5.7. Saphena junction ligations & crossectomy

- stripping of the pathological veins:
  - external stripping by Babcock procedure, stripping by invagination - Van der Stricht procedure, Brinzeu procedure;
  - extirpation of the saphena by long incision - Terier Alglave procedure;
  - phlebectomies (extirpation of varicose veins by mini incision as the Muller procedure). These methods produce an important modification of the venous hemodynamique. As a concept, it is important what happens with the insufficient perforating veins and with the other superficial remaining veins;

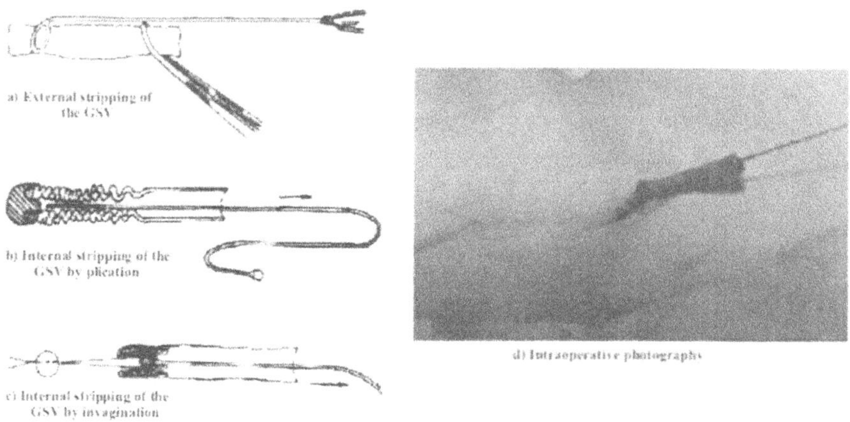

Fig.5.8. Stripping procedures of GSV

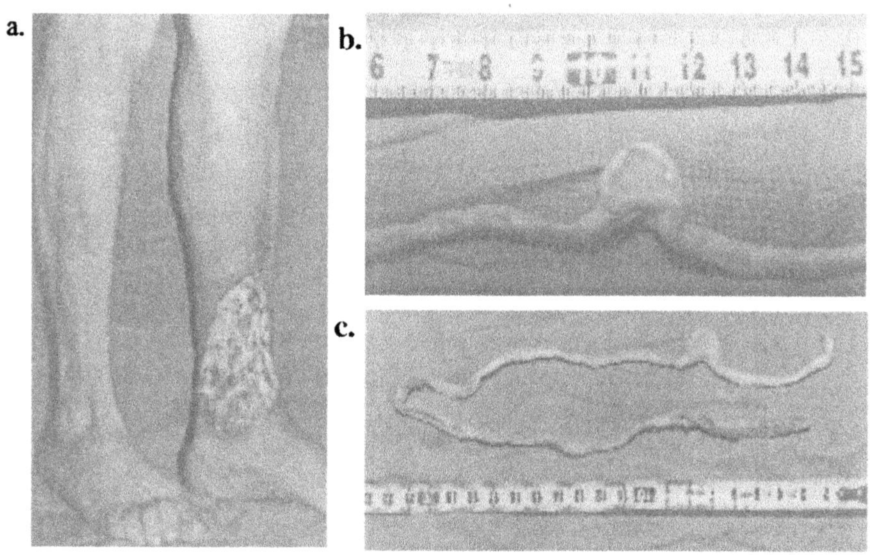

Fig.5.9. Primary neglected varicosis with chronic venous insufficiency: giant ulcer (a.) and the stripped GSV (b., c.)

- alternatives to stripping:
  - freezing technique,
  - sclerosing by operative high frequency catheter,
  - intraoperatory sclerosis with catheter.

Modern methods:

- vein revalvulations (Kistner technique of repairing the valves in primary vein insufficiency), Raju technique;
- vein endosurgery : recalibration, valve repair;
- cuffing of dilated superficial veins for diminishing the vein diameter and remaking the continence of the valves(Hetteny A., Corcos L);

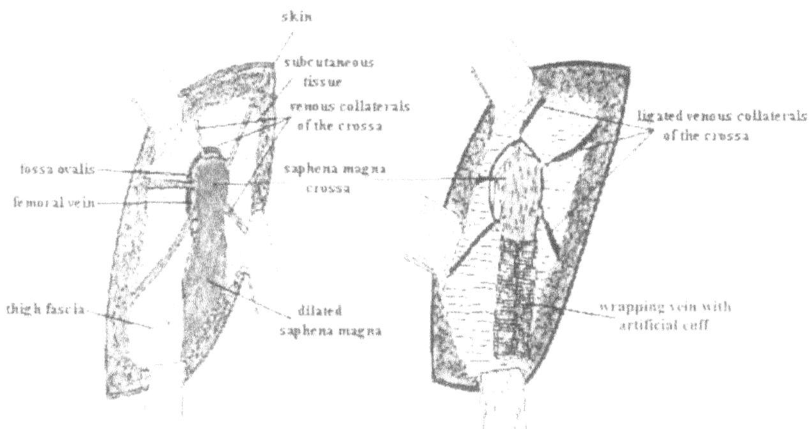

Fig.5.10. Wrapping procedure of GSV

- Chiva operation: Claude Franceschi introduced the conservative hemodynamic surgical treatment of venous insufficiency in ambulatory ("one day") surgery which is a preserving procedure. The saphenous cross is ligated, then you immediately put ligatures on the saphena from a distal position to an insufficient perforating vein which could allow and direct the blood reflux into the deep venous system. The late results are controversial and even contested at present.

Indications:

For the following reasons it is required surgical intervention:

- cosmetic reasons (profession requires, psychic comfort);
- functional disturbances for not improved varicose by medical treatment. Its major symptoms are: pain, cramps and tiredness;
- complications of the varicose disease (edema, superficial thrombophlebitis and ulcer).

The indications of sclerotherapy are at present extended by phlebologists. Thy are guided in their technique by the echo-Doppler to inject the sclerosing substance. Even thus the sclerosing of the crosses is a risky procedure. The results of surgical treatment are safer and less risky. It is said, "a good sclerotherapy is better than a bad surgery and viceversa".

Techniques:

The GSV saphenectomy – the usual intervention upon the inferior limb varicose – is carried out by spinal anesthesia, epidural anesthesia or recently by local anesthesia and sedatives in "one day surgery". The upper incision of 5-6 cm is usually performed obliquely next to the crural ligament (above the inguinal fold) centered on the junction of the internal saphena in femoralis vein detected by the echo-Doppler. We dissect and locate the saphena cross and we ligate it tangent to the femoralis vein (high ligature) in order to avoid a venous diverticulum that can favor the blood stasis and the thrombosis and we cut the vein at this level. We catheterize GSV with a special wire named stripper that has an oliva at one end. It can be catheterized backward to the proximal part of the calf (short stripping) or to the internal malleolus (long stripping). We can initially discover the saphena at the internal malleolus and we catheterize it upward to its proximal part. We cut the vein distally and the stripping of the vein is carried out by plicature (Babcock technique) or by invagination in its lumen (Van der Stricht technique).

The LSV saphenectomy: we make a small transversal incision in the popliteal space, the incision being centered upon the saphena's cross, the crossa will be ligatured and cut. Then we catheterize towards the distal part uncover it in its distal area and carry out the stripping.

Results of the saphenectomy:

The long-term results were noticed by many studies. Fischer performed a complete study and followed the patients a few decades after surgery. The results were:

- in short term the symptoms generally responded well to the operative procedures. The immediate improvement is 86 % for pain, 94 % for cramps, 78% for tired and heavy legs, 88% for edema and 100% for superficial thrombosis. In 30 years the cure rate decreased, the symptoms returned to a certain degree in the decades that followed. But the symptoms can be the result of other conditions, too. Therefore the patient has to be informed by the physician about this eventuality;
- the complications were cured in the majority of the cases and the number of relapsing was very low.

The treatment of the varicose thrombophlebitis consists in rest and avoidance of the orthostatic position, non-steroid anti-inflammatory medical treatment (phenylbutazone) and analgesics. We apply local wet bandages and ointments with heparinoid and hialuronidase. The anticoagulant treatment is excessive and contraindicated in the circumscribed forms and it becomes necessary in the extended forms of the varicose thrombophlebitis. If affects the entire saphena to the proximity of its junction or even the junction or the insufficient perforating veins. There is a high risk of thrombosis in the deep vein system and of pulmonary embolism. In this situation the anticoagulant treatment as in DVT is recommended.

The treatment of the varicose vein tears consists in rest (raising up the affected limb) and compressive bandage that is directly applied on the wound. In case of extended tear we initially compress the torn superficial varicose and then the definitive hemostasis is carried out with 2 ligatures through the skin above and below the bleeding area under the vein in the conditions of sterility. It is forbidden to apply the tourniquet next to the torn varicose in order to avoid an intense bleeding.

5.4. RECURRENT VARICES AFTER SURGERY (REVAS)

Definition:

REVAS is the presence of varicose veins in a lower limb after previous operation for varices. REVAS includes true recurrences, residual veins and varicose veins due to disease progression. The incidence is 20-80% depending on the duration of the follow-up assessment. (5 till 20 years)

Glass (31,32) communicated a relapsing rate of 25% after 4 or more years of following the process up. The medium time to REDO surgery is between 6 and 20 years after the first operation.

Etiology of REVAS:

- residual veins remaining after an incomplete primary treatment (tactical or technical errors) or incomplete operations: failure to justly identify the lesions or to perform adequate technique or to accomplish the primary plan of the operation;
- evolution or progression of varicose disease;
- some possible factors such as: sex, heredity, hormonal status (especially pregnancy), profession, sports, diet and deep venous reflux.

REVAS can be diagnosed using anamnesis, physical examination, continuous-wave Doppler (the most used method), duplex scanning (method of choice), venography (a valuable method), plethysmography and venous pressure measurements.

Pathomorphology in REVAS

The main findings are:

- collateral venous channels bypassing the correct ligated junction;
- incorrect ligated saphena junction: long, with permeable tributaries and reflux;
- neovascularization: new conection between deep veins and varices performed to tortuous and thin-walled neoveins, with variable thickness of media and avalvulate, without parietal innervation and very friable at dissection;
- cavernoma: a lot of fragile veins realizing venous shunts;
- disconnection at the junction and connection to other sites.

Classification

It uses the CEAP scale proposed by the Consensus Group (16) and modified as follows:

- C= clinical signs (grade 0-6) supplemented by A for asymptomatic and S for symptomatic presentation;
- E= etiologic classification (congenital =C, primary =P and secondary =S);
- A= anatomic distribution (superficial =S, deep =D, perforator =P, alone or in combination);

- P= pathophysiological dysfunction (reflux =R, obstruction =O, alone or in combination).

Anatomical classification has been adapted for REVAS as follows (85):

- T is for topographical site: g=groin, t=tight, p=popliteal fossa, l=lower leg including ankle and foot, o=other;
- S is for source of recurrence and reflux from deep system: 0=no reflux, 1=pelvic/abdominal, 2=saphena-femoral junction, 3=thigh perforators, 4=saphena-popliteal junction, 5=popliteal fossa perforator, 6=gastrocnemius veins, 7=lower leg perforators;
- R is for reflux: R+ for significant, R– for lack of clinical significance, R? for undefined clinical significance;
- N is for nature of source: Ss is for same site (1=technical failure, 2=tactical failure, 3=neovascularisation, 4=undefined, 5=mixed), Ds is for new site (1=present at the previous operation, 2=new, 3=uncertain or not known and insufficient information at the time of first operation);
- C is for contribution from persistent incompetent trunks: AK=GSV above knee, BK=GSV below knee, SSV=SSV present, Φ=without/other;
- F is for posible conributory factors: gF=general (family history, obesity, pregnancy, hormons), SF=specific (primary deep venous incompetence, postthrombotic syndrome, iliac vein compresion, congenital, lymphatic, calf pump dysfunction).

Disability score proposed by the Consensus Group is graded as follows: Φ=asymptomatic, 1=symptomatic but can walk normally without compression, 2=symptomatic and can walk normally only with leg compression, 3=total disability.

Treatment

It consists in compression, drugs and surgical procedures (sclerotherapy and REDO surgery). Surgical techniques are divided into two groups: procedures that eliminate reflux from the deep to superficial venous systems and procedures for eradicating varicose veins. (Perrin- 84)

Treatment consist in:

- compression: improves symptoms but without action on etiology;
- drugs: flavonoids ameliorate symptoms especially oedema and the venous tonus;

- sclerotherapy and ultrasound guided sclerotherapy have a variable degree of eficacity to obtain occlusion and durable constriction of the vein. The USA and Australian flebologist use higher concentration of sclerosants combined with compression. The French increase progressively the doses and quantities of sclerosants without compression. The scleroterapeuts inject first the principal and more proximal points of reflux. (Perrin – 84)
- surgery:
  - control of the stumps with flush ligature and resection; some surgeons recommended to put a barrier between the deep veins and the superficial tissues by suturing a patch, a muscle or a fascia over the femoral vein to prevent neovascularisation;
  - phlebectomy, resection of residual trunks;
  - ligatures of perforans veins.

The presence of deep venous insufficiency is a negative factor. When possible the primary or secondary deep insufficiency must be operated on.

The long-term results of re-operation for REVAS consist in 35% recurrence rate (Eklof, Juhan - 22). Probably the neovascularisation is responsable for the recurrence of the correct operated cases (Davy - 19, Nyameke - 78, Glass – 31,32). The postoperative sclerotherapy improves the late results.

CHAPTER 6

THROMBOEMBOLIC VENOUS DISEASE

TAKE HOME MESSAGES

- Decisive factors for DVT: parietal lesions, venous stasis and hyper coagulation (Virchow triad), influenced by internal and external predisposing factors. Thrombophilia is a predisposition to thrombosis caused by a genetic or an acquired defect. Inherited thrombophilia is responsible mainly for venous thrombosis
- Multiple clinical signs of DVT are insufficient for accurate diagnosis. There are different clinical, topographic and evolving forms of DVT. Doppler, D-dimer test, pletismography, phlebography, MRI are useful for diagnosis. Further tests must investigate the possible risk factors: neoplasm, infections, genetic defects and if possible to correct them.
- Complications of the DVT are postthrombotic syndrome followed by CVI, pulmonary embolism and venous gangrene.
- Prophylactic treatment is represented by LMWH administration and by external elastic compression. The curative treatment is more controversial: anticoagulation with unfractionated heparin / LMWH or fibrinolysis. The surgical venous thrombectomy with Fogarty catheter is recommended only in the iliofemoral thrombosis. The new trend is represented by the ambulatory anticoagulation and the early mobilization.

6.1. GENERALITIES

The extended thrombosis that develops in the major veins is of extremely high clinical importance. In 1846 Virchow recognized the association between venous thrombosis in the legs and pulmonary embolism. This disease is also called thrombophlebitis, deep venous thrombosis (DVT), phlebitis, thrombosis but the thromboembolic venous disease is the appropriate name. This name suggests the anatomopathological lesions, the development of the disease in veins and includes the major complication that aggravates the disease.

Definition:
DVT is a process of the blood coagulation in the deep vein axle, which is followed by a phlebitic inflammatory reaction. Practically it is the activation of coagulation in veins in areas of reduced blood flow. (102)

6.2. ETIOPATHOGENY

The formation, development and propagation of venous thrombi are the results of an imbalance between thrombogenesis and the body's protective mechanism, especially the circulating inhibitors of coagulation and the fibrinolitic system.

6.2.1. Predisposing Factors

- external: weather factors (foehn wind), stress, excess of lipids, drugs (vitamin K, anticonceptionals, diuretics), mechanical (traumas);
- internal: old age (patients over 60-70 years), female patients more frequently, heredity, cardiac decompensation, myocardial infarction, hemiplegia.

There are a lot of patients with unexplained venous thrombosis, or with recurrent venous thrombosis although they underwent a correct treatment, or unusual location of the thrombosis. In these situations we may suspect congenital or acquired hypercoagulability disorders. There are a lot of main causes of acquired hypercoagulability: smoking, heparin-induced thrombocytopenia, warfarin, antiphospholipid syndrome, pregnancy, oral contraceptives, diabetus mellitus, hyperlipidemia, polycythemia vera, vasculitis, hyperfibrinogenemia, nephrotic syndrome, malignant disease, surgery, thrombocytemia, homocystinemia. The venous thrombotic risk of oral contraceptives is high among women with coagulation abnormalities and with so-called third-generation contraceptives (containing desogestrel or gestodene). The risk is highest during the first year of use. The same situation is present in hormone replacement therapy. (Bauer - 4.)

6.2.2. Decisive Factors (Virchow Triad)

- vein wall lesion and endothelium disfunction are caused by external venous traumas, catheterizations, surgical operations and compression, inflammatory syndromes and age;
- vein stasis: is caused by prolonged rest in bed after traumas, plaster immobilization or surgical operation, extrinsic compression (tumoral process, Cockett syndrome, retroperitoneal fibrosis), external compression (clothes),superficial or/and deep venous insufficiency. It determines the decreasing of the calf muscles pump activity, hypovolemia. The following factors contribute to this process: the respiratory insufficiency, obesity, deficiency of the cardiac pump in heart diseases, cardiac rhythm disturbances and prolonged abdominal meteorism;
- hyper coagulation: the changes of the blood coagulation in the trauma shock, proliferative syndromes (polycythemias, neoplastic proliferations), dehydration, postpartum status, nephritic syndrome, cancer, some endocrine diseases, immunologic syndromes or because of thrombophilia (decrease of antithrombine III, protein S, deficiency of protein C, hiperhomocisteinemia, deficiency in factor V Leyden, hiperprothrombinemia, high levels of factor VIII).

Antithrombin III (AT) is a serine protease inhibitor, which inhibits the activated forms of factors IX, X, XI, XII and also inhibits thrombin and kallikrein. Antithrombin III deficiency is classified as type I when both concentration and activity levels are reduced and as type II when only the activity is reduced. Type I AT deficiency is associated with recurrent venous thrombosis and low levels of AT protein according to measurements by both functional and antigen assays. Clinical factors or genetic risk factors (factor V Leyden mutation and C677T mutation in the methylenetetrahydrofolate reductase gene) might interact with this deficiency and contribute to the appearance the thrombosis. (Arnaldi - 1)

Protein C is a vitamin K-dependent glycoprotein that is synthesized in the liver. Protein C is activated by thrombin and by the endothelial bound thrombin-thrombomodulin complex to APC that inactivates factors Va and VIIIa. In analogy with antithrombin III deficiency, protein C deficiency is classified in type I and type II. The resistance to APC is due to haplotype HR of the V factor gene or to the mutation Arg306Thr.

Protein S is also a vitamin K-dependent glycoprotein but is produced not only in the liver but also by the endothelium, megakaryocytes and Leydig cells in the testis. Protein S serves as a cofactor for APC, but also it may has an APC-independent inhibiting effect on the tenase complex (IXa-VIIIa). Type I protein S deficiency consists in low total and free concentration and low activity; type II or IIb consists in only a low activity and type III or IIIa consists in low activity accompanied by a reduction of free protein S concentration.

Homo/hetero mutation of factor V Leyden resistant at splitting and at activation by protein C consists in mutation of G1691A in exon 10 (Arg506Gln). Thrombophilia may be caused also by a homo/hetero mutation of prothrombin (G20210A).

The aminate acid homocystein results from metabolism of metionin; it is very toxic for the vascular wall. The high level of homocysteinemia determines thrombosis. Hyperhomocysteinemia may be an inherited state due to some mutations of cistation β-synthetase or of methilentetrahidrofolat reductase, or may be caused by a dietary deficiency in folate, cobalamin or pyridoxine.

High levels of factor VIII increase the risk of venous thromboembolism (more then five fold) but the mechanisms that cause high factor VIII levels are unclear. Present data showed that a single functional sequence variation in the factor VIII or VWF gene could not explain the majority of high factor VIII levels and thrombotic risk. (Ouriel- 80)

Decreased activity of protein C is present in 161 genetic mutations, decreased level of free protein S antigen – in 131 mutations and decreased activity of antithrombin – in 127 mutations.

6.3. ETIOLOGIC CLASSIFICATION OF DVT

Etiology: idiopathic -38.9%; postoperative-34.7%; malignancy-9.5%; trauma-7.9%; hypercoagulability-4.1%; neurological disorders-2.5%; prolonged immobilisation-2.5%. (Ouriel- 80)

The acquired hypercoagulable state that determine an increased risk of venous thromboembolism is caused by some factors as the following:

1. Iatrogenic conditions:
   - Surgery: general anesthesia and immobility per- and postoperatively slow down the blood flow. The vessels walls may be traumatized during surgery. A significant reduction of the level of antithrombin and protein C appears especially after total hip replacement, oncologic or gynecologic operations. Also after surgery it occurs acute phase reactions with increased fibrinogen, thrombocytosis and platelet activation with increased aggregability, high levels of factors II, VII VIII and XIII. Surgery lasting less than 30 minutes and local or regional anesthesia are not considered significant risk factors;
   - Estrogen treatment: oral contraceptives that contained 50-100mg estrogen/tablet produce a significant risk of venous thromboembolism. Hormone replacement therapy after menopause determines an increased risk of deep vein thrombosis and pulmonary embolism;
   - Protease inhibitors: at patients infected with HIV and treated by a combination of reverse transcriptase inhibitors and protease inhibitors it may appear as side effects a metabolic syndrome with hyperlipidaemia, decreased glucose tolerance and high levels inhibitor of plasminogen activator;
   - L-Asparaginase: it is used for the treatment of acute lymphatic leukemia and induces reduction of the antithrombin level via decreased synthesis in the liver;
   - Heparin-induced thrombocitopenia;
   - Indwelling intravenous catheters.
2. Venous thrombembolism secondary to another disease: cancer, myeloproliferative disorders, paroxysmal nocturnal haemoglobinuria, trauma and fractures, stroke, myocardial infarction and congestive heart failure, obesity, immobility due to infection, cardiolipin antibodies/lupus anticoagulant, Behcet's disease, Cushing's syndrome, nephrotic syndrome, inflammatory

bowel disease, hyperhomocysteinemia, hypofibrinolysis, varicose veins.
3. Physiological factors: age of 40 or over 40, pregnancy and puerperium, seasonal variation, long travels.

6.4. STAGES OF THE THROMBUS FORMATION

Thrombosis precedes the venous wall inflammation (phlebitis), which develops a few hours later. Seldom the phlebitis is the first step and than it triggers the thrombosis as in venous traumas or nearby infections.
The stages of the thrombus formation are:

- I - white thrombus
- II - red thrombus (mixed thrombus)
- III - the clot retraction
- IV - the organization of the clot: the fibroblastic proliferation and neoangiogenesis followed by venous recanalization with destruction of valves, stenosis, septa and adhesions obstructing the lumen

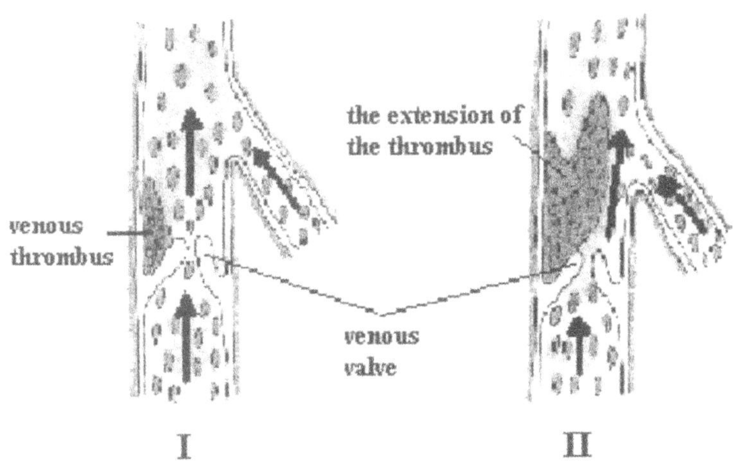

Fig.6.1. I. The beginning of the coagulation process & the appearance of the venous thrombus at the base of the venous valve.
II. The thrombus increases in volume & it occupies the most of the venous lumen.

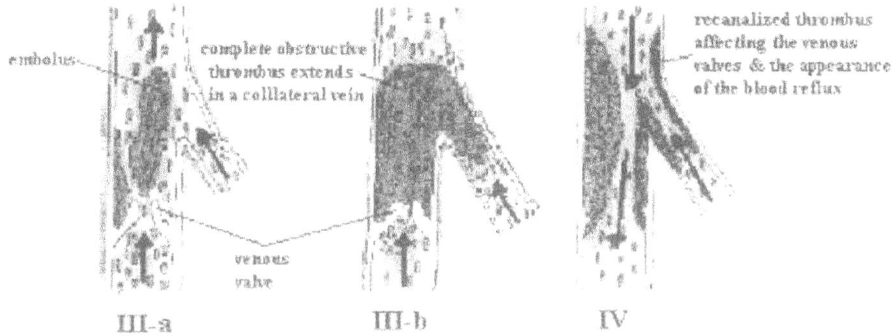

Fig.6.2. III-a. An important part of the venous thrombus splits from the venous wall & go away with the venous flux; it may determine embolic complication.
III-b. The thrombus extends in volume & it occupies all the venous lumen & also the first venous collateral.
IV. The venous lumen is recanalized; the venous valves are destroyed in this process & the reflux of the blood appears

There is a high risk of emboli in the I-III stages that correspond to 2-12 days after intervention and especially to 8-12 days (the stage III of retraction) when the risk of not adherent and disorganized thrombus coming off the vein wall is maximum.

The vein clot frequently appears in a sinus of a venous valve of the muscular veins of the calf or the pelvic veins. A part of the calf veins thrombi dissolves completely without external therapy by the fibrinolitic means of the organism. Approximately in 20% of cases the thrombus extends proximally and occupies the vein lumen. Then it grows in leaps, with stopping intervals that vary in function of the blood column immobilized by the stasis induced by the thrombus extended to the first bifurcation. The thrombus reaches the fork then it increases its volume and its length by accumulating the red cells, thrombocytes and fibrin, and it covers the orifice of the collateral vein. Thus the stasis appears in a new territory. The consequence is the coagulation of the stagnated blood and the extension in leaps of the thrombosis. Therefore the distal thrombi are frequently isolated and the extension has a jumping character up to the junction of the next collateral vein. The thrombotic process extends from the secondary veins to the main veins and then it propagates proximaly:

towards the calf veins, then popliteal, femoralis, iliac veins and vena cava. In case of a thrombosis located on the secondary veins the clinical symptomatology is minor and the evolution of the disease is positive. The patient will recover completely. In more extended thrombosis the vein flow is blocked up and this fact brings about the increase of the vein pressure in the distal part of the obstacle. The consequence is the edema of the extremity that is proportional with the importance of the vein blocking. The hyper pressure forces the perforans veins to dilate and permits the compensatory derivation of blood to the superficial system. So it appears the dilated compensatory pretibial veins described by Pratt as sentinel vein. The venous thrombus may determine a major edema in the proximal obstructions extended towards the iliac veins or vena cava inferior. In a few cases the DVT arises primarily in the ilio-femoral system as a result of direct venous wall injury as seen in orthopedic hip surgery or catheter induced DVT.

In case of central necrosis of the thrombus by an enzyme digestion it may appear bacterial colonization, which determines septic thrombosis. The same phenomenon occurs when prolonged venous catheter is maintained or when asepsis rules are neglected.

Little is known about the anatomic distribution of DVT. The distribution of thrombi increases from proximal (IVC-1.5%) to the distal venous segments (iliac-8.5%), femuropopliteal (53.1%) and calf (82.9%). Isolated calf veins thrombosis was found in 34.7%, isolated femoro-popliteal DVTs were found in 12.4% and iliac DVTs in 1.6%. There was a preponderance of left sided DVTs by a ratio 1.32:1, proximal 2.5:1 and distal 1.26:1. But when infrainguinal thrombi were unaccompanied by iliac involvements the left-to-right ratio continued to fall to the point where isolated left calf veins DVTs ratio was 0.94:1.

The presence of thrombus in a proximal segment was frequently found with the continuity of the thrombus in the distal adjacent segment. But the thrombus in one segment was not well correlated with the presence of the thrombus in the proximal adjacent segment.

In the left iliac stenosis the distal vein obstructions did not provide the opportunity to uncover the left iliac stenotic lesions of the May-Thurner syndrome.

It is probable that DVT begins more often distally and propagates proximally. But the reverse is possible when DVT begins proximally, especially in May-Thurner syndrome or malignancy and propagates distally. The stenotic iliac vein might predispose the distal vein to dilatation and stasis that determine endothelial hypoxia and trigger the distal thrombosis. When the iliac vein stenosis progresses to proximal thrombosis with complete obstruction, the thrombus propagates slowly distal. The iliac thrombosis may extend towards vena cava inferior. This process is followed by the extension of the DVT to the contra-lateral lower limb and the eventual appearance on the other side of edema, pain and cyanosis.

This anatomical data would suggest that the access through the calf, solear or distal superficial veins allow more effective clearing of popliteal thrombus.

Circumscribed thrombosis appears in surgery at the spot of the veins ligatures or in inflammatory lesions and it has no special clinical significance. The deep veins thrombosis arrived sometimes in leg amputation as a stump thrombosis.

6.5. CLINICAL EVOLUTION

The diagnostic of DVT is difficult because the physical findings are not sufficiently accurate to certify this illness and the silent DVTs are very frequent.

General symptoms

The temperature increases gradually up to 38° C (the Michaelis sign) without any other reasonable motivation. The antibiotics do not reduce fever in DVT. The anticoagulation drugs such as heparin reduces fever. High fever usually indicates other diagnosis as cellullitis or lymphangitis.

Functional signs

Anxiety, restlessness, spontaneous pain or cramp in calves.

Objective examination:

- the tegument is glossy, under pressure, discrete cyanosis, warmer than the opposite limb; the calf is heavy. In case of a deep swelling there can be noticed sub- and epifascial edemas. The edema is hard, it does not keep the pitting and it is associated with pains and functional disability. The increasing of the limb's diameter is initially proved only by measurements but in time it becomes self-evident. The bilateral measurements must be done repeatedly and precisely at the same level of the limb; a difference of more than 2 cm in circumference is suggestive for the thrombophlebitis;

- Pratt sign: the pretibial vein named also "sentinel vein" is dilated.
- Payr sign: the pain is felt when you compress the medial plantar muscles. This is important for the differential diagnosis with the rheumatic affections of the joints;
- Bisgaard sign: it hurts when you compress the muscle canal;
- Tschmarke sign: pain is felt when you compress the calf;
- Ducuing sign: pain is felt in case of shaking the calf muscles;
- Homans sign: pain is felt in calf when we carry out the passive forced dorsal flexion of the foot with the knee straight. The sign is not present in some cases of confirmed DVT and is false positive in 50% of calf pains;
- Lowenberg sign: pain is felt in case of compressing the calf with the cuff of the tensiometer under a pressure higher than 100 mm Hg;
- tenderness: the calf is affected by edema and thrombophlebitis; the calf is full and heavy and it has a diminished tenderness. The patient is in dorsal decubitus, his knees are flexed at 90° and we examine comparatively both calves.

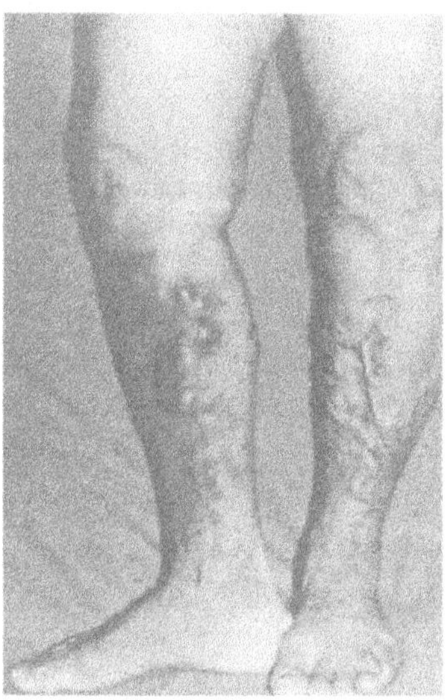

Fig.6.3. Thrombosis of the right GSV extended to crossa & femoral vein

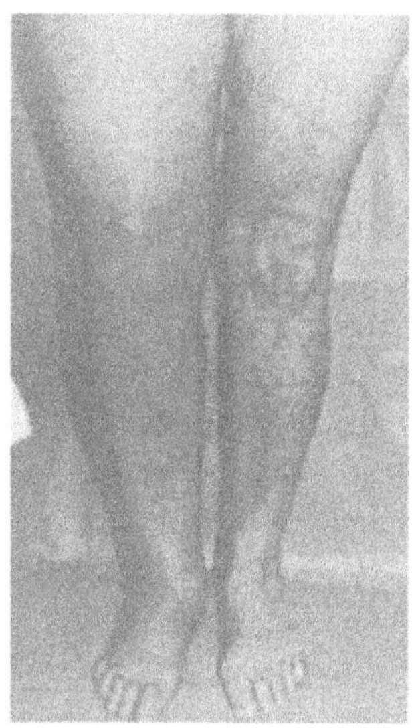

Fig.6.4. Right ilio-femoral posttraumatic thrombosis

Other signs:

- Rielander sign: pain is felt in the inguinal region;
- Louvel sign: pain is felt in the inferior limb at cough;
- pain felt on the canal of the adductor muscles;
- Meyer sign: pain is felt in the medial part of the tibia 8 cm distal from the knee joint.

Pain and edema are generally unilateral in DVT. Tenderness is characteristic to the calf muscles or above the region of the deep veins in the thigh in DVT. The presence of pain and tenderness away from this area probably indicates another diagnosis.

The presence of risk factors, of clinical signs and the alternative diagnosis are comprised in the Wells clinical prediction guide for DVT (117):

Table 6.1. The Wells score for DVT

Clinical parameter	Score
Active cancer: treatment ongoing or within 6 months or palliative treatment	1
Paralysis or recent plaster immobilization	1
Recent bedridden for >3 days or major surgery <4 weeks	1
Located tenderness along the deep venous system	1
Entire leg swelling	1
Calf swelling >3 cm compared to the asymptomatic leg	1
Pitting edema (greater in the symptomatic leg)	1
Collateral superficial veins recently appeared and non varicose veins	1
Probability of alternative diagnosis as likely or > that of DVT	-2

Total of Wells score:

- High probability: score 3 or more
- Moderate probability: score 1 or 2
- Low probability: score 0 or negative

6.6. CLINICAL FORMS

6.6.1. Topographic Clinical Forms

The thrombosis affects:

1) The inferior limb - the most frequent forms are:
   - circumscribed calf thrombosis: first the sinuses of the calf muscles are involved in, but the posterior tibial vein and the peroneal vein can also be affected: a swelling of the calf can be noticed, but not a very important edema;
   - short saphenous vein thrombosis is a not negligible complication of the insufficiency of short saphenous vein. Barrellier found it in 20% of cases of superficial thrombosis. Although the vein is encompassed in the aponeurotic lining we can palpate a sensitive vertical zone which is warmer and harder than normal and has some degree of edema in the retromalleolar region; tachycardia and fever do not occur; (Davy- 19)
   - the popliteal-femoralis thrombosis: an edema up to the knee level;
   - the ilio-femoralis thrombosis determines a white edema of the calf and thigh called phlegmatia alba dolens. The pale color of the extremity and the absent distal arterial pulses indicate the associated arterial spasm that determines acute arterial ischemia and pain. There are petechiae and dilated superficial veins too;
   - the very extended ilio-femoralis thrombosis: it obstructs all drainage veins and is called phlegmatia coerulea dolens (blue painful): the massive edema of the calf and thigh is associated with arterial ischemia due to arterial spasm, femoral arterial pulse reduced, cold and blue teguments, muscular ischemia, state of shock;
   - the thrombosis extended to hypogastric veins is recognized by: inferior abdominal pains, annular and rectal pains, disuria, urine retention, hypogastrium compression pains, uterus and parametrium mobilization pains in cases of vaginal touch and the increasing of the superficial venous drawing above the inguinal ligament;
   - the inferior cava vein thrombosis: it can be recognized by bilateral edemas of the inferior limbs, with collateral circulation of the cava-cava type, by decreasing of the blood pressure, the

presence of the shock. It may appear as a result of the extension of the thrombotic process from the peripheral regions (initial distal vein thrombosis of one limb) to the cava vein;
- bilateral thrombosis: usually it appears like a clinically obvious thrombosis of only one limb but the other limb is affected too and this can be proved by imaging studies; sometimes it gradually extends to a tip-lorry from the initial affected limb to the second limb.

2) The thrombosis of the superior limb.
3) The effort or compression thrombosis.
4) The migratory thrombophlebitis: patients with neoplasm(Trousseau sign), Burger disease, focal infections, rickettsiosis.
5) The thrombosis of the internal jugular vein is iatrogenic on indwelling central catheter, in hypercoagulable states or in association with extensive head or neck sepsis. Other etiology of this thrombosis is the presence of the ovarian hyper-stimulation syndrome, where there is a hipercoagulable state with different venous and arterial thrombosis. The explanation for this state is the hemoconcentration, subsequent high viscosity, venous stasis and increased levels of coagulation factor V, fibrinogen and profibrinogen and fibrinolisys inhibitors.
6) The thrombosis of some visceral veins (portal vein, lienal veins) in malignant hemathologic diseases. Pelvic veins thrombosis is frequent in septic genital diseases.

Clinical/topographic forms depend on the affected venous system:
- superficial forms;
- deep forms.

6.6.2. Evolutive Clinical Forms

- highly acute forms
- acute forms
- subacute forms
- latent recurrent forms
- recurrent forms

6.7. LABORATORY-IMAGING STUDIES

6.7.1. Laboratory Studies

DVT is often clinically silent. DVT is recorded for 45-70% of patients with proven pulmonary embolism. Hematological and coagulation studies are important after confirming the diagnosis by other methods and for checking the anticoagulant treatment.

Fibrin degradation products determination (D- dimmer test) establishes the DVT presence with 93 % sensitivity for proximal localization, but it is relatively nonspecific. The tests are not clot specific and are positive in other conditions as recent surgery trauma, pregnancy, myocardial infarction and cancer with metastasis. Different D-dimmer assays are available and especially a new qualitative ELISA test. The Simpli RED assay is a rapid qualitative RBC agglutination assay sensitive for proximal DVT, but less sensitive for calf DVT.

Protein S, protein C, antithrombin III, factor V Leyden, prothrombin 20210A mutation, antiphospholipid antibodies are important for young patients, in unusual sites of thrombosis, or DVT without clear etiology.

6.7.2. Imaging Studies

- Doppler continuous flow study determines the absence of venous flow in DVT. Actually Duplex-Doppler is very important, its specificity and sensitivity are 98 %. The direct criterion for detecting DVT is represented by failure to compress the vein, because of the presence of the thrombus in the lumen. The indirect signs are the absence of the normal phasic Doppler signal changes of the venous flow with respiration and compression. Doppler ultrasounds detect the femoral thrombosis and the thrombosis proximal from inguinal ligament or the calf DVT. Doppler cannot differentiate between old and recent clots. This diagnostic depends on the accuracy of the ultrasound device and on the doctor's skills and experience;
- plethysmography: in proximal DVT, venous outflow from the lower limb is slowed down and the venous capacity is increased. The recordings of the volume changes permit to differentiate between DVT and normal flow. There are limitations of this

method: its lack of sensitivity for calves DVT, for non-occluding proximal DVT and the ilio-femoral vein thrombosis above the inguinal ligament;

- phlebography;
- fibrinogen marked with radioactive iodine is no longer recommended for DVT because it is relatively insensitive for proximal vein thrombosis, the results are obtained after 24 hours and the specificity is low. Pulmonary scintigraphy is recommended in the embolic suspicion;
- MRI is an expensive method. Without contrast substance it was successfully used on angiology in the 80's. CE-3D MRA is the alternative for invasive catheter angiology for the diagnosis of angiological disease and for postoperative control of the surgical intervention. Contrast-enhanced magnetic resonance angiography (CE-MRA) is now a routine in some clinics. It obtains fast 3-dimensional (3D) sequences. This method together with applications of dedicated surface coils as well as bolus triggering permit CE-MRA to obtain a focused image of the arterial but venous system, with an excellent quality (high signal to noise ratio). MRI is useful for finding the iliac DVT and thrombosis of inferior cava vein. The sensitivity for calves DVT is better than in the case of other noninvasive methods. It can be used in the diagnosis of DVT in the second and third trimester of pregnancy;

6.8. EVOLUTION

The phases of the thrombosis consist of the onset, the development of thrombophlebitis, the period of remission, the convalescence (the edema disappears completely in clinostatic position but it appears in orthostatic position), the stabilizing period (the symptomatology disappears) and finally the late complication – postthrombotic syndrome.

The attitudes regarding prophylaxis, the definition of high risk groups patients and the proposed prophylactic methods are very different and variable with the geographical region.

DVT can lead to post-thrombotic syndrome (PTS). PTS has a high importance on the quality of life and health-care costs. (Boccalon)

The incidence of PTS has been found to be 35-69%, 3 years after DVT and 49-100% after 5-10 years depending on the extension of thrombosis.

6.9. COMPLICATIONS

- pulmonary embolism;
- venous gangrene;
- postthrombotic syndrome (postphlebitic);
- chronic venous insufficiency: calf ulcers, cellulitis, edemas.

6.9.1. Pulmonary Embolism (PE)

The PE is the most important cause of preventable mortality in hospital in the Western countries. Epidemiological data indicate that the frequency is 160 per 100000 for DVT, 20 per 100000 for symptomatic nonfatal pulmonary embolism and 50 per 100000 for fatal autopsy-detected pulmonary embolism. Pulmonary embolism continues to be a major cause of death for hospitalized patients in developed countries despite all the anticoagulation measures.

The most dramatic and serious complication is caused by the detachment of a thrombus from the peripheral venous system. It is moved by the blood stream to the heart and then to the pulmonary arteries or their branches and determines total or partial obstruction of these arteries. It results an increasing of the pulmonary arterial pressure and this may have consequences on the right cord and venous stasis; the central venous pressure increases and a volume deficit (mechanical complications) is present. There are added reflex artery- and broncho-constriction, obstruction, coronary-cardiac reflexes, syncope, even asphyxiation and death to those already mentioned. The most frequent starting point is represented by the calf thrombophlebitis and than the thigh or pelvic thrombosis. The maximum risk of appearance is 8-12 days after surgery. The emboli may be caused by the detachment of a thrombus from the right side of the heart. In the case of an interatrial or interventricular septum foramen, the thrombus may come from the left side of the heart. Other embolias, except the thromboembolic disease, are rare but possible (fat,

amniotic, gaseous, tumoral, foreign bodies, especially iatrogenic, cholesterol, septic material emboli). The incidence of the pulmonary emboli is 15% in general hospitals, 27,5% in case of cardiac patients, 50,3% in case of valvular patients, as it results at necropsy studies.
The risk of mobilization is enormous for the recent thrombi (red) that are not organized and not endothelized, so they do not adhere to the venous wall. The thrombi from the sinuses, junctions or venous valves are moved at a sudden change of the venous pressure, due to the late beginning of the patient's mobilization, sudden muscular contractions, sneeze, defecation, attempts of important fracture reduction. (80)

There are three types of emboli: small (under 1 mm), middle (which are 2-3mm in diameter) and big (which are 1-1.5cm in the diameter and 20-30 cm long). In case of big emboli the obstruction takes place on a pulmonary artery or an important branch, the right side of the heart cannot empty itself and thus it dilates so that the left side of the heart can fill itself only partially.

Pulmonary embolism with simultaneous symptom of DVT is likely to cause postthrombotic syndrome (71)

6.9.1.1. Anamnesis

It offers data regarding the favoring conditions for the phlebitis. The risk of pulmonary embolism is more frequent in urologic, orthopedic, gynecologic interventions, postpartum, general surgery interventions, fractures of femoral neck or pelvic bones, after a treatment with contraceptive pills, diabetes, arterial hypertension, policytemia, dehydration, after myocardial infarctions not anticoagulated, hemiplegias.

6.9.1.2. Symptomatology

P.E. appears suddenly, as a so called "lightning on clear sky" manifested with anxiety (increased by eventual small embolias in antecedents), thoracic retrosternal pain or violent precordial pain, cyanoses, dyspnea, tachycardia, an evolution to cardiogen shock or death in some minutes.

6.9.1.3. Clinical Examination

At the lung examination sometimes there may appear some little specific symptoms: rough or diminished vesicular murmur, circumscribed pleural friction, circumscribed ronckus, bronhospasm with wheezing. The symptoms of the cardiogen shock appear in the massive pulmonary emboli. In middle-sized P.E. there might happen a pulmonary infarction with pains at 24-48 h and small hemoptysis, with red blood or with hemorrhage sputum. Dyspnea is variable. The fever is present for 2-3 days with values up to 38° C. Clinically there can be observed a small or middle pleural flowing with the diminishing of the vesicular murmur even its disappearance. The symptomatology is persisting for 5-7 days and the flowing may be present up to 2 weeks.

In small and repeated P.E. there might appear short periods of dyspnea, tachycardia, disturbances of cardiac rhythm that regress quickly due to fibrinolisis. It is said, "for the diagnosis of P.E. the examination of the inferior limbs is more valuable than the cardio-pulmonary exam".

If the emboli are small there will appear more attenuated thoracic pains with a respiratory uneasiness, cough with hemorrhage sputum and the clinical aspect of corticopleuritis.

6.9.1.4. Positive Diagnosis:

- clinical signs and symptoms;
- EKG: the overload of the right side of the heart, tachyarithmias; the modifications can be transitory and it is necessary to repeat the EKG;
- standard thoracic X-rays: The decreasing of the pulmonary transparency, typical triangular atelectasis with the tip to the hilum and the base to periphery, the amputation of the pulmonary hilum, the decreasing mobility and the ascending of the hemidiaphragma, small pleural flow present after 2-3 days from the onset of P.E.;
- standard heart X-rays: The increased volume of the mediastinum by the dilation of the superior cava vein; the dilation of the right side of the heart and of the pulmonary arterial cone in hilum with sudden amputation in the territory with P.E.;
- echocardiography: the dilation of the right side of the heart and pulmonary artery;
- the values of the blood gases: severe hypoxemia;
- the pulmonary scintigraphy with micro-aggregates of serum albumin marked with Tc 99 shows "the cold areas," not irrigated with blood where the P.E. stops the blood perfusion;
- pulmonary angiography: indicated in severe forms which need surgery for treatment;
- CT;

- MRI.
- Laboratory examinations: moderate increasing values of BSR, leucocytosis 10-15.000, normal GOT and GPT but the total and indirect bilirubin increases moderately after 3 days from the onset.

6.9.1.5. Differential Diagnosis:

- myocardial infarction;
- dissecant aneurysm of aorta;
- pleuro-pulmonary affections of other etiology;
- bronchial asthma;
- fat or gaseous emboli.

The further complications of the untreated P.E. are chronic pulmonary hypertension determined by the persisting obstruction of the pulmonary artery branches. The evolution of the P.E. to exitus may happen immediately in supra-acute forms.

6.9.2. Vein Gangrene

It is a rare complication that appears in the complete blockage of the return circulation by extended thrombosis of the inferior limb veins affected by thrombophlebitis. It is recognized by a quick development of a massive edema of the ill inferior limb, with the appearance of hemorrhage flictenae, eschars which determine broad areas of ulceration with difficult healing after elimination.

6.9.3. Postthrombotic Syndrome (Postphlebitic)

The sequelae of DVT of lower limbs are frequently recognized as postthrombotic syndrome. Almost a third part of lower extremity fractures determines postthrombotic sequelae and venous thrombosis. When the popliteal or more proximal veins are involved in the thrombotic process it is more likely to result a postthrombotic syndrome. At this stage the thrombus is included in the fibroconjunctive organization process, after which it may result the following possibilities:

- fibroconjunctive organization - hard, thick obstructed girdle;
- one channel patency with the partial restoring of the venous lumen but with the alterations and destroying of the vein valves and resulting vein insufficiency;
- complete patency by adjacent non-valvular collateral channels of the vein;
- complete patency with the restoring of the permeability and maintaining the continuity - it is an exceptional situation (1-2%).

6.9.3.1. Physiopathology

The disturbances of the return circulation with venous stasis, orthostatic and orthodynamic venous hypertension determine the symptoms mentioned below and the tissular modifications. A blood derivation is produced through the collateral vessels that avoid the obstacle through perforans veins to the superficial vein system. The insufficiency of the valves determines vertical long reflux respectively horizontal short reflux. The permanent orthostatic venous hypertension determines an initial reducible edema that becomes afterwards irreducible. Cutaneous trophic lesions, hyperpigmentation, hypodermitis, cellulitis and finally calf ulcer may appear.

The following 5 types of postthrombotic syndrome are described as:

- obstructive: the obstruction of the venous axis persists or the patency is deficient and insufficient for the flow;
- reflux: the blood circulation inverts because of the venous avalvulation;
- substitutive: the dilation of the collateral veins in order to avoid and by-pass the obstacle;
- restrictive: the loss of the deep venous system compliance and capacity of venous storage;
- mixed: the association of the syndromes mentioned above.

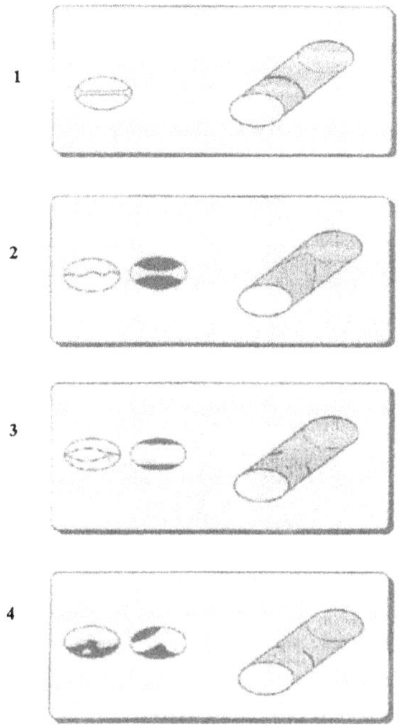

Fig.6.5. Types of venous valves:
1. normal valves
2. long valves
3. short valves
4. reshuffled valves

6.9.3.2. Symptomatology

Practically is similar to chronic venous insufficiency but at hydrostatic varices the decompensation and the appearance of the calf ulcer can be noticed after an evolution period of aproximative 20 years and at postthrombotic syndrome the CVI can be noticed in 1-2 years. This means that the PTS evolves faster and in a severe form of CVI with leg ulcer.

6.9.3.3. Positive Diagnosis

It is established according to anamnesis and symptomatology of a previous DVT (in the antecedents of the patient) and according to the appearance of the edema, the secondary varices, and the trophic lesions with ulcer after 1-2 years.

6.9.3.4. Differential Diagnosis

It is made between PTS and chronic venous insufficiency as a result of hydrostatic varicose (which is however formed slowly). We can also establish the differential diagnosis of the main symptoms:

- edema;
- calf ulcer: arterial ulcer, hypertensive ulcer (Martorell), Marjolin ulcer (malignancies on old burns), neoplastic ulcer, ulcer in impetigo, ectima, endured eritema Bazin, sclerodermia, exceptional luetic ulcer and in other countries ulcer in leper.

6.10. TREATMENT OF THE ACUTE VEIN THROMBOSIS AND OF THE COMPLICATIONS

Now the treatment of DVT is considerably different from the standard treatment in use 10 years ago. Unfractionated heparine was introduced in clinical practice in 1937 and played the main role in the management of DVT for a long time. The discovery of LMWHs 25 years ago (R.Rosenberg and U.Lindahl in 85,44) modified the treatment. Thus since 1982 it was introduced in clinical practice (85)

The prophylaxis is recommended for patients with risk of thrombosis, especially for obese patients, with important surgeries (especially orthopedic interventions, important urological intervention, gynecological interventions) or in case of prolonged immobilization in bed or in plaster and in neoplasia.

T.W.Wakefield (85) demonstrated experimentally that the treatment with recombinant P-selectin glycoprotein ligand Ig determines a significant inhibition of thrombosis and vein wall inflammation decreases cytokine expression in the vein wall and also determines the thrombus resolution.

6.10.1. Prophylactic Treatment

Consists in pharmacological and mechanical methods (Haas - 39):

6.10.1.1. Pharmacological Methods:

- unfractionated heparin in small doses (5.000 U.I. s.c./8 hours) according to Kakkar's method; the efficacy is accepted worldwide for the prevention of venous thromboembolism in surgical and orthopedic patients;
- LMWH is administrated in the preoperative period (started 12 hours before surgery) and then is continued in the postoperative period (12 to 24 hours after surgery till mobilization). The period of administration is controversial 9-14 days or even 4 weeks. It is as effective and as safe as unfractionated heparin;
- adjusted dose of warfarin with the target INR of 2.0-3.0 started preoperatively or immediately after surgery;
- the correction of the hydroelectrolites balance to prevent the increasing of the blood viscosity;
- aspirin 80-325 mg/day (contraindicated for patients with gastro-duodenal ulcer); it has a limited prophylactic effect;
- dextran (MW=40000) in perfusion (antiaggregating drug for the thrombocytes); it has only a partial effect.

6.10.1.2. Mechanical Methods:

- mobilization: passive movings also on the operation table for the blood mobilization from calf veins storage;
- graduated compression stockings or compressive bandages compulsory applied preoperative and maintained postoperative until the mobilization;
- intermittent pneumatic compression of the lower limb

6.10.2.Curative Treatment can be medical and surgical (in selected cases).

6.10.2.1.Medical Treatment

Developed in two different directions closely following the 2 methods that could limit the blood coagulation:

- decrease of the concentration of the coagulation factors that depend on vitamin K. This is put into medical practice by prescribing antivitamin K (cumarines) orally. The main problems in this case are the delayed efficiency and the possibility of hemorrhages when the substance is overdosed or it interacts with other medication or with food;

- blockage of the coagulation factors possible using two groups of substances. Hirudine is a direct inhibitor and it binds on the active site of an enzyme. Hirudine is a protein of 65 aminoacides and initially isolated from the salivary gland of leach. Nowadays it is produced by genetic engineering. The second one is represented by an indirect inhibitor, which can activate the antithrombin (AT)-the physiological inhibitor of coagulation. The substance in use is heparin class of drugs. Heparin activates AT producing a conformational change of AT. This class of drugs was discovered in 1917 by the student McLean, working in the laboratory of Howell and it was put into medical practice in 1937. Heparin was extracted it was initially from the bovine lungs but now from porcine intestinal mucosa. Heparin is a mixture of several polysaccharides associated with a variety of biological substances but only a third of them bound to AT determining anticoagulation. The main problems in case of using heparin for treatment are mediated autoimmune thrombocytopenia, hemorrhages and osteoporosis (on long term daily administration). Association with acid acetyl salicylic (ASA) must be avoided. ASA impairs the platelet release reaction and therefore combined with the anticoagulant effect of heparin may produce hemorrhages. In these cases with hemorrhages we can use protamine sulfate. The $T_{1/2}$ of the heparin is 30 minutes and we must use an adequate dose of protamine sulfate as antidote. Patients with liver disease are highly sensitive to heparin. The anticoagulation with heparin is adequate when the clotting time is 2-3 times the normal value measured by the Lee-White method. (85) Heparin molecule has an important negative electrostatic charge, which interacts with positively charged proteins and increases its elimination. Heparin bound with platelet factor 4 produces an allergic reaction resulting heparin induced thrombocitopenia. The first step in controlling the side effects of heparin was the decrease of the dose administrated. The second step was the introduction of LMWHs which is sustained by the following observations: antifactor Xa activity is independent by the molecular weight whereas antithrombin activity requires a polysaccharide with a minimum molecular weight of 6000 and composed of 20 monosaccharides chain about. LMWH is obtained from unfractionated heparins (UFH), has a molecular weight between 2000-10000Da, it inhibits through AT the factors IIa, IXa, Xa (multitargeted agent) and it has multiple mechanisms of action. LMWHs are better tolerated than UFH, they remain in circulation longer and also they are injected only one or two per day. LMWHs are the best medication in the prophylaxis of DVT and PE. Recently they are used for the treatment of DVT and PE. After i.v or s.c administration LMWHs induce the release of tissue factor pathway inhibitor (from its vascular pool). This effect contributes to their antithrombotic effect. Each type of LMWH has a different hemorrhagic risk. LMWHs have lower effect than UFH in inducing platelet aggregation, in releasing lipoprotein lipase and on the activity of hepatic lipase. LMWHs just like UFH and a special pentasaccharide have a concentration-dependent inhibitory effect on factor VIIa generation and activity. There are several types of LMWHs with different molecular weights such as: enoxaparin 3500-5500Da, nadroparin 4200-4800Da, dalteparin 5000Da, tinzaparin 4900Da, ardeparin 5500-6500Da. Elderly patients compared to healthy young volunteers respond better at LMWHs. In pregnant women long term treatment with LMWHs has a good tolerance and safety.

In 1981 it was obtained the structure of a pentasaccharide (PS) that bound to AT and activated the latter. The PS is an inhibitor of factor Xa and it is entirely obtained through chemical synthesis. Its molecules have a high affinity for AT because it has a specific binding site within the AT molecule.

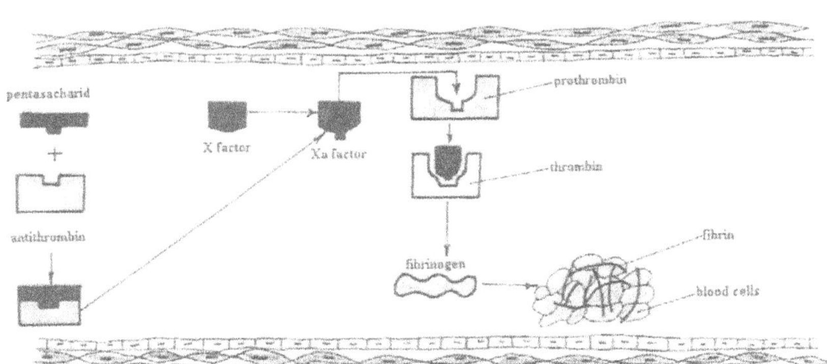

Fig.6.6. The thrombus formation & the anticoagulant action of the antithrombin – pentasacharid complex on the Xa factor.

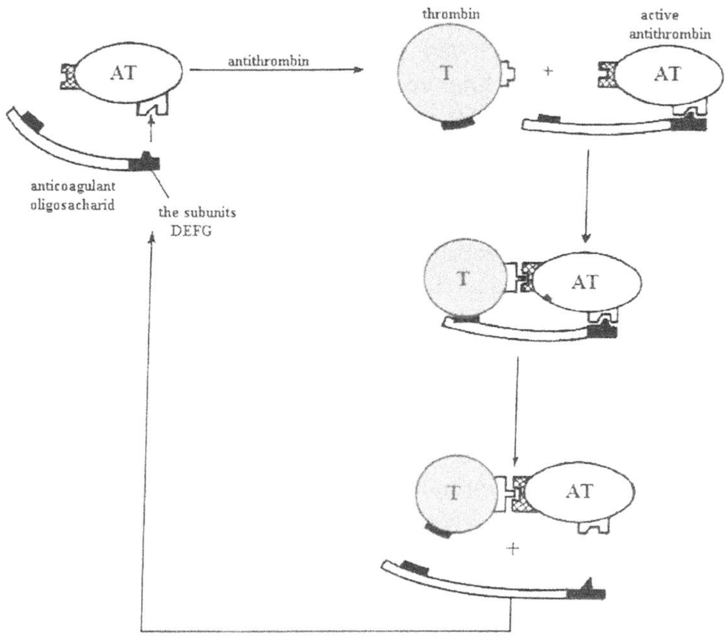

Fig.6.7. Recycling effect of anticoagulant oligosacharids

The advantages of using PS are:

- a small size, a low electrical charge therefore it hasn not the harmful side effects of heparin because it do not interact with platelet factor 4. The PS fixed on AT determines activation of thrombin; when thrombin is locked to AT and it is inhibited, the PS is released and can activate other antithrombin molecules by a recycling effect;
- single targeted agent (inhibition of factor Xa), with the activity automatically regulated by the quantity of AT in circulation so the overdose is avoided, a single injection per day being prescribed.

This anticoagulation followed by long-term oral anticoagulation therapy was directed to prevent thrombus propagation, re-thrombosis and pulmonary embolism.

Now the management of DVT involves the use of various modalities directed to:

- removal of the thrombus by mechanical thrombectomy;

- recanalization of the normal and anatomic pathway by catheter-directed thrombolitic therapy;
- restoring normal anatomic hemodynamics;
- prevention of clot extension and pulmonary embolism.

In the case of calf forms thrombosis: heparin 5.000 u.i. in bollus and then 500-1.000 u.i./h recommended continuously i.v. 7-10 days with APTT in limits of 50-75 seconds (2-3 times bigger than the normal one); then it is associated with dicumarins for 3 days at least (until Quick index is 20-30% and INR=2-2.5). You should use 5 ml sulfate of protamin i.v. and 10 mg of vitamin K i.v. in case of bleedings. In cases of calf thrombophlebitis it is recommended to rest in bed with the affected inferior limb in elevation 20-25 cm from the normal level, local wet compresses and general analgesics. After the decrease of edema the mobilization is done gradually. After this procedure the dicumarinic treatment should be continued for 3 months orally in cases when the cause is known and the thrombosis is reversible or even for 6 months when the cause is unknown and it persists.

Recent trials especially from Swiss, France, Austria and Germany have proved good results of the ambulatory treatment of the DVT. It is recommended to administer LMWH (for example tinzaparin 175 IU/kg once/day, 8 days, associated with elastic compression). From the second day to the end they associate tinzaparin with oral anticoagulation. The results were good on 827 cases. The relapse or the progression of DVT was 0 %. Pulmonary embolia was registered in 1,9 %, pain in 2 % and leg edema in 7,5 %. The patients with DVT treated in ambulatory were selected cases excluding the iliofemural localization, the important pain or edema, the presence of cancer and the lung embolia. H.Partsch demonstrated that the ambulatory treatment with LMWH and the early movement with Unna boots or elastic stockings relieve more quickly the pains and decrease the edema than the bed rest without compression. (82)

In the case of iliofemoralis forms on the first 10 days it may carry out surgical thrombectomy. There exists an alternative to this procedure - the fibrinolysis, which transforms the plasminogen in plasmina and dissolves the thrombus. There are some treatment schemes (for example the attack dose of streptokinase in bolus 250.000 u.i/30 min., then 100.000 u.i/h in perfusion for 1-3 days) with the control of thrombin index in the hospital; then heparin 300-1.000 u.i./hour i.v and dicumarins with the Quick index control. The risks of fibrinolysis are: allergy, hemorrhages and embolias with fragments of the thrombus. Urokinase isolated from human fetal kidneys cells grown in cultures is non antigenic. The initial dose is 4400u.i/kg i.v. bolus followed by 4400u.i/kg/h i.v. for 1-3 days.

Recombinant tissular plasminogen activator (rt-PA)/Altepase /Activase produced by genetic engineering, is the main activator of fibrinolysis in the blood. It has an elective lysing action on the formed thrombus but therapeutic doses of rt-PA affect hemostasis and induce hemorrhage complication like all the other thrombolitic agents. Prolonged fibrinolysis requires monitoring of coagulation factors as a precaution. Although currently there is no adequate method for monitoring this therapy, the prolongation of APTT and thrombin time (TT) reflects best the effects of rt-PA. Front-loaded regimen recommended for Altepase adult dose: 15 mg i.v. bolus initially followed by 50 mg i.v. over the next 30 min. and than 35 mg over the next one hour. Heparin i.v is necessary after putting an end to this treatment when APTT ratio is lower than 2. The treatment with rt-PA determined a reduction in the thrombotic mass, but there is no clear evidence of better results (in thromboembolic complications and development of CVI) compared with heparin treatment alone.

Fibrinolysis is recommended in:

- viability of limb is potentially compromised (venous gangrene);
- massive iliac-femoral or cava thrombosis;
- DVT occurred on the last 7 days;
- young patients with no contraindications;
- cases without absolute or relative hemorrhagic risk factors;
- cases with absolute contraindications to heparin;
- cases with type II heparin-induced thrombocytopenia (with a platelet count smaller than 40000-50000/mm^3).

The contraindications of fibrinolysis are: patients over 65 years because of the cerebral hemorrhage risk, recent surgical operations because of the hemorrhage risk by fibrinolysis on the surgery sutures, bleeding risk (ulcer, tumors, renal disturbances with hemorrhage).

On one hand the valvular insufficiency is less likely to develop at patients who undergo early lysis of the thrombus by anticoagulation therapy. On the other hand those who are treated with heparin develop PTS in 80% of cases compared to those who take thrombolytics and may develop PTS in only 36% of cases. (Rhodes)

6.10.2.2. Surgical Treatment

It consists in venous thrombectomy that may cause in some cases valvular incompetence. Another adjunctive method to venous thrombectomy is arteriovenous fistula that provides enough blood flow through the vein till the denudate endothelium can be regenerated. (Rhodes)

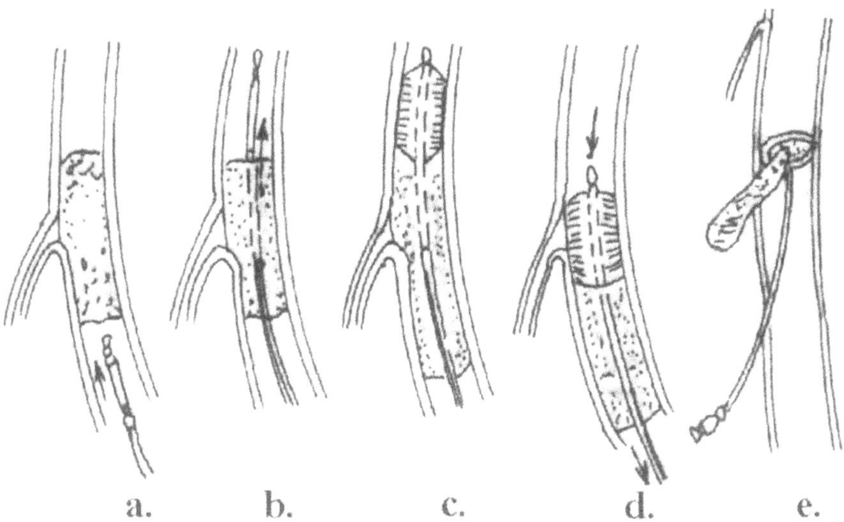

Fig.6.8. Venous thrombectomy with Fogarty catheter

The deep iliac thrombectomy is carried out with local anesthesia; today it is not necessary to dissect the other side of the femoral vein, and to introduce the Fogarty catheter for the cava vein blocking. Now we only discover the thrombosed femoral vein and we introduce the Fogarty catheter, which means that the withdrawing of the test is done with the distended balloon. By using the Valsalva method it can be noticed an increasing of the patient's abdominal pressure, which helps to the elimination of the thrombus and prevents its moving in the cava vein. This is a situation when the thrombus might become an embolus with the risk of getting into the pulmonary arteries. Nowadays it is not evident that venous thrombectomy or thrombolysis is better than anticoagulation treatment alone. More the postoperative re-thrombosis is possible. (Comerota - 15)

6.10.3. Treatment in Case of Complications

6.10.3.1. Treatment of Pulmonary Embolism

- morphine 10 mg i.v.;
- papaverin 50mg i.v.;
- oxygen with or without intubation;
- theophylline in bronchial spasm;
- the treatment of cardiogenic shock with vasopressor drugs;
- the treatment of cardiac rhythm disturbances;
- the surgical treatment.

N.B. If it is impossible to administrate continuously heparin the schedule is i.v. 5.000 u.i. sodic heparin in an 4 hour's interval (6 times in 24 hours) or even once in 6 hours (4 times in 24 hours).

In case of shock we should pay attention to the overloading with liquids because the blood volume is normal.

The etiologic treatment related to the stage of pulmonary emboli is:

- stage I: reduced symptomatology – heparin 5.000 u.i./4 hours, 6-10 days long or calciparin 2x12.500 u.i./day followed by dicumarins per os after 10-14 days;
- stage II: the symptomatology consists of anxiety, hyperventilation – administration of strepto- or urokinase, Trendelenburg embolectomy, an embolectomy with an extra corporeal circulation;
- stage III: the symptomatology consists of dyspnea and collapse. It requires a quick angiography and administration of fibrinolitic drugs on the catheter for fibrinolysis. If the obstruction of the pulmonary artery exceeds 50% it will be immediately necessary to do a surgical embolectomy;
- stage IV: consists of shock and dyspnea -- it requires immediate surgery;
- stage V: consists of shock and Cheyne-Stockes breathing and requires immediate surgery.

The usual surgical treatment consists of pulmonary thrombembolectomy: thoracotomy, spotting and then incision of the pulmonary artery, extraction of the embolus, control arteriography. The intervention is “heroic," especially its initial variant (without an outmode circulation). Trendelenburg introduced this technique but Kirschner was the first who succeeded in performing it in 1919. The endoscopic intervention consists of percutaneous introduction of catheters into the veins, then through the cava vein system and heart to the pulmonary artery and aspiration or destroying the thrombus by using a laser or lysine. Postoperative anticoagulant treatment is necessary.

The treatment in recurrent pulmonary embolias or in cases of contraindication of heparin therapy is the venous ligatures on femoral veins or cava inferior vein distal the renal veins in order to prevent the migration of the thrombi from this level. We can apply clips on the cava vein or we can use a filter type umbrella as Mobin-Udin, Greenfield or the filter like a wire ball that opens inside the vein lumen. The last methods allow the blood passage but they stop the emboli.

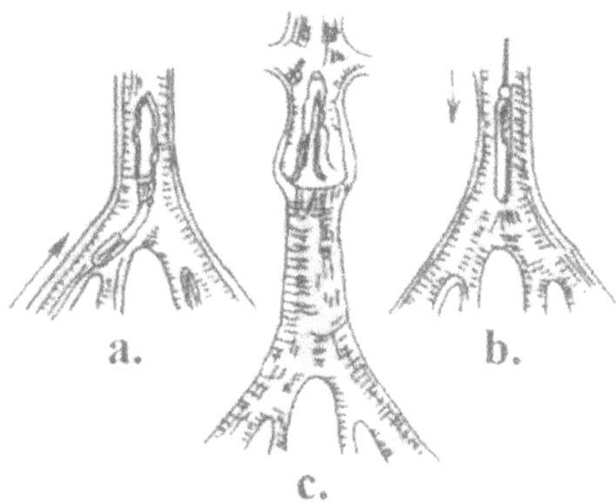

Fig.6.9. a, b – The placement of Greenfield catheter
c – Filter placed in inferior cava vein distal of the renal veins

6.10.3.2. Treatment of Postthrombotic Syndrome

The bedridden state and the postural drainage are very important. The compressive elastic or non-elastic bandages (elastic stockings or compressive cuff) are used. The administration of non-steroid anti-inflammatory drugs as phenylbutazone 200 mg/day in association with diuretic drugs (pay attention to diuretic drugs: the dehydration and the hemoconcentration favor the thrombosis) is useful.

Surgeons elect the operation depending on the two functional variants of the deep venous system:

- The permeable deep venous system: suppression of the reflux points and varicose veins;
- Obstructed deep venous system: valvulated venous transplant, valve transplant or the derivation of the venous flux for bypassing the obstacle ("Palma operation").

In case of broad varicose ulcer it can be used a free split skin graft cut with the dermatome.

6.11. PARTICULAR FORMS OF THROMBOPHLEBITIS

6.11.1. Migratory Thrombophlebitis

It is represented by the multicentric leaping recurrent superficial vein thrombophlebitis. This happens in case of local infections: dental, sinusal, cholecystic, appendices, etc. or in neoplasm (collateral effect of the neoplasic disease), collagen systemic diseases or blood dyscrasias. It may be the first symptom of Burger-Winiwarter thromboangeitis. The etiologic treatment of main disease (the neoplasm, etc) and symptomatic anti-inflammatory therapy with phenylbutazone 200 mg/day or prednisolon 50-60 mg/day associated with compression is done if it is possible.

6.11.2. Superior Limb Thrombophlebitis (Paget-Von Schroetter)

It a appears more frequently in cases of young patients. It consists of acute thrombosis of the axillary or subclavian veins.

It can be classified as:

- primitive: in cases of young people who made an important physical effort or practiced sport (tennis, bowling);
- secondary: axilar tumors or adenopathies, compressive scars, the presence of the compressive Lange muscular arch, the subclavian vein compression in the thoracic aperture; basilic vein catheterization for measuring the PVC (central venous pressure) for perfusions, direct traumas, radiotherapy, hypercoagulability.

There are many symptoms: the venous drainage in arm and shoulders decreases with the appearance of marmorated skin, edema of the arm and shoulder, pains at palpation of the deep or superficial venous tract.

Diagnosis

It is established by imagistic examinations: Doppler, phlebography and radioactive marked fibrinogen.

Evolution:

Often favorable under medical treatment.

Treatment:

- thrombectomy: is rarely indicated, only in serious forms that need desobstruction with Fogarty balloon catheter. The urgent surgery is a possible attitude. Lee V.A. suggests a delay for one month while he is using anticoagulation. The patients with stenotic veins on venography and with compression by thoracic outlet syndrome are recommended for operation.
- fibrinolytic treatment is indicated when the diagnosis is made soon after onset of thrombosis. Then anticoagulant drugs are needed with the control of prothrombin index and Quick index.
- external compression;
- etiologic treatment;
- anticoagulant treatment: indicated constantly.

6.11.3. Pelvic Varicose and Thrombophlebitis

When the reflux is not found in saphenofemoral junction or other deep or superficial veins in the lower limb, we may find it through the vulvar varices. Pelvic varices could be the cause of pelvic congestion syndrome and dyspareunia. Pelvic pains appear especially at multipara women. The pelvic varicose in women is known as "varicocele of the broad ligament".

The pelvic infections at women with septic abortion, pyosalpinx, puerperal infections determine the pelvic thrombophlebitis and septic embolias. The surgical treatment consists of evacuation of uterine cavity, excision or evacuation of the abscesses associated with highly effective antibiotherapy. For preventing the pulmonary embolias it is recommended to do the ligature of the ovarian veins and of the inferior cava or to place a filter in the cava vein.

The treatment of pelvic congestion syndrome consists of administration of medroxiprogesterone acetate 10mg, 3 times/day, 6 months. Small doses of danazol were proved to be useful alternatively. The intra-uterus system Mirena, which might offer protection for the symptomatology for a couple of years, was used recently for the treatment. The laparoscopic resection of the uterine nervous plexus was carried out sometimes at cases refractor at medical treatment. But the efficacy of this technique is still in discussion. The radical operation-total hysterectomy with bilateral anexectomy, is decided very rarely, at cases with long lasting complains, refractor at any treatment.

6.11.4. Suprahepatic Veins Thrombosis (Budd-Chiari Syndrome)

The suprahepatic veins obstruction is characterized by hepatomegaly, ascites and liver insufficiency. The Budd-Chiari syndrome is determined by the presence of a congenital ring, a perforated membrane or even complete membrane at the level of inferior cava vein, endophlebitis, increased coagulation in polycythemia vera. The treatment consists of porto-caval anastomosis in order to derivate the blood from the portal system. Recently the percutaneous transluminal angioplasty was done with stent or membranectomy through the catheter.

6.11.5. Traveler's Thrombosis (Jet-leg Thrombosis, Economy Class Syndrome) (TT)

The traveler's thrombosis is a new entity in phlebology. In comparison with the enormously high number of long lasting travels, the number of the DVT is low. The frequency of travels that triggered venous thromboembolism is 0.0014% of long flies, but over 40 years the frequency is 0.004%. The clinic latent thrombosis appears in 0.01%. Probably a lot of asymptomatic and oligosymptomatic thrombophlebitis remain unknown. (81)

Definition

Includes the following criteria:

- travel by plane, bus, car, train in sitting position;
- duration >3-5 hours;
- absence of venous thrombosis or thromboembolism at the beginning of the travel;
- interval between travel and thrombosis no more than 2 weeks.

Pathophysiology

The pathophysiology is complex. The main factors are:

- long-lasting immobilization in sitting with angulation of poplitea vein. On the plane the thrombosis is more frequent in the economy class fly;
- low oxygen pressure on the plane, equal to altitude of 2000-2500m. This reduces the fibrinolysis. The delivery of EDRF (endothelium derived relaxing factor) determines vasodilatation and venous stasis;
- dehydration of the passenger is pluricausal. It includes the low humidity in the plane, the increased diuresis determined by in-taking caffeine and alcohol, the relative insufficient intake of water;
- before travel venous alteration of the endothelium.

Risk factors

- history of venous thrombosis;
- existence of an evolving cancer, a calf fracture, a recent femoral catheterism, a heart insufficiency or a thrombophilia;
- estrogenic treatment;
- the age.

Favoring conditions

- smoking;
- alcohol drinking;
- using of hypnotic substances;
- dehydration.

Determinant conditions

They are induced by the technical details of the plane:

- relative hypoxia;

- immobilization and sitting position without the possibility to walk and so determining the compression of the popliteal vein for several hours.

The Wiener Consensus (1995) accepted 3 **risk groups**:

- group 1:Low risk: travel with high risk (many hours in sitting position);
- group 2:Medium risk: when there are at least 2 from the presented factors) age over 40, (latent) heart insufficiency ,chronic venous insufficiency and important varices, pregnancy, abundant adipose tissue, contraceptive pills;
- group 3: High risk: history of venous thrombosis without relation with the actual disease, malignant tumors, history of family thrombosis, orthopedic immobilization of lower limbs, recent operation with high risk of thrombosis.

Symptoms:

Swollen legs, calf pains, and eventually the signs of pulmonary embolia with dyspnea. There were recorded even deaths that were on debate.

Diagnostic

Follows the schedule of the DVT. The main location of the traveler's thrombosis is the popliteo-femoral vein (74%-H. Partsch - 81)

Prophylaxis consists of:

- movement of lower limbs, eventually raising up and walking around;
- wearing class I compression stockings (calf length) especially in the presence of varicose disease or risk factors;
- intake of 1 l drinks/5 hours of travel;
- reducing doses of sleeping and tranquilizer drugs.

The high-risk travelers need more aggressive prophylaxis:

- acetilsalicilique acide 100-160 mg /day, which has an anti-thrombotic effect;
- LMWH in prophylactic doses, administered with 2 hours before the flight. In circumstances of repeated flights, the anticoagulation must cover the whole travel period.

6.11.6. Thrombosis of the Inferior Cava Vein (ICV)

In 1644 Schenk was the first who described the thrombosis of the inferior vena cava. (109)
It appears in the following 3 situations:

- invading tumor in cava vein; frequently the renal cancer or hepatic cancer invade cava vein. If vena cava occlusion occurs slowly the long-term sequelae appear rarely because a good collateral circulation is developed. If vena cava occlusion occurs more quickly the edema will appear in the majority of the cases (up to 70%). In this situation we shall resect tumor in block and replace the cava vein. There are other possibilities to resolve this problem: excision of a part of vena cava and primary suture or patch closure, transcaval removal of tumor thrombus, resection of vena cava with ligature;
- iliac thrombosis extended to inferior cava vein;
- thrombosis of cava vein distal from a ligature, a Greenfield caval filter or a Mobin-Uddin umbrella etc. The filters can be blocked or obstructed by emboli or by a massive thrombosis.

The turbulence effects, thrombosis or other venous defects, diminish the accuracy of the native MRI for inferior cava vein. The " blood pool agents " method with high concentrations of paramagnetic substance achieves a high quality visualization of vena cava inferior. (R.Vossheinrich - 116).

The appearance of the acute thrombosis of the inferior cava vein causes functional hypovòlemia and hypertension.

The proximal extension of the inferior cava vein thrombosis can affect also the renal veins. Thus the thrombosis can be associated with the nephrotic syndrome. If a pulmonary embolus is detected it is necessary to connect a cava vein filter proximal to the renal veins.

6.11.7. Thrombosis of the Superior Cava Vein (SCV)

6.11.7.1. Etiology:

- malignant tumors: 90% of cases are represented by the superior lobar cancer of the right lung(3-5% of patients evolves to superior cava vein syndrome) followed by mediastinum tumors(thymomas,

Hodgkin disease, lymfosarcomas), thoracic metastasis(from breast and thyroidian cancers, melanomas);

- benign tumors: bulky mediastinum tumors, plunging bulky goiter or true goiter, atrial mixomas;
- thrombosis of SCV: idiopathic/secondary(polycitemia, mediastinitis) or exceptional iatrogenic(after catheterismes);
- traumas: compressive mediastinum hematoma, direct traumas on SCV
- inflammation: fibrous mediastinitis.

The thrombosis of SCV can be added to the compression or the tumoral invasion of SCV and thus it determines a sudden obstruction of a partial stenosis caused by a chronic partial compression. In this case taking into account the clinical aspects it appears a sudden aggravation of the symptomatology.

6.11.7.2. Physiopathology

The obstacle in SCV can appear:

- gradually associated with the development of some collateral ways for the blood drainage;
- suddenly, associated with an extended obstruction of SCV and its collaterals resulting an increased stasis upstream. This stasis determines a very high venous pressure at the arm level or cephalic extremity up to 500 cm H_2O accompanied even by cerebral edema that can be fatal in a few minutes.

The thrombosis may extend to the axillaris or unnamed veins. The permeability of the azygos vein attenuates the effect of the obstruction trebling the amount of the transported blood from 11% to 35%.

6.11.7.3. Symptomatology

The patient presents headaches, nausea, vomiting, visual disturbances, stupor or convulsions. The voice is hoarse. He may also present dyspnea because of the edema of the vocal chords and pulmonary edema accompanied by cough. At inspection we observe the edema of the face, neck, shoulders and arms ("mantle" edema) and the teguments are cyanotic or purple. The symptoms aggravate in dorsal decubitus and improve in sitting position. The veins of the neck, shoulders and arms are turgescent developing an abundant collateral circulation at the level of the anterior thorax and abdomen. In the case of the unnamed vein thrombosis if SCV is permeable the symptoms will be discreet because of the compensation of the venous drainage through the contra lateral cervical veins.

6.11.7.4. Investigations

- The venous pressure proximally from the obstacle is increased over 200 cm H_2O;
- The simple thoracic X-rays may diagnose the thoracic tumors;
- The phlebography done by venous puncture located distally from the obstacle (axillary, unnamed, superior cava, azygos veins) shows the locations, the extension and the types of the obstacle and also the compensatory collateral circulation;
- The echocardiography;
- The aortography is useful for the differential diagnosis of the aorta aneurisms;
- The bronchoscopy.

6.11.7.5. Differential Diagnosis

Angioneurosis edema, heart failures of different etiologies, effort thrombophlebitis of the superior limb, the obstruction of the unnamed vein by a compression with an arterial loop.

6.11.7.6. Complications

- The thrombosis of the superior cava vein is a complication that aggravates a partial chronic obstruction. Clinically it is noticed a paroxysmal aggravation of the symptoms of the superior cava vein syndrome;
- The tearing of the esophageal varices secondary to the venous hypertension in the superior cava vein territory causes the superior digestive hemorrhage.

6.11.7.7. Treatment

Diuretic treatment, liquids restriction, radiotherapy, chemotherapy are recommended in urgency in the case of malignant obstruction of the superior cava vein. In case of the thrombosis of the superior cava vein anticoagulant eventually fibrinolysis treatment is recommended. The malignant tumors invading the superior cava vein are usually too extended and the radical oncologic surgical treatment or even the palliative surgical treatment are no longer possible to perform. In case of benign obstruction the excision of the compressive tumors is recommended. In this case the surgical procedures are not codified and they adapt to the local situation (venous by-pass, resection of the tumor with the superior cava vein and replacing the vein by graft, recanalization of the superior cava vein lumen, thrombectomies).

6.11.7.8. Prognosis

The prognosis of the malignant etiology of the superior cava vein thrombosis is poor; the patient will live at most 6-8 months. In case of fibrosing mediastinitis successful operation will continuously improve the symptomatology and induce good and long lasting results.

CHAPTER 7

CHRONIC VENOUS INSUFFICIENCY OF THE INFERIOR LIMBS (C.V.I.)

TAKE HOME MESSAGES

- Mainly PTS, the neglected varicose disease and the compression syndrome determine the etiology of CVI. In PTS the venous insufficiency occurs early. The main signs for CVI are varices and the trophic lesions: lipodermatosclerosis, atrophie blanche, dermite ocre, calf ulcer
- Tisular modifications in CVI are complex, involving venous lumen and wall, the elastic fibers, the collagen, the proliferation of fibroblasts, the leucocytes migration and cellular destructions.
- Required investigations are echo/duplex Doppler, pletismography and phlebography for medical practice and research purpose.
- Particular forms of CVI are: Cockett, Martorell, calf muscular compartment, solear, popliteal vein entrapment syndromes.
- Medical treatment is complex and controversial. The trials demonstrated the utility of flavonoids, antiinflamatory drugs. Elastic compression is useful, together with exercises and adequate life style. Surgery suppresses the venous reflux (crossectomy, perforans veins ligatures, valvuloplasties), the dilated varicose veins or it bypasses the venous obstructions. Ulcer needs to be treated locally and ultimately needs skin graft.

7.1. DEFINITION

The chronic venous insufficiency is defined as the decompensated stage of the venous circulation in the inferior limbs with symptoms and signs produced by venous hypertension as a result of structural or functional abnormalities of the veins (A.N. Nicolaides - 76). Clinically it is characterized by advanced trophic lesions like edemas, subcutaneous cellulite, lipodermatosclerosis, dermatitis and calf ulcers, all being determined by the increasing of the venous pressure.

Also the venous insufficiency is a functional defect of venous return resulting from reflux, obstruction or both. The venous pump is inefficient in decreasing the venous pressure. The activity of the pump is determined by: competent venous valves, ankle joint mobility and functional calf muscle. (H. Partsch - 82)

7.2. ETIOLOGY

It is represented by:

- postphlebitic syndrome in most of the cases (about 50% of DVT);
- advanced, neglected hydrostatic varicose veins with the decompensation of the deep and superficial venous system After Basle Study 21% of patients with mild varicose veins and 50% of patients with severe varicose veins develop signs of CVI;
- congenital venous malformations;
- arterio-venous shunts of varied etiologies (traumatic, congenital, iatrogenous etc.).

7.3. PHYSIOPATOLOGY

The evolution of the postphlebitic syndrome is characterized by the persistence of the obstruction and the avalvulvar recanalization of the vein. In neglected hydrostatic varicose veins it happens that the superficial decompensation of the venous system overloads the perforating veins that become insufficient favoring the reflux in the deep venous system by a vicious circle. The overload of the deep veins determines their dilatation and the valves incontinence. The venous hypertension determines characteristic changes in the microcirculation and also in the elastic structures of veins and fascia. These changes produce a permanent high venous pressure approximately equal with the pressure determined by the blood column height from heart to malleoli (because it is not segmented by the insufficient valves). The value is approximately 100mmHg. Because of the decreased compliance at walking the muscle pump pushes the blood through the insufficient perforating veins at 130 mm Hg pressure in the superficial venous system. The plantar veins are the initial component of the venous pump pressed by the pumping mechanism at each step. The pressure in the dorsal foot vein is reduced during walking from 80-100 mmHg to 10-20 mmHg at healthy subjects. At patients with inefficient pump the foot vein pressure is not reduced to these low values. At patients with varicose disease the blood volume in legs in standing position may reach 1 l compared to healthy people where the blood volume is 0.3 l. The increase of the venous blood pressure is rather the initial process. The result is the inflammatory reaction in the veins. The vein hypertension is sent backwards to venules and it has bad effects on capillaries.

The endothelial damage leads to an increase in fibrinogen transudation resulting the formation of a pericapillary fibrin cuff. The capillary permeability is disturbed and thus results the liquid and proteins extravasations in the interstitial space. The local tissue ischemia has an important role in the nearby venous ulcer area, assessed by transcutaneous PO_2 measurement. The O_2 extraction is far less than the extraction in normal control regions. (14, 111)

The result of high pressure in the venous lumen is the formation of edema in the interstitial space (extravasation of plasma liquid, plasma proteins as fibrinogen and a little amount of erythrocytes). When these substances reach this space they sequestrate growth factors or matrix material decreasing their availability to their plastic function.

In CVI the vessels are tortuous, elongated, with important vascular resistance and therefore with low blood flow. In the same time the total flow in the diseased area is high. The venous stasis induces the dilatation and elongation of vessels. The high pressure determines the hypertrophy of the musculature and in places where the pressure is less high the venous wall is atrophied. Stasis also determines the increase in number of the arteriovenous anastomosis. (Ramelet - 93) Probably the explanation is a sequence of ischemia and reperfusion in critic area. These cycles facilitate the variation of the fluid shear stress and stretch and an inflammatory process that consists of the appearance of tissue injury and ulcer. The first step is the margination of the leukocytes, the second step is the attachment of leukocytes to the endothelium and the third is their migration into the tissue. This interaction is mediated by the red cells and all this process takes place in the postcapillary venules or at micro vascular bifurcations. It is known that in the normal blood stream the red cells are placed in the proximity of the vessel wall and the leukocytes are placed in the middle of the vessel. But in CVI the blood cells switch their positions in the blood stream in order to permit the attachment of the leukocytes to the endothelium (a weak adhesive interaction-rolling) and their recruitment. This process is due to the decrease less than 1 μm of the distance (the minimal distance for their reaction) between the leukocytes and their endothelial receptors. The activated endothelial cells produce P-selectine, E-selectine, VCAM and ICAM-1. The leukocytes extend pseudopodes between or even through the endothelial cells. They migrate in the interstitial space where they release oxidants and hydrolytic enzymes. These substances have cytotoxic effects. The activated leukocytes destroy the parietal barrier and permit the flooding of fluids and proteins into the interstitial space. The edema increases the oxygen and nutrient diffusion distance, raises the tissue pressure, reduces the capillary backward flow and the capillary exchanges.

Patients with chronic venous disease show increased leukocyte priming. The primed leukocytes show increased surface CD62L (involved in the initial "rolling"), CD11B (ligand for firm leukocytes adhesion and than transmigration). Ono T., Bergan J., Schmitd Schonbein and Takase S. put in evidence the inflammatory mechanism that explain the damage of the venous valve in CVI (3,14,111).

The fibrinolysis is also affected by venous hypertension, so that the perivascular fibrin cuffs persist and after that the oxygenating process and the tissues metabolism decrease. These cuffs act as a barrier to diffusion finally causing local tissue ischemia and macroscopic venous ulcer. The microthrombosis are caused by the oxidative explosion of the leukocytes and by the reduced fibrinolysis resulting from the epithelial damage that leads to activation of the blood platelets. Fibroblasts play an important role in wound healing involving motility, contraction, fibrosis and expression of the alpha smooth muscle actin cytoskeletal protein. Patients with chronic venous insufficiency are known to have dermal changes and impaired venous ulcer healing. Fibroblasts migrate in the interstitial spaces, rich in protein. That explains the fiber-conjunctive process with the thickening and liposclerosis of the subcutaneous tissue. One of the causes of hiperpigmentation and lipodermatoslerosis is the dilated, elongated and tortuous capillaries. Some red cells go through the altered vascular wall and they are destroyed in the interstitial space. The altered hemoglobin changes into hemosiderin, which is stocked as dark brown (till black) pigmentation that characterizes the altered skin in C.V.I. Probably melanin participates too. On the skin and subcutaneous tissue with deficient trophicity the infections occur, namely streptococci that obstruct and make the lymphatic drainage more difficult because of the acute lymphangitis. Thus the edema increases in volume. Sometimes an allergic dermatitis can be added. This dermatitis may be determined by the unguents and ointments that the patient has used (especially antibiotics). The pruritus and grattage lesions favor the continuous infecting process with pathogen germs.

Patients with postphlebitic syndrome and deep veins obstructions and with perforating veins insufficiency record an increase of venous pressure at walking (130-140 mm Hg). Thus it may look like an ischemia with pains at walking ("venous claudication").

The swollen and fibrosing teguments are usually located near the tibial malleoli, where the venous hypertension is high, the skin nutrition is precarious and the region is exposed to traumas. The calf ulcer occurred in these places. The ulcer is a destructive tissue lesion with a precarious cure.

The orthostatic and orthodynamic phlebohypertony is explained in the postphlebitic syndrome by 5 mechanisms:

- Venous obstruction: in the complete obstruction of a deep vein portion. The blood return to the affected inferior limb is performed with difficulty because of the collateral compensatory circulation and the perforans veins forced by dilation and by inversion of the circulation's direction. At walking and effort the vein pressure in the superficial distal veins will increase.
- Vein restriction: the blood evacuation capacity from the vein reservoir of the inferior limb is reduced by the alteration of the vein walls (rigidity, the decreasing of the elasticity and contractility). Thus the capacity of the veins is reduced. The blood is quickly accumulated in limb veins in the orthostatic position. The result of this process is the phlebohypertony because the veins do not damp anymore loosing their natural capacity of accumulating blood in orthostatic position.
- Blood reflux is the result of the vein avalvulation caused by real destructions in the postphlebitic syndrome, respectively by dilation and valvular insufficiency in hydrostatic varicose disease. The result is the permanent orthostatic and orthodynamic phlebohypertony.

- Substitution: the collateral veins derived the high pressure and bypass the obstructed deep vein
- Mixed mechanism.

7.4. CLASSIFICATION OF CVI

Table 7.1. Classification of CVI

CEAP Classification C=clinical signs	Widmer's Classification (Stages I-III)
C3 Edema	CVI I Corona phlebectatica paraplantaris, edemas
C4 Skin changes (pigmentation, eczema, lipodermatosclerosis)	CVI II Trophic lesion, hyper or hypopigmentation, dermite ocre, atrophie blanche, lipodermatosclerosis
C5 Healed ulcer	CVI IIIA Healed ulcer (scar)
C6 Active ulcer	CVI IIIB Active ulcer

7.5. SYMPTOMATOLOGY IN CVI

The anamnesis, the correct history of the disease and the clinic examination guide us on the postphlebitic, hydrostatic, or arterio-venous shunts etiology. CVI appears after a long period of time (15-20 years) in hydrostatic varices and very quickly (after 1-2 years) in postphlebitic syndrome. We are interested in the evolution of each symptom from CVI and the treatments followed by the patient.

The main complaints of the patient with CVI are: heavy legs, aching, itching, sensation of burning, the restless leg syndrome, pain accentuated in orthostatic position. At a local exam of the inferior limbs we can notice the following symptoms:

- Dilated varicose veins as corona phlebectatica or veins blow-up or even "caput medusae" in iliac or femoral vein obstruction
- Edema is extended. It persists also at rest and it is quickly aggravated in orthostatic position. In time it has a progressive character from the

distal parts to the proximal ones and it increases in diameter like an "inverted champagne bottle"

- Dermatitis: usually located in the inferior third of the calf. The teguments are glossy, red or pink, warm at palpation and sometimes with pain sensibility at touch;
- Eczema: it has a policyclic form, a vague outline often with an exudative character;
- Brown pigmentation: hemosiderin and melanine deposits in the tegument;
- White atrophy of the skin;
- Calf trophic ulcer that is an oval, trophic lesion with irregular edges. It gradually extends in surface and in depth. The bottom of the ulcer is red-brown, sometimes covered by serous and serosanguinolent secretions, possibly purulent or escariotic. In the indurated base of the ulcer an insufficient or thrombosed vein might be present. Next to this vein it might by noticed an insufficient perforating vein;

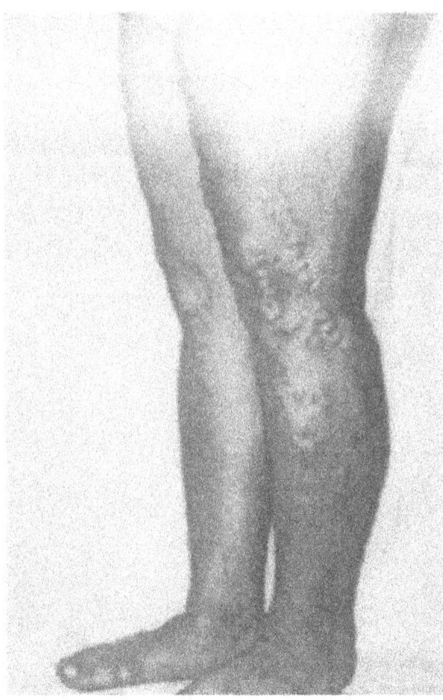

Fig.7.1. Primary varicosis "Dermite ocre"

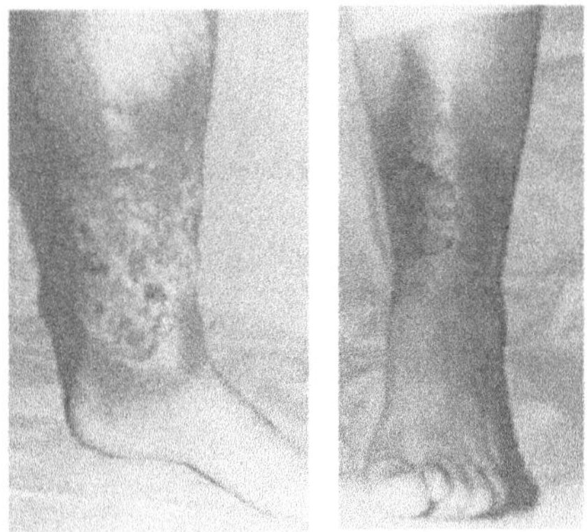

Fig.7.2. PTS: leg ulcer (2 casses)

- Superficial varicose veins are dilated, sinuous, with thick or very thin walls. Some of them represent collateral ways for drainage (in the postphlebitic syndrome). Clinically we can spot some insufficient perforating veins (see the clinical maneuvers of diagnosis). In case of indurative cellulite the varicose veins can be palpated like rigid grooves or "canyons" in the hard part of inflammation.
- Venous claudication: pain on walking with disappearance on resting but only when the legs are raised (seldom symptom).

The clinical tests for diagnosis are very useful. We can locate the insufficient perforating veins by a careful examination. With a certain probability we can also locate even lesions of the deep venous system. These tests are: Trendelenburg, Mahornery-Ochsner, Schwartz, Perthes. (see5.3.4)

7.6. INVESTIGATIONS

The investigations can record the anatomic expansion, pathology, cause and functional severity of obstruction and reflux.

7.6.1. Continuous Doppler Ultrasonography records:

- the lack of the vein flux;

- an increased flux at the compression of the muscles distal from the Doppler transducer (in case of the obstructive syndrome);
- the presence of the reflux longer than 0.5 sec. at Valsalva maneuver or at the compression of the limb muscle proximal to the ultrasonograph transducer (in the avalvular syndrome).

In addition to this we can locate the insufficient perforans veins using a correct clinical and echo Doppler examination.

7.6.2. Pulsate Echosonography Doppler

Pulsate echosonography Doppler is colored now. This shows the image of the superficial and deep venous system and exactly the location of the insufficient perforans veins respectively the existence of the deep veins valves.

7.6.3. Duplex Doppler

- Importance: it is a combination of scanning in mode B with a pulsate Doppler and it has been used since 1980 for the diagnosis of DVT (reflux) and recently extended to detect the obstruction or the reflux in CVI. It allows the vein visualization and the measurement of the vein flux at the same time. It might notice the permeability of the veins and the existence of some thrombi in their lumen (the normal veins are compressible, the thrombosed veins are incompressible). We can also notice the vein valves and their function. For the elucidation of the anatomy and pathology we can use color-flow duplex scanning which has multiple advantages: decreases the time and improves the accuracy of the examination and also provides instant visualization of the blood flow and its direction. It is the proper method for serial examinations to follow up the evolution of the thrombi.
- Technique: a multi-frequency transducer is placed on the saphenofemoral junction with the patient standing and holding the entire weight on the opposite limb. We can also examine the patient in the 15° reverse Trendelenburg position using the Valsalva maneuver to elicit reflux. For the investigation of LSV and popliteal veins the patient is examined in the standing position or in a sitting position on the edge of a couch with the foot on a chair.

- Results: a normal vein is seen as an echogenic intraluminar structure (red cells aggregates) that moves slowly in the cephalic direction; one can also see the movements of the venous valve cusps, the smooth lining of the venous wall; it can be approximated the anterior and posterior vein wall. Old thrombosis with or without recanalization appears as high echoes in the lumen with irregular walls. In this case you cannot fully approximate the vein walls. By sliding the transducer up and down the leg in cases of varicosities we can identify incompetent perforating veins. In the color-flow duplex imaging the reflux appears red and lasts for more than 0.5 seconds, the lumen appears black if the reflux is missing and in patent vessel with old thrombosis on the screen we see blue when we compress the distal limb and red when we release the compression.
- Limits: in cases of obese patients or patients with swollen legs and when we operate above the inguinal ligament the image is difficult to be obtained.

7.6.4. Plethysmography

Plethysmography shows especially the valvular incompetence and is more useful for the diagnosis of acute thrombosis.

Principle:

It is the method that records the changes in volume or other dimensions of the body in response to each heartbeat or temporary occlusion of venous return. The venous outflow plethysmography detect the obstruction of a deep vein by a lesser decrease of the venous flux after deflation of a pneumatic cuff that occludes temporarily the venous return in the proximal limb. Several devices are available: strain gauge plethysmography (SPG), impedance plethysmography (IPG), air plethysmography (APG) and photoplethysmography (PPG).

- SPG records the calf volume changes with the patient in the supine position. We use two tourniquets –one put proximal on the thigh and the other put distal on the thigh. The proximal cuff is inflated above the arterial systolic pressure to isolate the limb from the general circulation. The distal cuff is inflated up to 50 mmHg determining a downward direction of the venous blood through the incompetent veins. During the inflation of the distal cuff the strain gauge records the increase in calf circumference. In the cases of chronic venous insufficiency it is better to record the calf volume with the patient doing calf muscle exercises. This technique is used for screening and quantifying CVI, also for evaluating venous claudication and for differentiating between CVI and lymphedema.

- IPG measures the changes in electrical resistance; it uses 2 pairs of electrodes placed 10 cm apart on the calf; an increase in volume determines a decrease in resistance; a decrease in volume raises the resistance.
- APG uses a 36 cm polyurethane cuff that surrounds the leg from knee to ankle; it is inflated with air at 6 mmHg; this cuff is connected to a pressure transducer that will determine the volume of the calf; after stabilization of the calf size (about 2 minutes) the thigh cuff is rapidly deflated and so the changes in calf volume or circumference are recorded.
- PPG uses an infrared light that is absorbed in the skin; this absorption is dependent on the volume of the blood in the superficial dermal venous plexuses. The absorption is due to the hemoglobin from the red cells so when the quantity of the hemoglobin is high (when venous pressure is high), light absorption increases. This technique is used for screening to detect CVI or to determine the general function of the lower limb veins without using more expensive or invasive tests.

Results:

The values of the venous outflow depend upon the type of transducer used. Most of the techniques measure the increase of the calf volume and the rate of decrease in calf volume. In acute DVT with total occlusion when the thigh cuff is inflated the increase of the calf will be minimal. If there is only a partial occlusion it will appear only a small rise in calf volume with the thigh cuff inflated.

7.6.5. Phlebography

Phlebography is a minimal invasive investigation that shows exactly the extension of the venous stenosis and obstruction, the state of the venous system, of the valves and of the drainage ways. It was proposed in 1920 but the greatest development was registered later when the contrast substances were improved. There are more techniques with different indications.

7.6.5.1. Ascending Phlebography

- Importance: Cid dos Santos introduced this exam in 1938 and even now in the age of more sophisticated exams, it is considered the "gold standard" for detecting chronic venous obstruction (presence, site and anatomic extent) and for distinguishing between primary and secondary disease. It is also used for detecting incompetent perforating veins and for establishing the accuracy of new investigations.
- Technique: first we put a tourniquet above ankle then we inject contrast medium into a vein on the dorsum of the foot and so it will be directed into the deep veins. For slowing the ascendant movement of the contrast substance we may use a second cuff on the thigh or we may tilt the table. If we want to visualize the iliac veins and the inferior vena cava we have to inject supplementary the contrast substance in the femoral vein in the same time with Valsalva maneuver.
- Results: for diagnosing the DVT and venous chronic obstruction DeWeese and Rogoff established the following criteria:
  - the presence of well-defined filling defects in veins full with contrast substance demonstrated in more than 2 radiographs;
  - in cases with thrombotic obstruction we can not obtain a visualization of a calf vein or a good opacification of the proximal and distal parts of a proximal vein and also the presence of collateral vessels;
  - the thrombus can be completely or partially obstructive. Fresh thrombus is visualized as filling the most of the venous lumen but it is not adhesive to the venous wall, old thrombus with recanalization is visualized as irregularities of the venous wall and the loose thrombus is visualized as cylindrical filling defect surrounded by a thin white line of contrast medium.
- Disadvantages: the method cannot exactly quantify the function of the vein and it cannot visualize all the collaterals.

7.6.5.2. Descending Phlebography

- Importance: Luke introduced the method in 1941. This method shows the reflux in the superficial or deep veins, the localization and morphology of the venous valves, the extent of the reflux, the venous anatomy in complex cases and also differentiates between primary and secondary disease.

- Technique: we introduce a cannula through a brachial, femoral or popliteal vein and inject the contrast substance the patient being in orthostatic position using a tilting table. Valsalva maneuver is necessary for the valve closure.
- Results: according to this method there are 5 grades of reflux:
  - grade 0-no reflux below the confluence of the superficial femoral and profunda femoris veins;
  - grade 1-reflux into the superficial femoral vein but up to the middle of the thigh;
  - grade 2-reflux into the superficial femoral vein but not through the popliteal vein with competent popliteal valves;
  - grade 3-reflux to a level just below the knee with incompetent popliteal valves but the valves in the axial calf veins are competent;
  - grade 4-reflux into the axial veins (femoral, popliteal and calf) up to the level of the ankle.
- Disadvantages: it is invasive, costly, has potential complications and uses contrast agents that are heavier than blood.

7.6.5.3. Pelvic Phlebography

- Importance: visualization of the main pelvic veins;
- Technique:
  - backward catheter into external iliac vein with contrast medium injection till the internal iliac vein is visualized as far as the first competent valve then it is possible selective catheterization of the hypogastric vein and to obtain a good pelvic venography;
  - intrauterine: injection of the contrast medium into the fundus of uterus and then the iliac fossa is compressed, this showing the opacification of the other side of the ovarian vein.

7.6.5.4. Selective Ovarian and Internal Iliac Phlebography

- Importance: it is used when we suspect incompetence of the ovarian veins with reflux into the vulvar veins through the internal iliac vein.
- Technique: injection of the contrast medium through a catheter introduced in basilic, right femoral or internal jugular veins using a tilting table or Valsalva maneuver.

- Results: the technique shows: varices in both broad ligaments of the uterus, varices of the thigh (passing through the obturator and internal pudendal veins) and even the varices of the calf.

7.6.5.5. Intraosseous Phlebography (not used currently):

Intraosseous phlebography consists in direct injection of the contrast medium into the great trochanter and shows the hypogastric tributaries.

7.6.5.6. Upper Extremity Phlebography:

Used for patients with venous thrombosis localized at the subclavian and /or axillary veins and with thoracic outlet syndrome. The contrast medium is injected into the basilic vein and the progress of contrast medium is followed up but only the digital method visualizes the proximal extent of the thrombus and the status of more central veins.

7.6.5.7. Varicography

- Importance: it is additional to the ascending phlebography; very important in the cases of recurrent varicose veins and venous malformations and also facilitates the use of minimal incisions and precise surgery;
- Technique: direct injection of contrast medium through a canulla into the investigated superficial vein.

7.6.6. Liquid Crystal Thermography:

Liquid crystal thermography is an accurate, simple, relatively cheap and rapid screening test to localize incompetent perforators. The layer of liquid crystals applied on the skin of the thigh and leg determines hot spots where the incompetent perforans veins with warmer blood cross the fascia.

7.6.7. Femoral Vein Pressure Measurements

Used to determine the severity of the ilio-cava obstruction by inserting a needle or a catheter into the common femoral vein and measuring the pressure at rest and after exercise.

7.6.8. Arm/Foot Pressure Differential

This method is important because it selects the patients for venous reconstruction. A by-pass procedure is indicated if the patient has a high arm/foot pressure differential. Venous pressures are recorded simultaneously in a vein of the foot and a vein of the arm in the supine position and then during reactive hyperemia or after the injection of papaverine.

7.6.9. Foot Volumetry

It is represented by the measurement of volume changes of the foot during exercise.

Foot volumetry determines the degree of venous insufficiency, indicates its location (superficial, deep or both), evaluates the therapeutic interventions and determines the extent of valve damage.

7.6.10. Microcirculation Study

Some methods for microcirculation study are: skin biopsy, capillaroscopy, laser Doppler fluxmetry, transcutaneous oxygen tension, interstitial pressure measurements and fluorescent microlymphography.

- Skin biopsy is used to exclude the malignancy in leg ulcers or to establish the exact diagnosis in uncertain skin changes (vasculitis).
- Capillaroscopy is the method that studies the morphology and function of skin capillaries (capillary diameter and density, shape indices obtained with digital image processing). It has a limited value in the clinical management of CVI.

- Laser Doppler fluxmetry provides a continuous and noninvasive measure of local blood flow and evaluates the effect of compression therapy on local skin blood flow. The results showed that elastic compression for several weeks or intermittent pneumatic compression for several hours normalized the high red cell flux in CVI and induced normal vasomotion.
- Transcutaneous oxygen pressure ($TcPO_2$) is used only for studying the pathophysiology of the skin changes and ulceration appearing in CVI.
- Interstitial pressure measurements consist in determining the pressure in nail fold capillaries, microlymphatics and the interstitium. It is also a research method with no clinical application.
- Fluorescence microlymphography determines the presence of the lymphatic microangiopathy in lipodermatosclerosis and it is also used for clinical research into the pathophysiology of edema and skin changes in CVI, being the only method available for analyzing the structure and function of the lymphatics in the skin.

7.6.11. Laboratory Exams show:

- high plasma fibrinogen levels;
- elevated fibrinogen degradation products (rapid turnover of the macromolecules);
- increased level of inhibitor of plasminogen activator 1 (PAI I), which otherwise is considered a marker for damage to the skin microcirculation, causing a defect in fibrinolisis;
- high level of thrombomodulin suggesting endothelial dysfunction.

7.7. PARTICULAR CLINICAL FORMS OF CVI

7.7.1. Cockett Syndrome

Definition:

The Cockett syndrome (1965) is defined by the compression of the left iliac vein of varied etiology.

Etiopathogeny:

The main cause is the compression made by the right primitive iliac artery at the crossing with the left iliac vein. The osseous etiology (hyperlordosis, compression by discus protrusions or osteophytes) or the endovenous etiology (valves, bridles, partial membranous septi) is also possible. Under these circumstances an acute iliac thrombosis followed by a severe postphlebitic syndrome appear, and they are resistant at medical treatment.

7.7.2. Martorell Syndrome

It consists of thrombosis of the extern iliac vein (like in Cockett syndrome) but with the development of a very visible suprapubian derivative circulation. It may also occur in the thrombosis of the right iliac vein.

7.7.3. Calf Muscular Compartment Syndrome (Wilson 1912, Blandy and Fuller 1957, Reneman 1968)

It is usually located in the antero-lateral compartment of the calf. In case of thrombophlebitic syndrome, it produces a phlebohypertony having during walking intermittent venous claudication as clinical symptomatology.

7.7.4. Solear Syndrome (M. Servelle and J. Babilot 1969)

Solear Syndrome is determined by the compression of the popliteal vein by a tight solear ring. Clinically we notice a circumscribed calf edema, especially distal and relative small varices, resistant to sclerotherapeutical treatment. We establish the diagnosis by phlebography, Doppler ultrasonography and echo Doppler.

7.7.5. Popliteal Vein Entrapment Syndrome

Popliteal vein compression was found in approximately 42% of limbs undergoing ascending phlebography and in 22 % of the cases it was found bilaterally (Raju - 92). The clinical importance is controversial. The differential diagnosis of CVI includes the popliteal vein entrapment in patients in whom other more common etiologies have been excluded on the basis of the investigations.

The main causes of popliteal vein entrapment are anomalies of the medial head of the gastrocnemius muscle, which was found in 60 % of cases. Other causes are muscular and fibrous compression bands, additional third head of gastrocnemius muscle, soleus sling, anomalous course of the popliteal veins and artery (lateral to the lateral head of the gastrocnemius muscle), thick perivenous fascia, angulation of the popliteal vein by the LSV and the gastrocnemius veins (at their entry point during calf contraction).

The pathological changes observed at the popliteal vein are the following:

- Sclerosis of popliteal vein especially at the pressure points and above the insufficient valve
- Pre-stenotic dilatation
- Post-stenotic dilatation
- Post-thrombotic changes
- Insufficiency of popliteal venous valves

The clinical evaluation of the compression syndrome puts in evidence the CVI symptoms namely pain, edema and ulcers. The diagnostic of the syndrome is established by:

- ascending venography : aspects of hourglass appearance to diffuse compression. Important maneuvers are especially the active plantar flexion, but sometimes passive dorsal flexions of the leg too;
- echo-Doppler;
- measurement of the venous pressure in the popliteal vein with a special catheter . Raju (92) has demonstrated the compression by using an 18 gauge angiocatheter with ultrasound scanning guidance introduced in the posterior tibial vein near the ankle and a 2 F catheter with tip-mounted pressure transducer positioned in the popliteal vein at the level of the joint line with fluoroscopic control. The patient performed 10 toe stand exercises while the popliteal pressure was recorded. The ambulatory venous pressure is recorded simultaneously. If the ambulatory venous pressure decreases less than 15 % or the popliteal pressure increases with exercise it is considered to be representative for the presence of a significant outflow obstruction.

The compression of the popliteal vein can be removed by surgical procedures:

- Dividing the medial tendons of the gastrocnemius muscles;
- Dividing all muscular and fibrous compression bands;
- Phlebolysis and liberation of a thick perivenous fascia;
- Detachment of the lateral head of gastrocnemian muscle;
- Repairing of popliteal vein valves when they are insufficient.

The late result of surgery is the significant improvement of clinical symptoms in 60 – 70 % of cases and even excellent in 40 % of cases (Raju –92).

7.8. CVI TREATMENT

The varicose disease and the postphlebitic syndrome are evolutional affections and more over they determine CVI. There are a lot of measures that can lower the venous hypertension like the stripping of incompetent saphenous veins and ligatures of perforators, sclerotherapy of incompetent varicose veins, non-elastic high-pressure compression, cold stress and phlebotonic drugs.

7.8.1. Medical Treatment

It is the major therapy that is applied in the majority of cases with CVI. First the patient has to be instructed to understand the constant and insidious character of the affection and the importance of some simple therapeutic measures that must be applied during the entire life. In a different manner the patients do not easily understand the necessity of this prolonged treatment that has a good result and stops the evolution of the disease for a long time. The control of the phlebohypertony and edemas is simple: wearing permanently elastic stockings, avoiding the prolonged orthostatic position and frequently raising up the inferior limbs above the level of the heart.

The medical treatment consists of phlebothrophics:

a) Benzopirones:

   - α-coumarinic derivatives;

- γ-flavonoids:
  - flavones, flavonole: diosmin, diosmentin, hydroxy-etyl rutin (O-beta hydroxy-etyl rutin, troxerutin);
  - flavane, flavanone: hesperidin, picnogenol.

b) Saponines: aescin, Daflon/Detralex (mycronised flavonoides), Ginkor Fort, Antistax, Troxerutin are well known drugs.

The antibiotic treatment and the antibacterial solutions are indicated only in case of clear bacterial contamination and after the identification of the germs and antibiogram. In case of calf ulcer it is recommended to disinfect with light antiseptics (solution of chloramines, betadine solution, Castellani solution), moist pads, hydrophilic dextranomer (Debrisan) on exudative ulcers, proteolytic enzymes used for cleansing of necrotic material, silver sulfadiazine (Flamazine), exposing at air and postural drainage by bed rest with raised leg. Topical antibiotics and healing ointments have limited efficacy and a high risk of sensitization. Anti-inflammatory treatment is useful in subacute and chronic inflammations (hypodermitis, cellulite).

Other systemic treatments are: antiplatelet drugs, anticoagulant drugs, prostaglandines, Pentoxifilin and Stanozolol. The last is a synthetic steroid anabolic drug, which stimulate cellular and plasma synthesis.

7.8.2. Surgical Treatment

Surgical treatment of the CVI aims to restore the normal vein flux by different interventions. Progress has been noticed in the last few years in surgical treatment but some of the methods need "the time test" checking. The usual interventions are:

- suppressing of the vein reflux by crossectomy, saphenectomy (internal and/or external), the ligature of the perforans veins (direct, subfascial, laparoscopic); the deep vein ligatures are abandoned;
- extirpation and suppression of the dilated varicous superficial non functional veins by stripping or phlebotomies;
- reconstruction of the deep vein system by valvuloplasties (intern, extern, cuffings) valvulated vein grafts, transplant of artificial valves (2001);
- vein by-pass, the venous derivation (Palma operation);

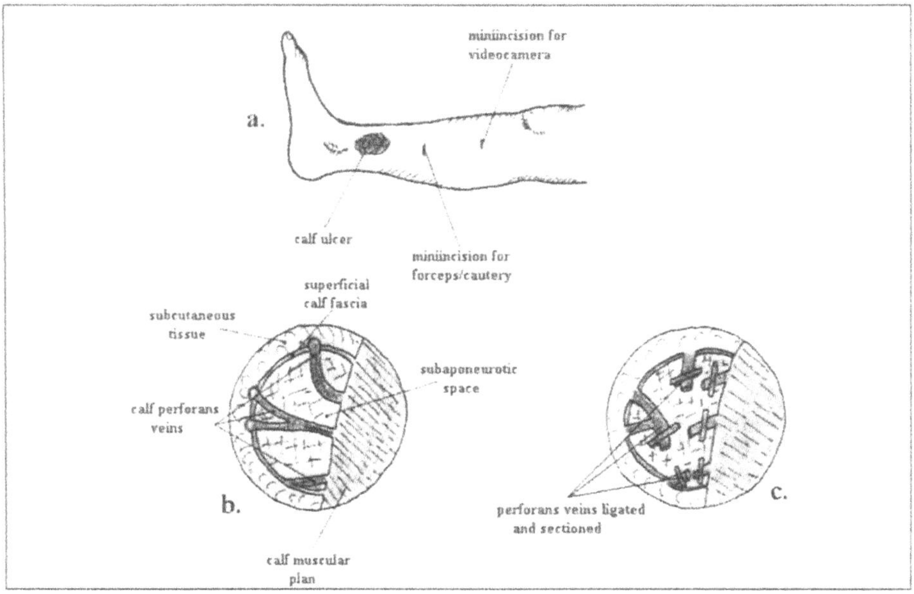

Fig.7.3. SEPS procedure
a. Leg ulcer
b. Perforating veins dissection
c. Ligatures & section of perforating veins

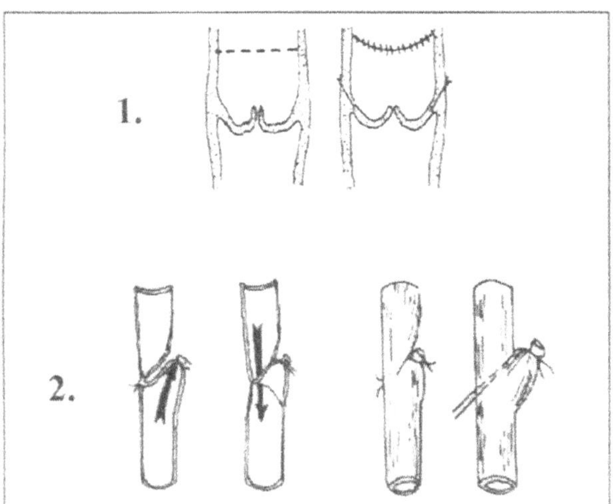

Fig.7.4. Valvuloplasties
1. Kistner-Raju
2. Brinzeu

- calf ulcer can be cleaned by simple curettage, by lasser, by water scalpel (and even by maggots!) and than covered by plasties with free split skin cut by the dermatome. Shave therapy consist in tangential excision of the ulcer with dermatome and than mesh skin graft on healthy tissue.

In the Cockett and Martorell syndromes the indications of surgical treatment are exceptional (derivations, decrossings). In the compartment syndrome the calf is decompressed by fasciotomy. The solear syndrome is diagnosed using laboratory tests and the surgical section of the solear ring treats it.

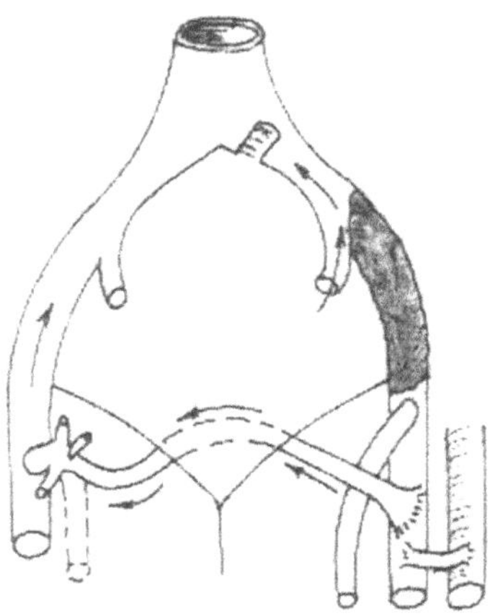

Fig.7.5. Palma operation: derivation of the venous flux from one external iliac vein to the other by a venous graft or reversed saphena

CHAPTER 8

CONGENITAL DISTURBANCES OF VASCULAR GENESIS

TAKE HOME MESSAGES

- Congenital disturbances of vascular genesis consist of hemangiomas, angiodysplasis and venous malformations. They are rare but are very different as symptomatology, prognostic and therapy as the other varices.
- Diagnosis is established by color echo-Doppler, phlebography, CT, MRI.
- Venous malformations are valve agenesis and hypoplasia, syndromes as: Klippel-Trenaunay, Proteo (Wiedermann), Maffucci, Bean, Parks-Weber. The treatment consists of sclerotherapy, surgical interventions (suppression of arteriovenous fistulas, venoplasties, valvuloplasties, removal of abnormal embryonal venous trunks, venous bypasses), cryotherapy with liquid CO_2, lasertherapy, interferon and corticotherapy.

8.1. GENERALITIES

The study of the congenital disturbances of vascular genesis began one 100 years ago (Hochstetter-1891; Lewis-1905). The growth factors and the integrines play an important part in these disturbances and influence the 3 stages of tumoral angiogenesis (21):

- first stage: stimulation induced by growth factors;
- second stage: proliferation with invasion;
- third stage: maturation stimulated by integrines.

The importance of medium, chromosomal disturbances or heredity influence is an unsolved problem yet.

8.2. CLASSIFICATION:

- hemangiomas ;
- vascular malformations (angiodysplasias).

Between those 2 types of congenital disturbances there were observed many differences regarding the appearance, development, diagnosis and treatment. Both disorders have a great variability of evolutionary forms.

8.2.1. Hemangiomas

They are benign endothelial tumors diagnosed in the very first year of life in 10-12% of the cases. Their expanding is in surface in 78% of cases and both in surface and in depth in 5%. In half of cases the hemangiomas have an autonomous proliferative phase on the first 6-8 weeks of life with possible spontaneous remissions in the first year of life. The remission is only partial in 30% of cases and is missing in 20%.

The types of hemangiomas are:

- simple hemangiomas (nevus vasculosus: segmental development on the dermatomes pattern, with frequent, spontaneous and complete regression);
- cavernosus hemangiomas (like a sponge with blood), can be superficial or deep. It may develop complications such as: ulcer, important hemorrhages and malign transformation;

- racemosum hemangiomas with multiple congenital arterial-venous fistulas surrounded by varices.

8.2.2. Vascular Malformations (Angiodysplasias)

The overall incidence of congenital vascular malformations in the population is 1.5% at birth (Eifert - 21). However sometimes they become detectable later, during childhood or adolescence. Generally they develop till puberty while later the expansion is very slowly. The venous malformations comprise 2/3 of all congenital vascular malformations and generally they affect the periphery.

The congenital vascular malformations are defined as " inborn errors of vascular morphogenesis developed in the embryonal stage leading to true structural anomalies; there are present at birth (congenital by definition) "(Mulliken - 74, Young - 114). The venous malformations occurred in the superficial, in the deep or in the two venous systems. They can be circumscribed or diffuse.

The present classification takes into account the location area of the malformation (at the trunk and out of the trunk), the clinical signs and the functional disturbances.

The vascular malformations are:

- arterial → aplasia, hypoplasia or obstruction, dilatation;
- venous → aplasia or obstruction,
  - dilatation,
  - avalvular veins,
  - hypertrophy and elongation of the venous valves,
  - persistence of anomalous embryonic veins,
  - phlebectasia: a diffuse dilatation of one or more venous segments,
  - aplasia or hypoplasia: an absence or under development of venous trunks,
  - aneurysm: a localized area of venous dilatation that communicates with a main venous structure by a single channel, which is not associated with arteriovenous malformations and it is not contained within a segment of varicose vein,
  - avalvulia: an absence of valve in the venous trunks of one or more extremities (Eifert - 21).

- lymphatic → aplasia or obstruction, dilatation;
- arterio-venous fistulas → superficial and profound;
- combined → arterial, venous or/and shunts.

From the medical point of view those malformations that determine functional disturbances (hypo/hypertrophy, chronic insufficiency) have great importance.

8.2.3. Venous Malformations (VM)

8.2.3.1. Pathogenesis of VM

Pathogenesis of VM depends on genetic anomalies of mediators (angiopoietin) and the membrane receptors. So they change the interaction between endothelial and smooth muscle cells. The result is an anomalous vein with a monolayer of flat endothelial cells on the wall replacing the smooth muscular tunic. VM may be present in sporadic forms or familiar hereditary forms. Also they can be represented as isolated malformations (in most cases), multifocal forms or even systemic disseminated forms. VM affect mainly the periphery: lower limbs or cranium and facial region (temporal, masseteric, frontal, palpebral, lingual, labial area) and less the chest and abdomen.

The effects of VM are:

- functional: motor deficiencies and sensory disorders;
- hemodynamic: venous stasis, CVI, thrombosis;
- coagulation: located thrombosis, consumption coagulopathy;
- psychological: depression (patients and family);
- esthetic: skin aspect, skeletal deformations.

The functional defects are very important and affects the social life:

- central: swallowing, speech, respiration, sight, hearing;
- peripheral: posture, walking and grasping disabilities.

The esthetic and psychological effects are very impressive, although they are not so important.

8.2.3.2. Anatomico-Clinical Classification of VM used two groups:

- simple: subcutaneous, intramuscular, intra-articular forms. The veins are abnormally dilated with very thin walls presenting a single layer of endothelial cells and a very hypoplastic smooth muscular coat;
- complex: combinations of hypo-,aplasia, congenital hypertrophy and incompetence of the valves, persistence of embryonal veins. The veins present a complete atresia of the venous valves cusps or dysplastic changes that produce mechanical defects in valve flap closure. The localization might be: superficial, deep, common femoral veins, internal iliac vein. The most frequent persisting femoral veins are the sciatic and marginal veins, which develop in the early stages and normally regress during the later phase of vascular genesis. In cases with persisting embryonal veins the changes are anomalous, twisted, irregular large-caliber venous trunks. Embryonal veins of the lower extremity extend into the acral regions towards the proximal part of the limb. Sometimes this persistence permits the derivation of the blood stream from the area of the hypo/aplastic femoral vein to the iliac territory.

8.2.3.3. Clinical Diagnosis

The superficial VM are visible as subcutaneous dilated, tortuous, soft and elastic veins with a bluish or purple-colored skin. The veins are easy depressed. They are expanded in the anti-gravity position. The local venous thrombosis is palpated as small hard nodules – phlebolith, “venous stones”. The intramuscular or intra-articular VM are not exposed to visual sight and are difficult to palpate and detect. The careful observation will generally show a typical asymmetry of the anatomical affected region. This is increased when the patient is lying down.

In complicated forms appear the classic signs of CVI:

- The Klippel-Trenaunay syndrome is defined as the association of three signs: cutaneous capillary malformation (nevus) as a port wine stain, unilateral anomalous development of the underlying bones and soft tissue hypertrophy of the limb and varices developed early in childhood. Sometimes in this syndrome a persistent sciatic vein (remnant of an embryonic axis) may be found in the sheath of the sciatic nerve and draining into the internal iliac vein or into the profunda femoris vein. Paradoxically the affected limb can be atrophic in some cases. The halux can be so hypertrophic that the patient cannot wear shoes and need to be amputated.

- The Proteo syndrome (Wiedermann H.R.) has multifocal capillary-venous and lymphatic malformations with anomalies of the muscles, skeleton and the peripheral nerves. It determines extreme hypertrophy and deformation of the affected limb.
- The Maffucci syndrome is an association of superficial VM with multiple enchondromatosis of the upper and lower extremities determining skeletal deformations with shortening of the limb and the possibility of developing chondrosarcoma.
- The Bean syndrome consists of multiple subcutaneous VM and disseminated VM in the gastrointestinal tract.
- The Parks-Weber syndrome is characterized by the presence of large arterio-venous fistulas that transmit the high arterial blood pressure into the veins. The result is the continuous dilation of the neighboring veins that become pulsate, varicose, with high pressure and reddish colored. The nevus is absent. The development of CVI and chronic arterial ischemia follow frequently.

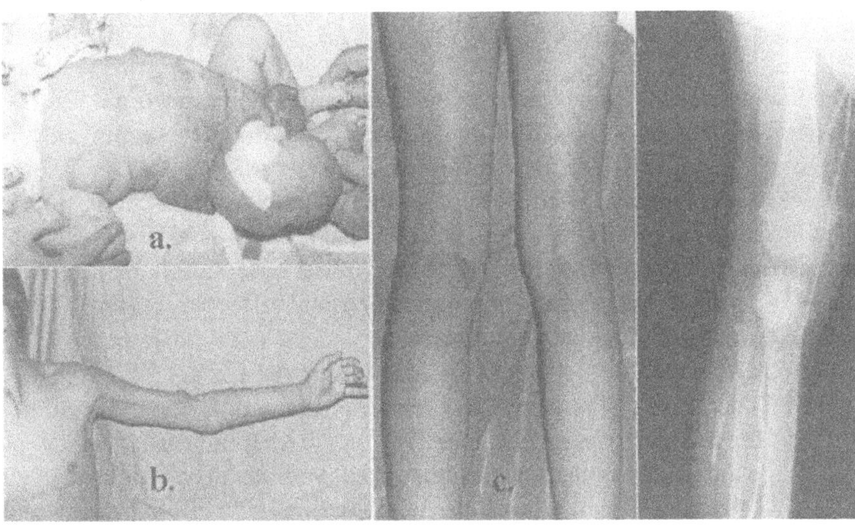

Fig.8.1.

a Complex venous malformations at new born

b Venous malformation of the superior limb at a child

c Venous hemangiomas in the popliteal region at a child (photo & angiography)

8.2.3.4. Imaging Diagnosis

It consists in standard X - ray, color echo-Doppler, computed tomography and magnetic resonance imaging. Phlebography is necessary to complete morphological and hemodynamic diagnosis and determine the superficial and deep extension. The association of ascending, descending and direct phlebography using tourniquets and hemostatic cuffs makes the complete picture of the VM. Arteriographies are sometimes useful.

8.2.3.5. Treatment

The preoperative exact evaluation of VM is decisive for establishing the therapeutic program. The treatment methods are:

1. Sclerotherapy: direct by palpation, echo guided, phlebo guided. The most used substance is 2-3% polidocanol (aetoxisclerol). The risks of the method are tissular necrosis, thrombophlebitis, granuloma and neurological lesions.
2. Surgery: eradication of the VM in association with abolition of the arterio-venous fistula. The congenital valvular incompetence can be repaired by external venoplasty, external valvuloplasty with endoscopic control or by direct surgical valvuloplasty. In the deep vein agenesia the removal of the compensatory dilated veins is dangerous and the surgery is contraindicated. In selected cases a bypass is required using the contra lateral LSV. An abnormal fibrous compression is easy to remove if it is present. The stripping of the persistent abnormal embryonal trunks is permitted only if the deep venous system is normal. Nowadays it is preferred the less invasive surgery with minimal skin incisions.
3. Criotherapy with liquid CO_2 is a cheap method used for the treatment of hemangiomas less than 1cm in diameter that are expanded in surface (not deeper than 2mm) especially in the facial region. The anesthesia is not necessary. The adverse effects are very rare.
4. Lasertherapy makes use of two different types of devices which have different biological actions:
   - laser with colored light impulses; it uses waves that are 585 nm long; they are completely absorbed by the hemoglobin and determine selective phototermolysis in the intradermal vessels. It is very efficient for the treatment of simple, flat hemangiomas;

- NeodymYAG laser; it uses waves that are 1064 nm long. It is recommended for the treatment of bulky hemangiomas that cannot be treated by cryotherapy or by laser with colored light impulses. This method stimulates the physiological regression of the hemangioma and it does not directly destroy it.

5. Medical treatment is indicated in fast-growing, wide-spread hemangiomas or in those located in vital areas for life (trachea and brain) and consists in interferon (IFN) or cortisone therapy:
   - IFN determines directly the inhibition of the proliferation and of the endothelial cells migration and also indirectly the inhibition of the production and the releasing of the endothelial cells growth factors. The main adverse effects are neurotoxicity (development retardation, spastic hemiparesis), neutropenia, and the increase of the transaminases, EKG and EEG modifications;
   - the corticotherapy determines the increase of the sensibility of the small arteries and capillaries for the vasoconstrictor mediators and the decreasing of their caliber. There are many well-known adverse effects. The main effects are osteoporosis, irritability, decreased resistance to infections and sleeping disturbances.

The treatment is individualized to the patient and the therapeutic strategy combines different methods. If it is possible we shall destroy the VM using resectable surgery, sclerosis or laser, if not we shall reduce the diameter of the VM by one or two methods and we combine them with medical therapy. In the first month "the wait and see attitude" is recommended. If the VM grows the therapy is necessary. In the case of complex vascular malformations with arterio-venous fistulas, the obstruction is performed by direct introduction of special liquid substances, sclerosing coils or surgical ligatures.

CHAPTER 9

MISCELLANEOUS VEINS PATHOLOGY

TAKE HOME MESSAGES

Veins and pregnancy

- Favoring factors for varices and thrombosis in pregnancy are: decrease of the venous muscular tonus produced by progesterone, increased blood level of the haemostatic factors I, II, VII, IX, XII and fibrinogen, compression of pelvic veins by pregnant uterus.
- Treatment of thrombosis consists of anticoagulation and later after delivery surgical intervention for varices.

Veins in reconstructive surgery and vein cuffs

- Autogenous saphenous vein is the best material used for aorto-coronarian and infrainguinal by-pass surgery.
- Veins placed in arterial system: complex, adaptative changes.

Venous aneurysm of the lower limb

- Saccular or fusiform dilation of a vein, mainly popliteal vein.
- Venous aneurysm is frequently asymptomatic; thrombosed it causes pain and edema. Pulmonary embolia: important alarm sign.
- Treatment: aneurysm resection with vein reconstruction.

Venous traumas of the inferior limbs

- Clinic: hematoma or external hemorrhage, hypovolemic shock, posttraumatic edema with limb cyanosis.
- Treatment: ligations/reconstructions followed by anticoagulation.

9.1. VEINS AND PREGNANCY

9.1.1. Generalities

In USA, Sweden and United Kingdom the pulmonary embolism is the main cause of maternal death due to medical complications. The morbidity represented by CVI as a result of DVT at pregnant women is 35%.

9.1.2. Etiopathogeny

The pregnancy determines major hemodynamic changes and a hypercoagulation state that affect the veins and their pathology. The favoring factors for the appearance of varices and thrombosis are:

- The oral contraceptives that reduce the level of protein S with 20% associated with smoking increase the risk of thrombosis with different locations.
- The decrease of venous muscular tone produced by the increased level of progesterone. The results are the increase of the capacity and the reduced venous flow with stasis. The compensatory mechanism is the hyperhydremia of the pregnant woman.
- The hyper-coagulation of blood that assures the uterine and placenta hemostasis at delivery. It is established a new balance with the increase of haemostatic factors I, II, VII, IX, XII but associated with a higher fibrinolysis. The level of the fibrinogen at the end of pregnancy is three times higher (Gerbasy 1990). The endothelium delivers the EDRF (endothelial delivered releasing factor) and PGI 2 (prostacyclin) and so it participates to the process. The number of thrombocytes is increased only postpartum. The complex thrombin- antithrombin increases, and fibrinolytic inhibitors become five times higher. The antithrombin III is normal in pregnancy, except the following: preeclampsy, CID, hepatic steatosis, thrombosis. The protein C is normal, but the level of protein S is lower from the middle pregnancy period till a few days postpartum.
- The compression of pelvic, iliac or cava inferior veins is produced by the pregnant uterus, especially in lying down position. The results are "supine hypotension syndrome" and especially the important venous stasis in the lower limbs. The compression of the left iliac veins by the right iliac artery is an associated factor.

The direct factors for thrombosis in pregnancy and postpartum time are:

- complications of pregnancy and delivery (as abortion, hyperemesis, placenta praevia, gestosis), the long lasting bed rest and immobilization (cesarion section, difficult instrumental delivery);
- vascular trauma at delivery, cesarion section at decollated placenta or infection;
- dehydration: hyperemesis, excessive diuretic drugs;
- use of antifibrinolitic drugs (in genital hemorrhages) or high doses of oestrogens (at the suppression of the lactation);
- the increase of venous stasis: β-receptors stimulation in tocolysis;
- uterine infection postabortum or placenta infection (the postpartum period determines the thrombosis of endometrial veins and the proliferation of anaerob agents).The septic pelvic mycrothrombosis is followed by fever and shivers. The septic thrombosis is usually present in the ovarian veins and extends to the iliac veins.

The risk of DVT and pulmonary embolism is 5 times higher in pregnancy and postpartum period than in non-pregnant women. The frequency of DVT and pulmonary embolism at a pregnant woman was 0.5-1.9‰ or even 0.5-3‰ compared with only 0.1-0.2‰ registered at non-pregnant women. (Bauersachs 1998)

The thrombosis of pregnant and postpartum women has frequently a proximal site, as the iliac veins. Therefore the thrombus is bulky and easy to be detached by important and direct pressure changes in the abdominal pressure. The embolus obstructs important pulmonary arteries and so the hemodynamic results are very dangerous and the mortality rate is high.

In Romania, in Timisoara the analysis of 10 years of casuistry of DVT before and after birth establishes its incidence of 5.12‰, respectively 16.9‰ after cesarion operation. The diagnosis of DVT was established in 69.3% cases in postpartum (Păscuţ - 83).

The presence of hereditary thrombophilia is an important favoring factor:

- deficit in antithrombin III, protein C, protein S, heparin co-factor II, thrombomodulin;
- mutation of factor V Leyden, prothrombine G20210A;
- hiperhomocysteinemia.

The point mutation of the factor V Leyden (G1691A) slows down the inactivation of factor Va by APC. This mutation is common in the caucasian population and virtually absent in other races. The presence of this mutation among pregnant women explains the significantly lower risk of intrapartum bleeding complications.

Hyperprothrombinemia, another cause of thrombophilia, is observed in caucasians and especially in Southern Europe.
The anomalous reduced fibrinolysis produces 50 % of thrombosis. The mechanisms are:

- the absence of the plasmin tisullar activator (PI);
- the absence of plasminogen;
- the excess of inhibitor of plasmin tisullar activator (PAI) registered in obesity or congenitally.

The risk of recurrent thrombosis during the pregnancy is 7-12 % (83).

9.1.3. Diagnosis

Clinic diagnosis is insufficient and consists in the following symptoms: the presence of edema at the lower extremities, the calf cramping, tenderness and Homans sign that are present only in some cases. Moreover the pregnant woman has some pains, easy to be assigned to thrombosis. Therefore the clinic diagnosis is insufficient in these special circumstances and it needs more exams:

- Doppler ultrasonography and pelvic echography: establish the presence of thrombosis and the location of the uterus;
- pletismography;
- ascending phlebography (postpartum);
- CT scan with contrast substance: postpartum;
- Xe 133 ventilation / perfusion scanning: useful even at the pregnant woman because the radiation of the fetus is very low, lesser than 0.2 GY. Pulmonary angiography permits a better visualization of the pulmonary artery obstruction. Postpartum 20% of women have perfusions defects probably due to throphoblastic embolisations.

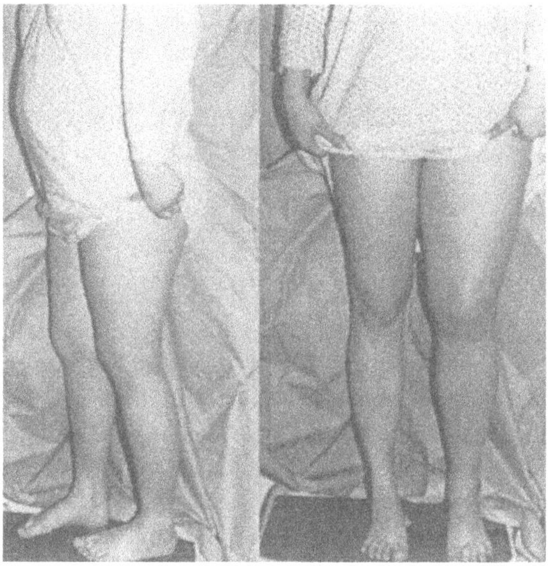

Fig.9.1. Deep thrombophlebitis of the inferior limb at a pregnant women

9.1.4. Treatment

The treatment of the superficial venous thrombosis consists in bed rest, analgesics, moist compresses, leg elevation, without any anticoagulation.

DVT: The anticoagulant of choice is represented by therapeutic doses of heparin because it does not cross the barrier of placenta. The pregnant woman with a confirmed DVT or pulmonary embolism during a previous pregnancy is a risk patient. She needs to start prophylactic anticoagulation 4-6 weeks before the moment when the previous DVT occurred. The ultrasonography checks the deep vein permeability on 20-th and 28-th week of pregnancy. If DVT is found, the therapeutic anticoagulation is recommended and the fibrinolysis is possible. Therapy is continued during the postpartum period until the deambulation. Recurrent pulmonary embolism needs percutaneous insertion of a Mobin-Udin, Greenfield or other devices to stop the embolia just bellow the renal veins.

The warfarin is contraindicated in pregnancy because its administration on the first trimester produces an embriopathy similar to pointed chondromalacy. On the second and the third trimester warfarin

must be avoided because of the cerebral affectation. The rate of spontaneous abortion and "in uterus" death is high, probably due to hemorrhage.
At women in lactation period warfarin seems to be safe because is mostly linked to proteins and therefore it diffuses a little or not at all into the milk.

9.2. THE VEINS IN RECONSTRUCTIVE SURGERY

The autogenous saphenous vein is the best material for aorto-coronarian and infrainguinal bypass and thus many surgeons prefer it when it is available. In this situation the normal saphena must be preserved, the stripping of the GSV and LSV must be limited to advanced varicose disease with dilation and venous wall damages not compatible with graft. But these veins were often used in a previous bypass grafting operation or were removed by stripping or they have already been varicose and futile.
There are many techniques of reconstructions with veins:

- classic surgical bypass with reversed vein graft;
- conventional in situ saphenous bypass graft (vein in normal position but with destroyed valves);
- endovascular assisted method of valvulotomy and side branch occlusion with angioscopic control and in situ bypass of the saphenous vein.

The absence of an adequate ipsilateral GSV has been reported at 40-45 % of cases that require the lower limb revascularisation. There are some possibilities of replacement such as:

- GSV (better to preserve for reconstruction of the other limbs) frequently needed;
- LSV;
- deep veins of the leg;
- inferior epigastric veins;
- arm veins (basilic and cephalic) and eventually veno-venous anastomosis;
- the remained part of GSV.

Harvesting of femuro-popliteal vein is a discussed possibility. Perloff, Thiede and Axtheln demonstrated in 1979 and 1981 that venous allografts were more immunogenic than other allograft tissues. When a graft is placed, an early inflammation occurs. The subsequent endothelial sloughing creates an attack and penetration of the surface. The smooth muscle and fibrous tissues of the inner elastic lamina of the vein graft are exposed and attacked. This process allowed host immune recognition of the inner wall structure with humoral and cell mediated reaction. (Johnson - 54)

Nonautogenous alternatives are the use of glutaraldehide stabilized umbilical vein, cryopreserved saphenous vein allograft, composite prostetic autogenous conduit. Cryopreservation maintaines intact and functional the endothelial and smooth muscle cells. The cryopreserved graft may function simple as a matrix repopulated with host cells. Probably during an initial rejection response to the allotype graft, the repopulation by host endothelial, smooth muscle and immune cells begins to occur. Probably those cells migrate from the anastomotic end of the graft. At 1 – 3 weeks after implantation, there were a variety of cells and after this period a complete absence of donor cells was observed. The reduced number of donor cells diminishes the immune reactions of the recipient. The use of prosthetic grafts needs adjunctive measures such as distal vein cuff and arterio-venous fistula in distal limbs arterial reconstruction. (Johnson -54).

Santilli (98) has demonstrated that it can be safely harvested 50 – 60 cm of femuro-popliteal vein. The harvested superficial femoro-popliteal vein is a theoretic alternative in the reconstructive arterio-venous surgery. All the superficial femoral vein and 15 cm of popliteal vein in men and 12 cm in women can be harvested distal to the adductor hiatus preserving one valve distally. After harvesting the superficial femuro-popliteal vein, the collateral veins assure a good flow when there are competent distal valves and when an important collateral vein is preserved in the popliteal stump for maintaining the link with the profound femoral vein. Mavor and Galloway studied the venous anatomy of lower limbs and demonstrated that in more than 90% of the cases there is a communication between the popliteal vein or venae comitans of the popliteal artery and the common femoral or profound femoral vein. Wells reported minimal clinical morbidity after superficial femoral and popliteal veins harvesting. Therefore the morbidity in the postthrombotic syndrome depends of the extension of obstruction and the intensity of the associated reflux.

9.3. VEIN CUFFS

Autologous vein graft, particularly on infrageniculated popliteal or crural arteries, has cumulative second patency rates of 80 % per 2 years (How - 48). The patency rate of prosthetic grafts was less than 50 % of the vein graft patency. When a vein cuff is interposed between a prosthetic graft and the artery the graft patency improves. The main cause of obstruction is the myointimal hyperplasia (MIH). The interposion of a vein cuff at the distal end of the prosthetic graft determines a reallocation of MIH into the vein cuff and a decreased MIH at the outflow artery. Thus the probability for a significant stenosis of the anastomosis decreases. It was demonstrated that MIH develops inverse proportional with WSS (wall shear stress) values, meaning that a reduced MIH is associated with a high WSS. The location of MIH depends also on the configuration of the anastomosis. This was proved experimentally and in clinic observations. The vein wall absorbs the impact of the prosthetic graft and transfers the response of reactive MIH from the host artery to the arterialized vein. The MIH consists of proliferation and migration of smooth muscle cells from the media to the intima and accumulation of extracellular matrix in response to injury. These events in the presence of veins cuffs were investigated studying the distribution and sites of various cytokines known to modulate anastomotic MIH development. TGF-beta 1 and PDGF –BB are two cytokines that play a major role in tissue remodelling and MIH process. The study confirms the presence and apparent upregulation of these cytokines in the intima and media of the host artery and the vein cuff. The suppression of smooth muscle cells cytokines production may limit the progression of MIH in the vein cuff because the cytokines are in the same location as cells that stained positively to smooth alpha actin. So the vein cuff may be a potential site for gene therapy directed MIH inhibition. (Kissin - 58) Although WSS was not measured within the vein cuff, it was demonstrated by velocity vector plots that there are some areas with low velocity that means low WSS. This low velocity occurs at the proximal cuff wall area and at the toe of the graft cuff anastomosis. (How - 48) The reorientation of MIH into the vein cuff and away from the host artery is a complex process. Probably the vein cuff has intrinsic biologic properties for protection of the anastomosis. The equivalent prosthetic cuff has not these properties and do not protect against MIH. (Hanna - 42)

Vein bypass grafting in response to arterial pressure and pulsate flow undergoes an adaptable remodeling process to strengthen the normally thin vein wall.

9.4. VENOUS ANEURYSM

The venous aneurysms of the lower limbs are the most important localization (Janbon - 52). The first venous aneurysm have been published in 1774 .May and Nissl reported in 1968 a popliteal venous aneurysm (PVA) observed on phlebography carried out for a post thrombotic syndrome. In 1976 Dahl has reported PVA complicated with repeated pulmonary embolia and he has operated it successfully. PVA with paradox embolia with acute peripherical ischemia was reported subsequently.

The popliteal aneurysms are probably not yet recognized as a diagnosis. 51 cases have been found till 1997 although Rubin (52) has reported an incidence of 0,2 % of cases examined with ecodoppler in the popliteal area. Janbon has observed an incidence of 0.01 %.

The PVA is defined as a dilation of the popliteal vein. It can be a fusiform or a saccular aneurysm. The fusiform type is over 1.5-2 times bigger than the proximal or distal veins respectively than the other side popliteal vein. The saccular aneurysm is a lateral sac that is connected to the vein by a colet. The definition for the fusiform PVA is difficult to formulate. The fusiform aneurysms are more frequently found but often they are asymptomatic. The saccular aneurysms are more rare. They are located on the external side of the vein and are often complicated with pulmonary embolia.

Etiological factors

They are not accurately established. Some possible etiological factors are the congenital dysplasia and the flexion-extension area of the popliteal vein.

PVAs are reported at women and also at men; left-right ratio is approximately 1.

It was found a hypoplasia of the smooth muscle from the middle layer of the vein wall and a decrease in number of the elastic fibres or a muscular hypoplasia with hypertrophic fibrosis. The popliteal vein has the thickest wall of all veins and it has a strong elastic layer. PVAs are determined by congenital favoring factors and mechanical factors. There is an embryological junction area at the proximal popliteal vein level that makes the communication between the primitive sciatic veins system and the second flow of the popliteal vein. PVA may also appear under the adductor ring where there is a venous valve respectively under the infragemelar valve, which decreases the rigidity of the popliteal vein walls and permits the ectasia of the vein to the aneurismal dimensions.

Clinical signs

Clinical signs are:

- local: -asymptomatic;
  -pain and swelling in the popliteal region caused by partial or complete thrombosis, edemas (25% of cases).
- pulmonary embolia (69% of cases, often serious relapsing even determining death);
- paradoxical embolia through re-opening of the foramen ovale in pulmonary hypertension and an increased pressure in the right atrium.

PVAs are the most frequent venous aneurisms. The average is 52-53 years with limits between 17-82 years.

The popliteal aneurisms have 2-5 cm in diameter and 8-10 cm in length. Their favorite place is the proximal popliteal veins.

Differential diagnosis

Differential diagnosis can be done with venous ectasias and segmental dysplasias of the veins.

Radiological diagnosis

It is established by a ascendent phlebography and echo Doppler that puts in evidence the diameter of the aneurism, its walls and its content with thrombi.

Treatment

The asymptomatic aneurisms especially the fusiform type must be supervised.

The symptomatic aneurisms and those complicated with pulmonary embolia must be treated as follows:

- anticoagulant treatment: it is insufficient and is indicated to be done 3-6 months after surgery;
- anti-embolia barrage with vena cava clips or vena cava filters;
- partial interruption of the cava vein: at elder, high-risk patients with pulmonary embolia;
- resection without reconstruction: carried out at completely thrombosed aneurisms;
- the vein reconstruction: resection with end to end anastomosis determine better results as conservative or filter placement (Sessa, Perrin - 104);
- wrapping with prosthetic tissue: risky in the condition of the vein flexion;
- venous graft or tangent resection with lateral suture (eventually using a venous patch-Aldridge technique).

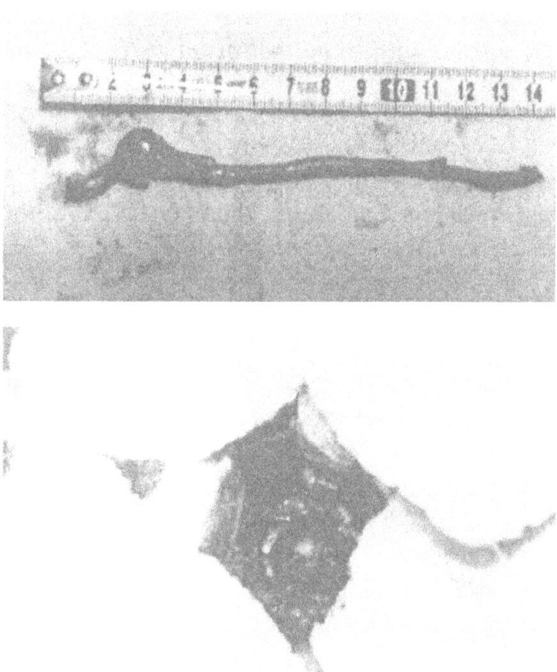

Fig.9.2. Aneurismal dilatation of the saphenous crossa in situ, extirpated

9.5. VENOUS TRAUMAS OF INFERIOR LIMBS

The venous traumas of the inferior limbs alone are very rare (under 14% in war conditions). They are frequently associated with arterial, nervous, osseous and muscular lesions. The venous wounds and the venous contusions represent the venous traumas.
The causes are:

- aggressions with weapons and gun shot;
- circulation, work and sport accidents;
- iatrogenous.

Clinical diagnosis

Clinical diagnosis is based on the following signs:

- an important hematoma;
- a hemorrhage with dark red blood and with a continuous flow;
- hypovolemic shock;
- posttraumatic edema with important cyanosis of the limb observed in the first 24 hours.

Diagnosis

Diagnosis is confirmed by the echo-Doppler exam and eventually by phlebography that shows the hematoma, the interruption of the venous axle, the hemorrhage. The clinical exam and the surgical exploration are generally sufficient and there is not enough time for another complex investigations.

Surgical treatment

Surgical treatment of the venous traumas consists in:

- ligatures of the injured veins;
- venous reconstructions by simple sutures, angioplasties with patches, end to end sutures with or without resections, reconstruction with endogenous or synthetic grafts interposed;
- incisions in the aponeurosis for the muscular compartments decompression;
- the arterio-venous fistula (this procedure is sometimes associated to maintain the patency of the reconstructed vein).

The ligature of the injured vein is recommended at high-risk patients or when we cannot carry out a reconstructive intervention. If the popliteal,

superficial femoral or extern iliac veins are injured we prefer the reconstructive surgery. If we carry out an arterial reconstruction we shall do also the venous reconstruction to avoid a thrombosis followed by an acute ischemia. The osseous-articular lesions require an osteosynthesis operation usually using extern stabilization. It is recommended that the duration of the circulation interruption should be as short as possible so we may use temporary intraoperatory shunts.
The venous ligatures determine complex secondary effects:

- the decrease of the arterial flow in the corresponding arteries with 50-75%;
- distal venous hypertension;
- the increase of the peripheral vascular resistance.

A collateral venous network develops after 48 hours and it makes the venous drainage. Some anatomical conditions are favorable like a double vein, a good collateral circulation and a patent superficial venous system.

The results of the venous reconstructions are superior that the ligatures. The risk of pulmonary embolism is almost zero after a reconstructive surgery and it is present after the venous ligatures that are followed by the venous stump thrombosis.

Evolution

Evolution of the patients with venous traumas may be favorable-asymptomatic patients who can do their activity again. It may appear complications too.

Immediate complications

Immediate complications are the infections of the lacerated tissues, hemorrhages, infections due to the septic materials from the wound.

The postoperative complications are the chronic venous insufficiency with varices, edemas of the inferior limbs, calf ulcers, venous gangrene that may require even the amputation, deep thrombosis, superficial thrombophlebitis, death (especially in case of important veins traumas), pulmonary embolism.

REFERENCES

1. Arnaldi L.A., Pretti F.A.: Antithrombin deficiency in brasilian patients with venous thrombosis. Molecular characterization of a single splice site mutation, an insertion "de novo point mutation"; Thromb Res; 104(6); 397-403; 2001
2. Ascher E., Jacob T., Hingorani A., Tsemekhin B., Gunduz Y.: J Vasc Surg 2001 May; 33(5): 1080-6
3. Avram J., Siska Ioana: The level of superoxide dismutase and glutathion in the blood of varicose saphenous veins; Phlebologie; 2; 155-159; 1999
4. Bauer K.A.: Hormon replacement therapy and the factor V Leyden mutation; Arterioscler Thromb; 22; 879-880; 2002
5. Blanchemaison P.: Pathophysiology; Phlebologie; Special issue; 41-41, 1999
6. Bradbury A., Evans C., Allan P., Lee A., Rucley C.V., Fowkes F.G.R.; What are the symptoms of varicose vein? Edinburg vein study cross-sectional population survey; BMJ; 318; 353-356; 1999
7. Brand F.N., Dannenberg A.L., Abbott R.D.: The epidemiology of varicose veins: the Framingham study. Am J Prev Med 1988; 4: 96-101
8. Brunner U., H.P.Friedl, A.Kohler, M.Lachat: Consideration chirurgicales en cas de lacerations traumatiques de la veine poplitee. Phlebologie, 50, 1, 83-85,1997
9. Caggiati A.: Fascial relationship of the long saphenous vein, Circulation, 1999, 100, 2547-2549.
10. Calvignac J.L.: Anevrysmes veineux poplites: Techniques chirurgicales. Phlebologie, 50,1, 39-43, 1997
11. Castellani L.: Chiva Operation, Cerc. exp. med-chir., III, 9-12 1998
12. Castellani L.: Progress in therapy of venous disease, Conference, Congress of angiology, Timisoara, 2002
13. Chiche L., Darrieus H.: Aspects particuliers des traumatismes veineux des members inferieurs en pratique de guerre. Phlebologie, 50, 1,79-82, 1997
14. Coleridge Smith P.D.: The microcirculation in venous hypertension; Cardiovasc Res; 32; 789-795; 1996
15. Comerota A.J., Throm R.C., Mathias D.S., Hamilton S., Mewissen M.: Catheter-directed thrombolysis for iliofemoral deep venous thrombosis improves health-related quality of life; J Vasc Surg; 32; 130-137, 2000
16. Consensus Group: Classification and grading of chronic venous disease in the lower limbs. A consensus statement. Vascular surgery, 1996, 30, 5-11
17. Cornu-Thenard A., Boivin P., Baud J.M.: Importance of the familial factor in varicose disease; J Dermatol Surg Oncol; 20; 318-326; 1994
18. Danielsson G., Eklof B., Kistner R.L.: What is the role of incompetent perforator veins in chronic venous disease; Journal of Phlebology; 2001; 1; 1; 67-70
19. Davy A., Ouvry P.: Possible explanation for recurrence of varicose veins. Phlebology, 1986, 1, 15-21
20. Davy A.: Supposed idiopathic insufficiency of the short saphenous vein, Phlebologie; 52 Special issue; 45-47; 1999
21. Eifert Sandra, Villavicencio J. L., Tzu-Cheg Kao, Taute Bettina M., Rich N. M., J Vasc Surg 2000; 31; 3; 462-469
22. Eklof B., Juhan C.: Recurrent of primary varicose veins in "Controversies in the management of venous disorders", Eklof B., Gores J.E., Thulesius O., Bergqist O., Ed. Butterworths, London, 1989, 220-223

23. Farah I., Villemur B., Voirin L.: Aspects chirurgicaux des traumatismes veineux des members inferieurs a la phase initial. Phlebologie, 50, 1, 71-78, 1997
24. Faries P.L., Pomposelli F.B. jr, Pulling M.C., Smakowski P., Rohan D.I., Gibbons G.W., Campbel D.R., LoGerfo F.W.: The use of arm vein in lower extremity revascularization: Results of 520 procedures performed in eight years, J Vasc Surg, vol 31, 1, 50-59, 2000.
25. Fegan W.G.: Conservative treatment of varicose veins; Progr. Surg.; 1973; 11; 37-45
26. Fischer R., Linde N., Duff C.: Cure and Reappearance of Symptoms of Varicose Veins after Stripping Operation- A 34 Years Follow-up; Journal of Phlebology; 2001; 1; 1; 49-54
27. Fowkes F.G., Evans C.J., Lee A.J.: Angiology 2001 Aug; 52 Suppl 1: S5-15
28. Fronek A., Minn C., Kim R.: Venous outflow and inflow resistance in health and venous disease, J Vasc Surg, vol 31, 3, 472-476, 2000.
29. Gerlach H., Blatter W.: Ergebnisse einer Multizenter studie zur kontrollierten ambulanten Behandlung der tiefen Beinen thrombose mit Tinzaparin. Vasomed, 4, 2001, 152
30. Gillot V.: Veines plantaires et pompe veineuse , Phlebelogie; 48; 49-70; 1995
31. Glass G.M.: Neovascularisation in recurrent saphena-femoral incompetence of varicose veins: surgical anatomy and morphology, Phlebology, 1995, 10, 136-142
32. Glass G.M.: Prevention of recurrent saphena-femoral incompetence through neovascularisation after surgery for varicose veins. British J of Surg, 1999, 76, 1210
33. Gloviczki P.: Subfascial endoscopic perforator vein surgery: indications and results. Vasc Med; 1999; 4(3); 173-80
34. Gloviczki P., Bergan J., Rhodes J.M.: Mid-term results of endoscopic perforator vein interruption for chronic venous insufficiency: lessons learned from the North American subfascial endoscopic perforator surgery registry. The North American Study Group. J Vasc Surg; 1999; 29(3); 489-502
35. Gobin J.P., Grossetete C.: Indications therapeutiques dans les anevrysmes veineux. Phlebologie, 50, 1, 61-66, 1997
36. Gosselin J., J.Marin, M.T.Barrellier: L'Anevrysme veineux poplite: historique et mise au point a partir d'une revue de la literature, Phlebologie, 50, 1, 17-22, 1997
37. Gupta A., McCarthy S., Pelvic varices as cause for pelvic pain: MRI appearance. Magn. Reson. Imaging. 1994, 12, 679-681
38. Haarst Van E., Liasis N., B.Van Ramshorst: The development of valvular incompetence after deep vein thrombosis, a 7 years follow-up study with duplex scanning; Eur J Vasc Endovasc Surg; 1996; 12; 295-9
39. Haas Sylvia: Recommendations for Prophylaxis of Venous Thromboembolism: International Consensus and the American College of Chest Physician-Sixth Consensus Conference on Antithrombotic Therapy; 2001
40. Haimovici H: Vascular Surgery, Ed. Blackwell Science 1996
41. Ham N.: Compression therapy with medical elastic stockings for venous diseases; Dermatol Surg; 24; 765-770; 1998
42. Hanna Abigail K., Duran W.N., Isabelle Leconte, Fox J.C., Neschis D.G., Hobson II R.W., Golden M. A.: Adenoviral-mediated expression of antisense RNA fibroblast growth factor reduces tangential stress in arterialized vein grafts, J Vasc Surg; 2000; 31; 4; 770-780
43. Henriet J.P.: Experience durant trois annees de la mousse de polidocanol dans le traitrement des varices reticulaires et des varicosites, Phlebologie 1999, 52, 3, 277-282

44. Herbert J.M., Petitou M., Lormeau J.C., Cariou R., Necciari J., Magnani H.N., Zandberg P., Amsterdam van R.G.M., Boeckel van C.A.A., Meuleman D.G.: A Novel Anti-Factor Xa Antithrombotic Agent, Cardiovascular Drug Reviews, vol 15, 1, 1-26, 1997
45. Hiltbrand B.: Traitement medical des sequelles des traumatismes veineux non-iatrogenes des members inferieurs. Phlebologie, 50, 1, 97-99, 1997
46. Hirai M.: Prevalence and characteristics of muscle cramps in patients with varicose veins; VASA, 29, 269-273, 2000
47. Hobbs J.: Surgery and sclerotherapy in the treatment of the varicose veins. Random trial. Archives of surgery 1974, 109,793-796
48. How T.V., Rowe C.S., Gilling-Smith G.L., Harris P.L.: Interposition vein cuff anastomosis alters wall shear stress distribution in the recipient artery, J Vasc Surg; 2000; 31; 5; 1008-1016
49. Ionita H.: Starile trombofilice, Conference, Congress of angiology; Timisoara 2002
50. Italian College of Phlebologie: Guidelines for the prevention and treatment of thromboembolic disease; 2001; 20; 2; 41-52
51. Jacob M.P., Badier-Commander C., Fontaine V., Benazzoug Y., Feldman L., Michel J.B.: Pathol Biol (Paris) 2001 May; 49(4): 326-330
52. Janbon C., Meynadier E., Quere I.: Anevrysme veineux poplite: Epidemiologie, Phlebologie, 50, 1, 23-25, 1997
53. Jantet G. and the RELIEF study group: Chronic venous insufficiency – results of the RELIEF study: a large, international, validated, quality of life investigation. Paper presented at UIP World Congress; Sept., 2001, Rome, Italy
54. Johnson T.R., Tomaszewski J.E., Carpenter J.P.: Cellular repopulation of human vein allograft bypass grafts, J Vasc Surg, vol 31, 5, 994-1002, 2000.
55. Juhan C., Alimi Y.:Sequelles tardives des traumatismes veineux: traitement chirurgical. Phlebologie, 50, 1, 101-103, 1997
56. Juhan C., Haupert S., Miltgen G., Barthelemy P., Eklof B.: Recurrent varicose veins, Phlebology, 1990, 5, 201-211
57. Kamphuisen P.W., Eikenboom J.C.: High factor VIII antigen levels increase the risk of venous thrombosis but are not associated with polymorphisms in the von Willebrand and factor VIII gene; Br J Haematol; 115(1); 156-158; 2001
58. Kissin M., Kansal N., Pappas P.J., DeFouw D.O.,.Duran W.N, Hobson R.W., J Vasc Surg; 2000; 31; 1; 1; 69-83
59. Kluken N.: Importanta clinica a anevrismelor arteriale si venoase, Cercetari experimentale medico-chirurgicale, 1, 21-26, 1995
60. Labas P., Ohradka B., Cambal M.: Surgical treatment of venous leg ulcers; Journal of Phlebology; 2001; 1; 1; 61-66
61. Labropoulos N., Mansour M.A., Kang S.S.: New insights into perforator vein incompetence. Eur J Vasc Endovasc Surg 1999; 18(3): 228-34
62. Lechter A. Alvarez A., Lopez G.: Pelvic varices and gonadal veins. Phlebology, 1987, 2, 181-188
63. Lee A.J., Evans C.J., Hau C.M., Fowkes F.G.: J Clin Epidemiol 2001 Apr; 54(4): 423-9
64. Lee A.J., Lowe G.D., Rumley A., Ruckley C.V., Fowkes F.G.: Blood Coagul Fibrinolysis 2000 Dec; 11(8): 775-81
65. Lee W.A., Hill B.B., Harris E.J. Jr., Semba C.P., Olcott IV C.: Surgical intervention is not required for all patients with subclavian vein thrombosis; J Vasc Surg, 32, 57-67, 2000
66. Lundqvist K, Schmidtchen A.: Br J Dermatol 2001 Feb; 144(2): 254-9

67. Luozzo Di G., Bhargava J., Powell R.J.: Vascular smooth muscle cell effect on endothelial cell endothelin-1 production, J Vasc Surg; 2000; 31; 4; 781-789
68. Mager J.J., Westerman C.J.J.: Value of capillary microscopy in the diagnosis of hereditary hemorrhagic telangiectasia; Arch Dermatol; 136; 732-734; 2000
69. Makarova N.P., Lurie F., Hmelniker S.M.: Does surgical correction of the superficial femoral vein change the course of varicose disease? J Vasc Surg, 33, 361-368, 2001
70. Maleti O., Lugli M., Collura M.: Anevrysmes veineux poplites: Experience personnelle. Phlebologie, 50, 1, 53-59, 1997
71. Mohr D.N., Silverstein M.D., Heit J.A., Petterson T.M., O'Fallon W.M., Melton III L.J.: The Venous Stasis Syndrome after Deep Vein Thrombosis and Pulmonary Embolism: a population-based study; 75, 1249-1256, 2000
72. Moyses C., Cederholm W.S.A., Michel C.C.: Hemoconcentration and accumulation of white cells in the feet during venous stasis J Microvasc Exp, 5, 319-20, 1987
73. Mulliken J.B., Glowacki J.: Hemangiomas and vascular malformation in infants and children: a classification based on endothelial characteristics. Plast Reconstr Surg 1982; 69: 412-420
74. Natali J., Farman T.: Implication medico-legales au cours du traitement sclerosant des varices; Cercetari experimentale medico-chirurgicale; 2-3; 111-115; 1999
75. Nelzen O.: Prospective study of safety, patient satisfaction and leg ulcer healing following saphenous and subfascial endoscopic perforator surgery. Br J Surg; 2000; 87(1); 86-91
76. Nicolaides A.N.: Chronic venous disease of the lower limb. Medicographia; 1994; 1; 3-6
77. Nohe N., Kurnik K., Grantzow R.: Systemische Therapie von Hämangiomen – Vasomed 2001, 1, 17
78. Nyamekge I., Shephard N.A., Davies B., Heather B.P., Earnshaw J.J.: Clinicopathological evidence that neovascularisation is a cause of recurrent varicose veins. Euro J of Vasc and Endovasc Surg, 1998, 15, 412-415
79. Ono T., Bergan J.J., Schonbein S.G.W., Takase S.: Monocytes infiltration in the venous valve J Vasc Surg 1998; 27; 158-166
80. Ouriel K., Green R.M., Greenberg R.K., Clair D.G.: The anatomy of deep venous thrombosis of the lower extremity, J Vasc Surg, vol 31, 5, 895-900,2000.
81. Partsch H.: Die Reisethrombose, Vasomed, 2001, 3, 108-111
82. Partsch H., Blatter W.: Vergleich von Bettruhe, fixem Verband und elastischem Strumpf in der Akutbehandlung der DVT Vasomed, 2001, 4, 153
83. Pascut D., Lighezan I., Pascut Magda: Particularitati si conroverse in boala tromboembolica din perioada sarcinii; Cercetari experimentale medico-chirurgicale; 6; 2-3; 154-161; 1999
84. Perrin M., Guex J.J, Ruckley C.V.: Recurrent varices after surgery (REVAS), Cardiovasc. Surg. 2000; 8: 233-45.
85. Petitou M., Herbert J.M.: Synthetic anticoagulants, Pour le science 2000, 274, 28-34
86. Pierik E.G., Urk Van H., Wittens C.H.: Efficacy of subfascial endoscopy in eradicating perforating veins of the lower leg and its relation with venous ulcer healing. J Vasc Surg 1997; 26: 255-9
87. Porter J.M., Moneta J.L.: International Consensus Committee on chronic venous disease, J Vasc Surg, 1995, 21, 635-645
88. Rabe E.: Symposion "News in CVI Therapy" Rome Sept. 2001
89. Rabe E., Pannier-Fischer F.: The importance of conservative and operative phlebologic treatment of ulcus cruris; Z Hautkrankheiten; 11; 651-655; 1999

90. Raffetto J.D., Mendez M.V., Marien B.J., Byers H.R., Phillips T.J., Park H.Y., Menzoian JO.: J Vasc Surg 2001 Jun; 33(6): 1233-41
91. Raju S., Fredericks R.: Valve reconstruction procedures for non obstructive venous insufficiency: rational, techniques and results in 107 procedures with two-to eight-year follow-up; J Vasc Surg; 1988; 7; 310-100
92. Raju S., Neglen P.: Popliteal vein entrapment: A benign feature or pathologic entity? J Vasc Surg; 2000; 31; 4; 631-641
93. Ramelet A.A., Monti M.: Phlebology-The Guide, Ed. Masson, Paris, 1999
94. Rehman A., Rallapalle V.S.P., Iqbal R., Grimley R.P., Jayatunga A.P.: A simple technique to reduce blood loss and improve cosmetics in varicose vein surgery; Phlebologie; 13; 153-156; 1998
95. Rembrandt Investigators: Treatment of Proximal Deep Vein Trombosis With a Novel Synthetic Compound With Pure Anti-Factor Xa Activity, 2000
96. Rosental P.L., Arous E.J., Friedman S.G., Ingengo M.D., Johnson B.L., Kraiss L.W., Martin J.D., Moritz M.W., Piano G., Rigdon E.E., Self S.B., Pallos L.L: Endovascular-assisted versus conventional in situ saphenous vein by-pass grafting: Cumulative patency, limb salvage, and cost results in a 39-month multicenter study, J Vasc Surg, vol 31, 1, 60-68, 2000.
97. Rothfuss M., Spathelf S., Häfner H..M., Nohé B., Jünger M.: Endothel-Leukozyten-Adhäsion induziert durch erhöhten Druck in vitro, Vasomed, 2001, 4, 150
98. Santilli S.M., Lee E.S., Wernsing S.E., Diedrich D.A., Kuskowski M.A., Shew R.L.: Superficial femoral popliteal vein: An anatomic study, J Vasc.Surg, vol 31, 3, 450-455, 2000.
99. Sarin S., Scurr J.H., Smith C.: Medial calf perforators in venous disease: the significance of outward flow; J Vasc Surg; 1992; 16(1); 40-6
100. Satiukova G.S., Kurguzov O.: Morfologiia 2000; 118(5): 29-35
101. Schreiber D.: Deep venous thrombosis and thrombophlebitis, Med J,Emergency Medicine-Cardiovascular, Ed. Boston Medical Publishing Corp., vol 2, 2001, 6, 1-23
102. Schultz-Ehrenburg, Weindorf N., Von Uslar D., Hirche H.: Prospektive epidemiologische Studie über die Entstehungsweise der Krampfadern bei Kinder und Jugendlichen. Phlebol Proktol 1989; 18: 3-11
103. Sessa C., Perrin M., Porcu P.: Popliteal venous aneurysms: two-center experience with 21 cases and review of the literature; Int J Angiol, 9, 164-170, 2000
104. Shoab S.S., Porter J.B., Scurr J.H., Coleridge-Smith P.D.: Effect of oral micronized purified flavonoid fraction treatment on leukocyte adhesion molecule expression in patients with chronic venous disease: A pilot study, J Vasc Surg, vol 31, 3, 456-461, 2000.
105. Schmeller W., Gaber Y.: Surgical removal of ulcer and lipodermatosclerosis followed by split skin grafting (shave therapy) yields good long-term results in "non-healing" venous leg ulcers; Acta Dermatological Venereol; 80; 267-27; 2000
106. Sobaszek A., Frimat P., Tiberguent A., Domont A., Chevalier H., Catilina P.: Venous insufficiency of the lower limbs and working condition; Phlebology; 13; 133-141; 1999
107. Sorensen H.T., Mellelkjaer L., Olsen J.H., Baron J.A.: Prognosis of cancers associated with venous thromboembolism; N Engl J Med; 343; 1846-1850; 2000
108. Schmid Schönbein G.W., Fung Y.C., Zweifach B.W.: Vascular endothelium leukocyte interaction, Circ Res ; 36; 173-184; 1975
109. Stuart W.P., Adam D.J., Allan P.L.: The relationship between the number, competence and diameter of medial calf perforating veins and the clinical status in healthy subjects and patients with lower-limb venous disease. J Vasc Surg 2000; 32(1): 138-43

110. Takase S., Bergan J.J., Schmid- Schönbein G.: Ann Vasc Surg 2000 Sep; 14(5): 427-35
111. Takeda Y., Agui T., Tanaka K., Okuzawa N., Tanigawa N.: Sclerotherapy with ligation of incompetent veins for a stasis ulcer due to varix cruris: minimal invasive therapy for varix cruris; Jpn J Surg; 29; 1154-1157; 1999
112. Thierry L.: What is the medical, social and economical impact of chronic venous insufficiency (CVI); Medicographia; 1994; 16; 7-11
113. Villemur B., Farah I., Perrin M.: Resultats de la chirurgie veineuse après traumatismes veineux des members inferieurs:aspects cliniques et hemodinamiques. Phlebologie, 50, 1, 89-96, 1997
114. Voirin L., Perrin M., Magne J.L.: Les anevrysmes veineux de la fosse poplitee: resultats de la chirurgie. Phlebologie, 50, 1, 45-51, 1997
115. Voshenrich R., Fischer U., Grabbe E.: MR- Angiographie heute und in Zukunft, Vasomed 2001, 4, 134
116. Weber J.: Angeborene Gefässmissbildungen: Hämangiome und Malformationen, Vasomed 2001, 1, 6
117. Wells P.S., Anderson D.R.: Value of assesment of pretest probability of deep vein thrombosis in clinical management; Lancet; 350; 1795-1798; 1997
118. Young A.E.: Pathogenesis of vascular malformation. In: Mulliken J.B., Young A.E., editors. Vascular birthmarks: hemangiomas and malformations. Philadelphia: W.B. Sauders Co, 1988; 107-113

INDEX

www.ingramcontent.com/pod-product-compliance
Ingram Content Group UK Ltd.
Pitfield, Milton Keynes, MK11 3LW, UK
UKHW021828170926
475607UK00007B/52

* 9 7 8 1 4 0 2 0 7 4 1 1 0 *